D0643940

Medical Tests
SOURCEBOOK

Health Reference Series

First Edition

Medical
Tests
SOURCEBOOK

*Basic Consumer Health Information about Medical
Tests, Including Periodic Health Exams, General
Screening Tests, Tests You Can Do at Home,
Findings of the U.S. Preventive Services Task Force,
X-ray and Radiology Tests, Electrical Tests, Tests of
Blood and Other Body Fluids and Tissues, Scope
Tests, Lung Tests, Genetic Tests, Pregnancy Tests,
Newborn Screening Tests, Sexually Transmitted
Disease Tests, and Computer Aided Diagnoses;
Along with a Section on Paying for Medical Tests,
a Glossary, and Resource Listings*

Edited by
Joyce Brennfleck Shannon

Omnigraphics, Inc.

Penobscot Building / Detroit, MI 48226

Bibliographic Note

Because this page cannot legibly accommodate all the copyright notices, the Bibliographic Note portion of the Preface constitutes an extension of the copyright notice.

Beginning with books published in 1999, each new volume of the *Health Reference Series* will be individually titled and called a "First Edition." Subsequent updates will carry sequential edition numbers. To help avoid confusion and to provide maximum flexibility in our ability to respond to informational needs, the practice of consecutively numbering each volume will be discontinued.

Edited by Joyce Brennfleck Shannon

Health Reference Series

Karen Bellenir, *Series Editor*
Peter D. Dresser, *Managing Editor*
Joan Margeson, *Research Associate*
Dawn Matthews, *Verification Assistant*
Margaret Mary Missar, *Research Coordinator*
Jenifer Swanson, *Research Associate*

Omnigraphics, Inc.

Matthew P. Barbour, *Vice President, Operations*
Laurie Lanzen Harris, *Vice President, Editorial Director*
Thomas J. Murphy, *Vice President, Finance and Comptroller*
Peter E. Ruffner, *Senior Vice President*
Jane J. Steele, *Marketing Consultant*

Frederick G. Ruffner, Jr., Publisher

Library of Congress Cataloging-in-Publication Data

Medical tests sourcebook : basic consumer health information about medical tests, including periodic health exams, general screening tests, tests you can do at home, findings of the U.S. Preventive Services Task Force, X-ray and radiology tests, electrical tests, tests of blood and other body fluids and tissues, scope tests, lung tests, genetic tests, pregnancy tests, newborn screening tests, sexually transmitted disease tests, and computer aided diagnoses ; along with a section on paying for medical tests, a glossary, and resource listings / edited by Joyce Brennfleck Shannon. — 1st ed.
    p. cm. — (Health reference series)
    Includes bibliographical references and index.
    ISBN 0-7808-0243-8 (lib. bdg. : alk. paper)
    1. Diagnosis Popular works. 2. Diagnosis, Laboratory Popular works. 3. Medicine, Popular. I. Shannon, Joyce Brennfleck. II. Series : Health reference series (Unnumbered)
RC71.3.M45 1999
616.07'5—dc21
                                                 99-35456
                                               CIP

∞

This book is printed on acid-free paper meeting the ANSI Z39.48 Standard. The infinity symbol that appears above indicates that the paper in this book meets that standard.

Printed in the United States

Table of Contents

Part II: Screening Tests You Can Do at Home

Part III: Findings of the U.S. Preventive Services Task Force

Part IV: X-ray and Radiology Tests

Part VII: Scope Tests

Part VIII: Lung (Pulmonary) Tests

Part IX: Genetic Testing

Part X: Pregnancy Tests and Newborn Care

Part XI: Sexually Transmitted Disease (STD) Tests

Part XII: Payment of Medical Tests

Part XIII: Additional Help and Information

Preface

About This Book

Medical tests offer health consumers and their physicians an immense amount of information about the internal workings of the body. Screening tests can warn of the need to change habits thereby improving health and longevity. Diagnostic medical tests allow early detection of disease so that proper treatments can be initiated. Test results, however, can be inaccurate. Some tests may be risky, and many tests are costly. The best decisions about necessary medical tests will be made as individuals work in partnership with their physicians clearly communicating health needs and concerns.

This book is designed to aid health care consumers in making informed decisions about medical tests. Specific tests are described in layman's terms, including procedures, benefits, limits, and possible risks. Tests that can be performed by the individual at home are described. Recent advances in genetic testing are explained. Information about health insurance and government agencies offering financial assistance for medical needs is included, and a glossary and resource directory provide additional help and information.

How to Use This Book

This book is divided into parts and chapters. Parts focus on broad areas of interest. Chapters are devoted to single topics within a part.

Part I: Periodic Health Exams and General Screening Tests provides an overview of health exams and screenings which are important for maintaining optimal physical health. These are listed by disease category.

Part II: Screening Tests You Can Do at Home describes tests that enable health consumers to monitor disease symptoms or detect conditions which require further testing, medical supervision, or counseling.

Part III: Findings of the U.S. Preventive Services Task Force emphasizes those preventive services that are beneficial in the context of routine health care. The age specific charts make recommendations of preventive services that have been proven effective in controlled studies.

Part IV: X-ray and Radiology Tests describes medical imaging tests including x-ray, ultrasound, computed tomography (CT) scanning, angiography, nuclear imaging, and magnetic resonance imaging (MRI) which can help doctors narrow down the causes of a patient's symptoms without surgery and sometimes diagnose an illness before symptoms even appear.

Part V: Electrical Tests presents the special tests which measure electrical impulses in the brain and heart. These tests are valuable diagnostic aids for epilepsy, sleep disorders, seizure activity, and heart function.

Part VI: Tests of Blood and Other Body Fluids and Tissues looks at the common tests used to determine if someone has a disease or health problem based on evaluation of blood, urine, or other tissue.

Part VII: Scope Tests describes the tests where the doctor literally looks inside the body using tubes, lights, and cameras to identify and treat injury or disease.

Part VIII: Lung (Pulmonary) Tests reviews spirometry and pulmonary function tests used to diagnose asthma and other lung diseases.

Part IX: Genetic Testing describes these specialized tests and the reasons for which they are used, including carrier screening, prenatal diagnostic testing, newborn screening, presymptomatic testing and risk assessment for such adult-onset disorders as Huntington's disease, some types of cancer, and Alzheimer's disease, and for forensic/ identity testing.

Part X: Pregnancy Tests presents the routine tests used to monitor the health of both mother and baby and the tests which may be suggested if there are indications of distress. Risk assessments for the tests are also included.

Part XI: Sexually Transmitted Disease (STD) Tests presents information about the types of tests used to allow early identification and effective treatment of many of the most common STDs.

Part XII: Payment of Medical Tests provides important information concerning health insurance, Medicare, and the Hill-Burton Free Care Program.

Part XIII: Additional Help and Information includes a glossary, a description of modern tools available to doctors and their patients for providing health care over long distances, and a resource listing of organizations by disease category.

Bibliographic Note

This volume contains documents and excerpts from publications issued by the following U.S. government agencies: Center for Biologics Evaluation and Research (CBER); Centers for Disease Control and Prevention (CDC); Food and Drug Administration (FDA); Health Resources and Services Administration (HRSA); National Cancer Institute (NCI); National Eye Institute (NEI); National Heart, Lung, and Blood Institute (NHLBI); National Institute of Allergy and Infectious Diseases (NIAID); National Institute of Arthritis and Musculoskeletal and Skin Diseases (NIAMS); National Institute of Child Health and Human Development (NICHD); National Institute of Diabetes, Digestive, and Kidney Diseases (NIDDK); National Institute Radiation Safety; Preventive Services Task Force; and Warren Grant Magnuson Clinical Center.

In addition, this volume contains copyrighted documents from the following organizations and individuals: American Cancer Society; American Diabetes Association; American Institute of Ultrasound in Medicine; American Medical Association; Steven H. Brick, MD and James Spies, MD of GCM Radiology; Denise Casey; Carol Greene, MD,

Peter Lane, MD, Benjamin Wilford, MD, and C. Holly Nyerges, MSN, CPNP, *Genetic Drift Newsletter*; Rosario Guarino, MD, Neurologist Online; Seline Haines, Washington University in St. Louis; Health Insurance Association of America; Healthwise, Inc; International Diabetes Center; The Johns Hopkins University; Mayo Health Information; Mt. Sinai School of Medicine; The Nemours Foundation; Brian Plant, MD, Department of Otolaryngology, University of Washington; Society of Nuclear Medicine; and Springhouse Corporation. Copyrighted articles from *Cancer Weekly Plus, Diabetes Forecast, Getting the Most of Your Medical Dollar, Health After 50, Health Beat,* and *Medical Update* are also included.

Full citation information is provided on the first page of each chapter. Every effort has been made to secure all necessary rights to reprint the copyrighted material. If any omissions have been made, please contact Omnigraphics to make corrections for future editions.

Acknowledgements

In addition to the many organizations and agencies who contributed the material that is included in this book, special thanks go to Jenifer Swanson for her research and internet expertise and to Karen Bellenir for her editorial guidance and assistance.

Note from the Editor

This book is part of Omnigraphics' *Health Reference Series*. The series provides basic information about a broad range of medical concerns. It is not intended to serve as a tool for diagnosing illness, in prescribing treatments, or as a substitute for the physician/patient relationship. All persons concerned about medical symptoms or the possibility of disease are encouraged to seek professional care from an appropriate health care provider.

Our Advisory Board

The *Health Reference Series* is reviewed by an Advisory Board comprised of librarians from public, academic, and medical libraries. We would like to thank the following board members for providing guidance to the development of this series:

Nancy Bulgarelli, William Beaumont Hospital Library, Royal Oak, MI

Karen Morgan, Mardigian Library, University of Michigan, Dearborn, MI

Rosemary Orlando, St. Clair Shores Public Library, St. Clair Shores, MI

Health Reference Series *Update Policy*

The inaugural book in the *Health Reference Series* was the first edition of *Cancer Sourcebook* published in 1992. Since then, the *Series* has been enthusiastically received by librarians and in the medical community. In order to maintain the standard of providing high-quality health information for the lay person the editorial staff at Omnigraphics felt it was necessary to implement a policy of updating volumes when warranted.

Medical researchers have been making tremendous strides, and the challenge to stay current with the most recent advances is one our editors take seriously. Each decision to update a volume will be made on an individual basis. Some of the considerations will include how much new information is available and the feedback we receive from people who use the books. If there's a topic you would like to see added to the update list, or an area of medical concern you feel has not been adequately addressed, please write to:

Editor
Health Reference Series
Omnigraphics, Inc.
2500 Penobscot Bldg.
Detroit, MI 48226

The commitment to providing on-going coverage of important medical developments has also led to some technical changes in the *Health Reference Series*. Beginning with books published in 1999, each new volume will be individually titled and called a "First Edition." Subsequent updates will carry sequential edition numbers. To help avoid confusion and to provide maximum flexibility in our ability to respond to informational needs, the practice of consecutively numbering each volume will be discontinued.

Part One

Periodic Health Exams and General Screening Tests

Chapter 1

The Not-So-Routine Physical

The annual medical checkup, once a cornerstone of American health care, is fading into medical history. Like Mercurochrome and the iron lung, the routine annual physical for people who aren't sick came and went in less than a century, replaced by an approach to periodic health screening based on a new awareness of the importance of risk analysis and targeted preventive services. That may sound like impersonal, high-tech medicine, but it isn't. Today's far-from-routine health checkup is grounded on a highly personalized concept: the idea that every individual is unique, that each of us has a medical history and lifestyle that strongly influence how healthy, or unhealthy, we are now and may be in the future.

Something Old, Something New

Today's health checkup draws on the best aspects of horse-and-buggy medicine, back when the family doctor was likely to be a long-time neighbor and friend. But it adds the product of research on factors that influence a person's risk of serious illness, factors that range from family history to eating habits. Using that knowledge, physicians can zero in on specific preventive strategies for individual patients, selecting those, like smoking cessation or nutrition counseling, that have a good chance of helping the patient avoid serious illness or injury and omitting others, such as chest x-rays, that are of little or no benefit to healthy people.

FDA Consumer, July/August 1992, reviewed November 1998.

At a time of high and rising health-care costs when health insurance providers are reluctant to cover the cost of routine checkups for people who aren't sick, moves to forego procedures of little or no value can save enormous amounts of money. At the same time, physicians are generally on the lookout for ways to make their limited time with individual patients as helpful as possible. Getting away from routine tests of dubious effectiveness and devoting more time to patient counseling that can pay off in better health have a powerful appeal for many health-care professionals.

The routine physical became firmly rooted in standard American health care almost half a century ago. In 1947 the American Medical Association recommended that every healthy person 35 or older pay a yearly visit to the doctor to get a battery of tests, a head-to-toe physical examination, and a conference to discuss anything that might concern either doctor or patient. That was a bold move on the part of organized medicine: People were being advised to see their doctors not just when they were sick, but when, presumably, they were well.

The idea was radical, but it wasn't new. The annual physical for seemingly well patients had been proposed at an AMA meeting as early as 1900. And a lot earlier still, as long ago as the 25th century BC, Chinese Emperor Huang Ti wrote: "The superior physician helps before the early budding of the disease," not when it has already developed. The modern health checkup takes that ancient wisdom one giant step further. Physicians today are able not just to offer help before disease develops, but to keep some diseases and disabilities from occurring in the first place.

For example, counseling a patient to quit smoking, better yet, persuading a youngster never to start, is a prime example of disease prevention that is now seen as a valuable part of a periodic health exam. Tobacco smoking contributes to 1 out of every 6 deaths in the United States, including 130,000 deaths each year from cancer, 115,000 from coronary artery disease, and 60,000 from chronic obstructive lung disease.

The same kind of hard statistical evidence makes the case for physicians helping their patients cut down on fat intake, use seat belts, curb alcohol consumption, get more exercise, and otherwise adopt a lifestyle that can lower the risk of disease and injury.

But a number of questions face physicians and health organizations, as well as patients who want the periodic health checkup to be as beneficial as possible. Which tests, what sort of counseling, and what immunizations or medicines are most effective in preventing or minimizing serious illness? Which ones are appropriate for some patients

4

but not all, for some age groups but not others? Which should be carried out every year, every three years, five years? How do you decide that a test is no longer needed or, conversely, that it ought to be done more often? The answers to such questions are less than certain, but patients and physicians alike have a good deal more to go on than they did a decade ago.

An Ounce (or Two) of Prevention

Two major government-sponsored inquiries sparked the reassessment of the routine annual physical. In 1979, the *Canadian Task Force on the Periodic Health Examination* published an evaluation of the effectiveness of preventive services performed routinely by Canadian physicians. A similar effort was launched in 1984 by the U.S. Department of Health and Human Services, of which the Food and Drug Administration is a part. The U.S. Preventive Services Task Force, a 20-member panel of non-federal physicians, other health-care providers, and preventive medicine experts, closely followed the Canadian scheme for ranking preventive services.

The U.S. task force's report, *Guide to Clinical Preventive Services*, published in 1989, focused on 169 measures targeted at 60 different illnesses and conditions. It has been called "the bible" of preventive medicine. If it is, then the "gospel" is; Schedule and structure periodic health checkups to match an individual patient's individual health profile.

Given that point of departure, the list of preventive services the task force found appropriate for all symptom-free patients is fairly short. The only components of the old "routine" physical exam recommended for every patient are measurements of height, weight, and blood pressure. On the other hand, the approach to prevention envisioned in the task force report attaches great importance to screening measures to identify patients at special risk of illness or injury.

Physicians are advised to take a full, detailed medical history, to identify occupational and behavioral factors that affect health, to find out about a patient's eating habits, use of alcohol and other drugs, use of tobacco, and sexual activity, anything that may put the patient at high risk for a specific disease or disability. The physician can then make informed choices among available preventive services, emphasizing the ones most likely to benefit an individual patient. Many of these measures involve the use of devices, tests and vaccines regulated by FDA.

For example, the task force recommends periodic blood pressure testing for everyone 3 or older. High blood pressure affects close to 60 million Americans, many of whom have no symptoms. It's a major risk factor for coronary artery disease, congestive heart failure, stroke, and kidney disease. High blood pressure is easy to detect, and it can be controlled with diet, exercise and drugs, preventing serious illness and death. On the other hand, the Preventive Services Task Force found no scientific basis for routine urine testing of all asymptomatic patients. Instead, the task force recommended periodic "dipstick" urinalysis for pregnant women and people with diabetes. Urine testing, the task force suggested, may also be appropriate for preschool children and people over 60.

Serious urinary tract disorders are uncommon, urinalysis is not especially reliable as a screening test for such disorders, and the effectiveness of early detection and treatment of urinary tract problems is unproved. Hence, doing a urinalysis routinely and repeatedly among symptom-free people can't be justified.

By the same token, electrocardiography (ECG) to screen for unsuspected coronary artery disease is recommended only for certain high-risk groups and for people, such as airline pilots, whose sudden heart attack could endanger public safety. "High-risk" in this instance means people who have two or more risk factors for coronary artery disease; cigarette smoking, high blood pressure or high serum cholesterol levels, diabetes, or a family history of coronary disease before age 55. The task force found no basis to recommend routine ECG screening of all individuals with no hint of coronary artery disease.

Again, the reason for the recommendation is straightforward: Studies have shown that routine screening of symptom-free people in whom the probability of coronary artery disease is low has been found to generate a large proportion of false-positive results. Studies of the more reliable stress ECG (or "stress test"), in which the patient is tested while exercising to raise the heart rate toward its upper limit, indicate that most symptom-free people with abnormal test results don't have coronary artery disease. According to the task force report, neither the regular nor stress ECG is recommended for children, adolescents, or young adults who show no evidence of heart disease and plan to start a strenuous athletic program.

Not Another Cookbook

While there is broad consensus among health authorities that an annual, more-or-less uniform checkup of symptom-free, presumably healthy people is inappropriate, experts and professional organizations don't entirely agree about exactly what should take its place.

In 1991, the American College of Physicians, whose members are specialists in internal medicine, published a lengthy report comparing its own preventive service and screening recommendations with those of the U.S. Preventive Services Task Force, the Canadian Task Force on Periodic Health Examination, and other organizations. There was general agreement on routine blood pressure screening and on counseling adults about tobacco use, nutrition, exercise, sexual behavior, substance abuse, injury prevention, and dental care. All groups also recommended tetanus-diphtheria booster shots every 10 years and influenza immunization for persons 65 and older. U.S. organizations also recommended pneumococcal immunization at age 65.

The groups generally agreed that women should have an annual Pap smear beginning at ages 18 to 20 and every third year from age 20 through the mid 30s. They did not entirely agree on how often and for how long older women with no symptoms of or risk factors for uterine cancer (including a family history of uterine cancer or a succession of abnormal Pap test results) should continue to have periodic Pap tests. However, the U.S. groups recommended Pap tests at least every three years through age 65.

An annual mammogram to screen for early breast cancer was uniformly recommended for women from age 50 on, but not all the organizations surveyed agreed on how often women under 50 should have mammography screening. The American Cancer Society (ACS) specifically advises women between 40 and 49 to have a mammogram every one or two years. All agreed, however, that women should have a clinical breast exam annually beginning at age 40.

A check of serum cholesterol every five years was recommended for all men between the ages of 20 and 70 (the Canadians narrowed that to between 30 and 59). The U.S. task force suggested that cholesterol screening of women, younger men, and the elderly was "clinically prudent," meaning that the physician should base a decision on factors such as a patient's fat consumption, known high cholesterol problem, or other coronary artery disease risk factors.

After age 50, ACS recommends yearly stool screening for occult blood, but the U.S. and Canadian task forces said there was insufficient evidence to recommend for or against this test.

Also after age 50, ACS recommended procedures to check for diseases of the colon: sigmoidoscopy every three to five years or air-contrast barium enema every five years. Again, neither the Canadian nor the U.S. task force recommended for or against these tests.

A Vote for Low Tech

Many experts think the new face of the periodic health examination is at least as important as new medical technology in safeguarding people's health. Americans seem to agree. A recent Gallup poll conducted for the Pharmaceutical Manufacturers Association Foundation found that 28 percent of heads of households thought that of all health-related efforts, lifestyle modifications, such as diet, exercise, and smoking cessation, had benefited them most. Diagnostic tools, x-rays, CAT scans, and heart monitors, for example, were judged most beneficial by 25 percent of those surveyed, and 25 percent placed drugs and vaccines at the top of the list. Improved surgical techniques scored best with only 16 percent of the sample. All of which supports the idea that active participation by patients and health-care providers has a critical role in efforts not just to treat, but to prevent, human illness.

A Physical Glance

- An annual overall physical for healthy adults of all ages is no longer recommended by most medical experts.

- Counseling about lifestyle and health is now considered an important part of a periodic exam.

- During a periodic exam, depending on your age and gender, your doctor may suggest one or more of the following tests and immunizations: blood pressure, cholesterol level, occult blood in stool, sigmoidoscopy or air-contrast barium enema, clinical breast exam, mammography, Pap smear, tetanus-diphtheria booster, flu immunization, or pneumonia immunization.

—Ken Flieger

Ken Flieger is a freelance writer in Washington, DC.

This article was reviewed for currency in 1998 by Debra S. Lazzaro, M.D., Diplomate of the American Board of Family Practice. Dr. Lazzaro is a Family Physician at Caylor Nickel Clinic, Bluffton, Indiana.

Chapter 2

Make the Most of Your Visit to the Doctor—Communicate

Communication is an important part of any relationship—sharing thoughts, asking questions and listening. Since relations between doctor and patient can be as limited as a yearly office visit, effective communication is especially important to ensure patients and physicians understand each other well.

"There are many questions and decisions that revolve around health care," says Dr. Thomas Taylor, associate professor and director of research in family medicine at the University of Washington School of Medicine. "Finding answers and making sense of what's best for your health is a process that takes time and commitment on a patient's part and relies on strong communication between a patient and doctor."

Changes in today's health care system and the increasing proliferation of health information available through media, the World Wide Web and other resources have affected doctor/patient relations.

"Patients today, in general, are much more assertive. They are more responsible for the costs of their health care and more aware of what they're getting for their money," Taylor explains. "Patients expect to be collaborators in their care."

Since patients are often looking for specific information about their health, even during a routine examination, Taylor said it's important to decide why the visit is important and convey this message to the doctor from the start.

Reprinted with permission. © March 18, 1997, Health Beat, Health Sciences/ Medical Affairs, News and Community Relations, University of Washington.

To do this, Taylor suggests taking time before the visit to make a list of questions about your health. "Look at the list and then select the top two items to discuss with your doctor," he explains. "That way you know what to focus on, and your physician, in turn, will probably be pleased that you are making a positive use of his or her time."

Taylor also recommends bringing supplemental information. If you've read information in the news or located a research study that you have questions about, bring a copy of it with you.

Since expectations for a physician vary from patient to patient, not every doctor is right for every patient. While most patients agree that competency is at the top of the list, from there, expectations vary. Because of this, Taylor says selecting a physician on advice from a friend or on referral from another physician may not always work.

"Some patients are looking to help make decisions, others only want information, and some would like a person to take charge," Taylor notes. "Decide what's most important to you."

As in all relationships, communication is a two-way street. While patients may expect certain qualities from their physician, they should also make efforts to be good patients.

So what are doctors looking for from patients? During initial consultations, physicians are in need of complete patient information—medical history, family history, medications, etc. During follow-up visits, doctors want to know if a patient's health has improved or deteriorated; and if so, in what way and when.

Taylor explains that a doctor's agenda is primarily focused on identifying, addressing and treating changes in a person's health condition. In addition, the doctor is assessing what the patient is seeking, whether it be information, reassurance or advice.

"Some patients want affirmation, others want to ventilate their feelings and others want someone to simply tell them what to do", Taylor says. "If you aren't happy with a physician, you should be prepared to find another."

Of course not all doctor/patient matches are perfect—many patients must compromise their image of a "perfect" doctor to achieve what in the end will be the best result.

"There are times in life when the technical quality of care is much more important than compassion or listening skills," says Taylor.

Chapter 3

Questions to Ask about Medical Tests

About the Test:

Before you agree to any medical test, ask the following questions. These questions are particularly important for expensive or risky tests.

1. What is the name of the test?

2. Why do you need it?

3. Are the test results likely to change your treatment? If not, the cost, inconvenience, or discomfort of the test may not be worth the information.

4. How accurate is the test? What are the rates of false positives / false negatives?

5. What can you do to improve the accuracy of the test? Should you restrict food, alcohol, medications, exercise, or other activities before the test?

6. What are the risks? Are there less risky tests that could be done first or that might determine the same thing?

7. What are the costs in money, time, and discomfort? Are there less costly tests you could do first?

8. What are the consequences of delaying or avoiding this test?

If several tests are recommended all at once, ask about the risk of delaying some of the tests.

- Is there some advantage to doing tests all at once?

- Could tests be done in stages, starting with the most important ones first?

- Given the doctor's suspicions about what is wrong, which tests are the most important?

About the Results:

1. When and how will you get the test results?

2. What is the next step if the results are positive?

3. What is the next step if the results are negative?

What Your Doctor Needs to Know:

1. Your concerns about the test(s).

2. Any medications you are taking or conditions you have that might interfere with the test results.

3. Previous test results.

Keep in mind that no test can be done without your permission.

Chapter 4

Cancer Detection Guidelines

Cancer-Related Checkup

A cancer-related checkup is recommended every 3 years for people aged 20-40 and every year for people age 40 and older. This exam should include health counseling and depending on a person's age might include examinations for cancers of the thyroid, oral cavity, skin, lymph nodes, testes, and ovaries as well as for some non-malignant diseases.

Special tests for certain cancer sites are recommended as outlined below.

Breast Cancer

- Breast self-exam monthly for women aged 20 and over.

- Breast clinical physical examination for women aged 20-40, every 3 years; over 40, every year. This exam should be done close to the time of the scheduled mammogram.

- Mammography for women aged 40 and over, every year.

Colon and Rectum Cancer

Beginning at age 50, both men and women should follow this testing schedule:

Reprinted with permission © 1998 "Cancer Facts and Figures," American Cancer Society, Atlanta, Georgia.

- Yearly fecal occult blood test plus flexible sigmoidoscopy and digital rectal examination every 5 years,* or

- Colonoscopy and digital rectal examination every 10 years,* or

- Double-contrast barium enema and digital rectal examination every 5-10 years.*

* The digital rectal examination should be done at the same time as sigmoidoscopy, colonoscopy, or double-contrast barium enema.

People should begin colorectal cancer screening earlier and/or undergo screening more often if they have any of the following colorectal cancer risk factors.

- A personal history of colorectal cancer or adenomatous polyps,

- A strong family history of colorectal cancer or polyps (cancer or polyps in a first degree relative younger than 60 or in two first degree relatives of any age),

- A personal history of chronic inflammatory bowel disease,

- Families with hereditary colorectal cancer syndromes (familial adenomatous polyposis and hereditary non-polyposis colon cancer).

Cervical Cancer

Pap test and pelvic examination for women who are or have been sexually active or have reached age 18, every year; after 3 or more consecutive satisfactory normal annual exams, the Pap test may be performed less frequently at the discretion of the physician.

Endometrium Cancer

Women at high risk for cancer of the endometrium should have a sample of endometrial tissue examined when menopause begins.

Prostate Cancer

Guideline Statement: Both Prostate-Specific Antigen (PSA) and Digital Rectal Examination (DRE) should be offered annually, beginning at age 50 years, to men who have at least a 10-year life expectancy, and to younger men who are at high risk. Information should be provided to patients regarding potential risks and benefits of intervention.

- Men who choose to undergo screening should begin at age 50 years. However, men in high risk groups, such as those with a strong familial predisposition (e.g., two or more affected first degree relatives) or African Americans may begin at a younger age (e.g. 45 years). More data on the precise age to start prostate cancer screening are needed for men at high risk.

- Screening for prostate cancer in asymptomatic men can detect tumors at a more favorable stage (anatomic extent of disease). There has been a reduction in mortality from prostate cancer, but it has not been established that this is a direct result of screening.

- An abnormal Prostate-Specific Antigen (PSA) test result has been defined as a value of above 4.0 ng/ml. Some elevations in PSA may be due to benign conditions of the prostate.

- The Digital Rectal Examination (DRE) of the prostate should be performed by health care workers skilled in recognizing subtle prostate abnormalities, including those of symmetry and consistency, as well as the more classic findings of marked induration or nodules. DRE is less effective in detecting prostate carcinoma compared with PSA.

Signs and Symptoms of Cancer

A symptom is an indication of disease, illness, injury, or that something is not right in the body. Symptoms are felt or noticed by a patient, but not easily observed by anyone else. For example chills, weakness, achiness, shortness of breath, and a cough are symptoms that might indicate pneumonia.

A sign is also an indication of illness, injury, or that something is not right in the body. But, signs are defined as observations made by a physician, nurse or other health care professional. Fever, rapid breathing rate, abnormal breathing sounds heard through a stethoscope are signs that may indicate pneumonia.

The presence of one symptom or sign may not provide enough information to suggest a cause. For example a rash in a child could be a symptom of a number of things including poison ivy, a generalized infection like rubella, an infection limited to the skin, or a food allergy. But, if the rash is associated with a high fever, chills, achiness and a sore throat, then all of the symptoms together provide a better picture of the illness.

In many cases, a patient's signs and symptoms do not provide enough clues to determine the cause of an illness, and medical tests such as x-rays, blood tests, or a biopsy may be needed.

How Does Cancer Produce Symptoms?

Cancer is a group of diseases that may cause virtually any sign or symptom. As cancer progresses, it goes through many stages, producing symptoms as it goes. The symptom produced will depend on the size of the cancer, the location of the cancer, and the surrounding organs or structures. If a cancer metastasizes (spreads), then symptoms will be very different, again depending of size, location, and surrounding structures.

As a cancer grows, it begins to exert pressure on nearby organs, blood vessels and nerves. This pressure creates some of the signs and symptoms of cancer. If the cancer is in a critical area, such as certain parts of the brain, even the smallest tumor can produce early symptoms.

Sometimes cancers form in locations where symptoms may not be produced until the cancer has grown quite large. For example, some pancreatic cancers do not produce symptoms until they begin to grow around nearby nerves, causing a backache. Unfortunately by the time a pancreatic cancer causes back pain, it has usually reached an advanced stage.

A cancer may cause generalized symptoms such as fever, fatigue, weight loss, etc. The cancer cells may release substances that alter metabolism. Or, the cancer may cause the immune system to react in ways that produce these symptoms.

Sometimes, cancer cells release substances into the bloodstream that cause symptoms not generally thought to result from cancers. For example, some cancers of the pancreas can release substances which affect blood clotting and cause blood clots to develop in veins of the legs. Some lung cancers produce hormone-like substances that affect blood calcium levels, affecting nerves and muscles and causing weakness and dizziness.

Why Is It Important to Recognize Symptoms?

The treatment of cancer is most successful when the cancer is detected as early as possible. It is possible to detect some cancers before symptoms occur. The American Cancer Society, and other organizations, encourage the early detection of certain cancers before symptoms occur by recommending a cancer-related checkup and specific early detection tests for people who do not have any symptoms. However, these recommended early detection tests do not diminish the importance of reporting any symptoms to your doctor.

Sometimes symptoms are ignored because the person is either frightened by their implications and refuses to seek medical help or does not recognize the symptom as being significant. It is very easy for individuals to think that a backache or fatigue is a "part of life" or that a breast mass is probably a cyst that will go away by itself. Whenever a symptom occurs, it should not be discounted or overlooked.

General Cancer Symptoms

It is important to know what some of the general (nonspecific) signs and symptoms of cancer are. They include unexplained weight loss, fever, fatigue, pain, changes in the skin.

- **Unexplained weight loss**: Most people with cancer will experience weight loss at some time with their disease. An unexplained weight loss of about 10 pounds may be the first sign of cancer, particularly cancers of the pancreas, stomach, esophagus, or lung.

- **Fever**: Fever is very common with cancer. Almost all patients with cancer will experience fever at some time, particularly if the cancer or its treatment affects the immune system and reduces resistance to infection. Less often, fever may be an early sign of cancer, such as with Hodgkin's disease.

- **Fatigue**: Fatigue may be a significant symptom as the cancer progresses. It may occur early, especially if the cancer is causing a chronic loss of blood as in some colon cancer or stomach cancers.

- **Pain**: Pain may be an early sign with some cancers, such as bone cancers or testicular cancer. Most often, pain is a symptom of advanced disease.

- **Skin clues**: In additions to cancers of the skin, some internal cancers can produce visible skin signs such as darkening of the skin, or hyperpigmentation; reddening, or erythema; itching; and excessive hair growth.

Specific Cancer Symptoms

In addition to the above general symptoms, the American Cancer Society has established the following seven common symptoms that could lead to a diagnosis of cancer.

1. A change in bowel habits or bladder function. Chronic consti-
    pation, diarrhea, or a change in the size of the stool may indi-
    cate colon cancer. Pain with urination, blood in the urine, or
    change in bladder function could be related to bladder or pros-
    tate cancer. Any changes in bladder or bowel function should
    be reported to your doctor.

2. Sores that do not heal. Skin cancers may bleed and resemble
    sores that do not heal. A persistent sore in the mouth could
    be an oral cancer and should be dealt with promptly, espe-
    cially for patients who smoke, chew tobacco, or frequently
    drink alcohol. Sores on the penis or vagina should not be
    overlooked.

3. Unusual bleeding or discharge. Unusual bleeding can occur in
    early or advanced cancer. Blood in the sputum is a sign of
    lung cancer. Blood in the stool could be a sign of colon cancer.
    Cancer of the lining of the uterus (endometrial cancer) or cer-
    vix can cause vaginal bleeding. Blood in the urine is a sign of
    possible bladder or kidney cancer. A bloody discharge from the
    nipple may be a sign of breast cancer.

4. Thickening or lump in breast or other parts of the body. Many
    cancers can be felt through the skin, particularly in the
    breast, testicle, lymph nodes (glands), and the soft tissues of
    the body. A lump or thickening may be an early or late sign of
    cancer. Any lump or thickening should be reported to your
    doctor. You may be feeling a lump that is an early cancer that
    could be treated successfully.

5. Indigestion or difficulty swallowing. These symptoms may in-
    dicate cancer of the esophagus, stomach, or pharynx (throat).

6. Recent change in a wart or mole. A change in color, loss of
    definite borders, or an increase in size should be reported to
    your doctor without delay. The skin lesion may be a melanoma
    which, if diagnosed early, can be treated successfully.

7. A nagging cough or hoarseness. A persistent cough that does
    not go away is a sign of lung cancer. Hoarseness can be a sign
    of cancer of the larynx (voice box) or thyroid. These are often
    late signs of cancer.

Chapter 5

Is Your Heart at Risk?
Heart Health Checkup

Cardiovascular System Diagnostic Tests and Procedures

Even if you do everything right, your cardiovascular system can still go wrong. That's why it's especially important to have your heart health evaluated by a trained physician. Most experts agree that if you are healthy, you should get a regular checkup at least:

- Twice in your 20s (every 5 years)
- Three times in your 30s (every 3 to 4 years)
- Four times in your 40s (every 2 to 3 years)
- Five times in your 50s (every 2 years)
- Every year if you are 60 or older

During an exam, your doctor will want to know if you have any specific complaints (such as chest pain), and get a medical history including information about all prior illnesses, hospitalizations, accidents, operations and allergies. Your doctor will also inquire about any medications you may be taking—so don't forget to mention over-the-counter drugs and dietary supplements such as vitamins. The doctor will also want information about your lifestyle or living habits that may have an impact on heart disease, such as smoking, alcohol use, illegal drug use and stress at work.

Reprinted with permission © November 1997 The Johns Hopkins University 1996-1999. InteliHealth available at www.intelihealth.com.

Your cardiovascular physical examination will include measuring your blood pressure, heart rate and rhythm, checking all the pulses, inspecting the veins of your neck, determining whether there is swelling, and listening to breathing and heart sounds. The doctor will check:

- **Heart rate and rhythm.** Your doctor will feel the pulse at the wrist.

- **Pulses.** Your doctor will also feel the pulses in your neck, groin and feet and listen over the arteries in the neck. Weak or absent pulses, or a murmur in the neck, suggest an obstruction to blood flow.

- **Swelling.** Doctors routinely look for excess fluid by examining the legs and ankles for swelling. Swelling, or edema, may develop with heart or kidney failure, liver disease, or if there's a blockage in a vein carrying blood back to the heart. Your doctor will press on the skin and watch how far it can be indented.

- **Breath sounds.** Using a stethoscope, your doctor will try to determine whether fluid has leaked into the air sacs of the lungs. Presence of this fluid, which makes a crackling or wet sound, may be an early sign of heart failure.

- **Heart sounds.** Your doctor will check for a regular heartbeat and listen for a murmur to determine any abnormal function of the heart valves.

Diagnostic Tests for Heart Disease:

Blood Tests

The most common blood tests related to heart disease measure blood cholesterol, triglyceride and HDL cholesterol levels, cardiac enzymes, oxygen content and prothrombin time, and check for thyroid disorders.

- Measurement of total cholesterol, HDL cholesterol and triglycerides allows a calculation of LDL cholesterol, and the ratio of LDL cholesterol to HDL cholesterol. Blood levels of triglycerides vary according to recent food intake. To get a true reading, be sure to fast for 12 hours before the blood is drawn.

- Cardiac enzymes: Enzymes found in the heart may leak into blood from damaged heart cells after a heart attack. If you experience chest pain, your doctor may test your blood for the enzymes creatine kinase (CK) and lactate dehydrogenase (LDH).

• Oxygen content: Measurement of blood oxygen helps to determine whether your overall circulation is sufficient, whether the lungs are providing enough oxygen to the bloodstream, and whether there is evidence of poor blood flow from the heart to the lungs. Oxygen is measured in blood drawn from an artery whereas standard blood tests use blood from a vein, usually drawn at the bend of the elbow.

• Prothrombin time (clotting time): Medications that slow blood clotting are anticoagulants, warfarin (Coumadin), for example, or antiplatelet drugs, such as plain old everyday aspirin. Although they are referred to as "blood thinners," they don't actually "thin" the blood; instead anticoagulants alter proteins in the blood that are responsible for clotting, while antiplatelet drugs prevent platelets from clumping and forming clots. Because people respond differently to anticoagulants, blood tests that measure prothrombin time are used to determine whether the drug dose is correct—effective, yet safe (too high a dose can cause bleeding). Prothrombin time is measured in people taking an anticoagulant, not in those taking aspirin.

• Doctors often check for thyroid disease because an abnormally functioning thyroid gland can lead to a racing heartbeat. One of the most common thyroid disorders is known as Grave's disease. The disorder results from an overactive thyroid gland that produces excessive amounts of thyroid hormones.

Chest X-ray

A chest x-ray produces an image on film that outlines your heart, lungs, and other structures in your chest. Chest films can give important information about the size and shape of your heart, calcium deposits that may be blocking blood flow and the condition of your lungs. A positive, or suspicious chest x-ray may lead your doctor to order a more specific heart scan.

Electrocardiogram (ECG)

An electrocardiogram records the electrical activity of your heart and is indispensable for evaluating many forms of heart disease. The tracing can be displayed either on a strip of paper or on a monitor. It can also be recorded on tape and transmitted over telephone wires.

An ECG tracing breaks down your heartbeat into a series of waves that give information about your heart rate, the rhythm of your heart, the presence of heart damage or inadequate blood and oxygen supply to the heart muscle, and abnormalities of heart structure.

Different waves represent the different areas of your heart through which tiny electrical currents flow, causing it to contract and relax. Briefly, the P wave represents the current in the atria; the QRS complex, the current in the ventricles; and the T wave, the electrical recovery period of the ventricles.

An ECG may be done to identify all types of abnormally fast and slow rhythms; distinguish between a heart attack that occurred in the past and one in progress at the time the ECG is taken; determine whether chest pain is being caused by inadequate blood flow in the coronary arteries and the site of this blockage; and provide clues about heart abnormalities, such as congenital conditions and thickening of the heart walls.

During an ECG, 9 to 12 electrodes will be attached to various parts of your body, including one on each arm and leg, six across the left side of the chest and at times one or more at other sites on the chest, neck, and back. The electrodes are attached with sticky pads while you are lying down. The machine then records the electrical activity from various contact points over a period of between 30 to 60 seconds. You won't feel anything.

There are two problems with the standard ECG test: it is taken while you are resting quietly, and so may miss abnormalities that occur with exertion; and because the test is so brief, some sporadic rhythm abnormalities may be missed. So other techniques have been developed to increase the likelihood of detecting an abnormality. These include:

- Exercise ECG is a reading obtained while you walk on a treadmill or pedal a stationary bicycle. This technique, also called a "stress test", is more likely to spot abnormal heart patterns and insufficient blood and oxygen supplies to the heart muscle during exercise.

- Ambulatory ECG (Holter monitoring) records your heart patterns, usually over a 24-hour period. Small electrodes that stick to your skin are connected to a portable recording device on a shoulder strap or belt worn under your clothing, while you go about your daily activities. The taped information can then be analyzed by a computer and printed out much like a standard ECG.

• Telephone-transmitted ECG is used to transmit your heart patterns to a hospital or doctor while you are having symptoms. When a symptom develops, you dial a telephone number and transmit the readings over a phone line.

Chapter 6

Hypertension, A Silent Killer

It's Important to Know about High Blood Pressure

High Blood Pressure, also called hypertension, is a risk factor for heart and kidney diseases and stroke. This means that having high blood pressure increases your chance (or risk) of getting heart or kidney disease, or of having a stroke. This is serious business: heart disease is the number one killer in the United States, and stroke is the third most common cause of death.

About one in every four American adults has high blood pressure. High blood pressure is especially dangerous because it often gives no warning signs or symptoms. Fortunately, though, you can find out if you have high blood pressure by having your blood pressure checked regularly. If it is high, you can take steps to lower it. Just as important, **if your blood pressure is normal, you can learn how to keep it from becoming high.**

What Is Blood Pressure and What Happens When It Is High?

Since blood is carried from the heart to all of your body's tissue and organs in vessels called arteries, blood pressure is the force of the blood pushing against the walls of those arteries. In fact, each time the heart beats (about 60-70 times a minute at rest), it pumps out

Excerpts from *Preventing High Blood Pressure*, a publication of the National Heart, Lung, and Blood Institute (NHLBI).

25

blood into the arteries. Your blood pressure is at its greatest when the heart contracts and is pumping the blood. This is called **systolic pressure.** When the heart is at rest, in between beats, your blood pressure falls. This is the **diastolic pressure.**

Blood pressure is always given as these two numbers, systolic and diastolic pressures. Both are important. Usually they are written one above or before the other, such as 120/80 mm Hg, with the top number the systolic, and the bottom the diastolic.

Different actions make your blood pressure go up or down. For example, if you run for a bus, your blood pressure goes up. When you sleep at night, your blood pressure goes down. These changes in blood pressure are normal.

Some people have blood pressure that stays up all or most of the time. Their blood pushes against the walls of their arteries with higher-than-normal force. If untreated this can lead to serious medical problems like these:

- **Arteriosclerosis** ("hardening of the arteries"). High blood pressure harms the arteries by making them thick and stiff. This speeds the build up of cholesterol and fats in the blood vessels like rust in a pipe, which prevents the blood from flowing through the body, and in time can lead to a heart attack or stroke.

- **Heart Attack.** Blood carries oxygen to the body. When the arteries that bring blood to the heart muscle become blocked, the heart cannot get enough oxygen. Reduced blood flow can cause chest pain (angina). Eventually, the flow may be stopped completely, causing a heart attack.

- **Enlarged heart.** High blood pressure causes the heart to work harder. Over time, this causes the heart to thicken and stretch. Eventually the heart fails to function normally causing fluids to back up into the lungs. Controlling high blood pressure can prevent this from happening.

- **Kidney Damage.** The kidney acts as a filter to rid the body of wastes. Over a number of years, high blood pressure can narrow and thicken the blood vessels of the kidney. The kidney filters less fluid, and waste builds up in the blood. The kidneys may fail altogether. When this happens, medical treatment (dialysis) or a kidney transplant may be needed.

- **Stroke.** High blood pressure can harm the arteries, causing them to narrow faster. So, less blood can get to the brain. If a blood clot blocks one of the narrowed arteries, a stroke (thrombotic stroke) may occur. A stroke can also occur when very high pressure causes a break in a weakened blood vessel in the brain (hemorrhagic stroke).

Who's Likely To Develop High Blood Pressure?

Anyone can develop high blood pressure, but some people are more likely to develop it than others. For example, high blood pressure is more common—it develops earlier and is more severe—in African-Americans than in whites.

In the early and middle adult years, men have high blood pressure more often than women. But as men and women age, the reverse is true. More women after menopause have high blood pressure then men of the same age. And the number of **both** men and women with high blood pressure increases rapidly in older age groups. More than half of all Americans over age 65 have high blood pressure. And older African-American women who live in the Southeast are more likely to have high blood pressure than are those in other regions of the United States.

In fact, the southeastern states have some of the highest rates of death from stroke. High blood pressure is the key risk factor for stroke. Other risk factors include cigarette smoking and excess weight. These 11 states–Alabama, Arkansas, Georgia, Indiana, Kentucky, Louisiana, Mississippi, North Carolina, South Carolina, Tennessee, and Virginia– have such high rates of stroke among persons of all races and in both sexes that they are called the "Stroke Belt States."

Finally, heredity can make some families more likely than others to get high blood pressure. If your parents or grandparents had high blood pressure, your risk may be increased. While it is mainly a disease of adults, high blood pressure can occur in children as well. Even if everyone is healthy, be sure you and your family get your blood pressure checked. **Remember, high blood pressure has no signs or symptoms.**

How Is Blood Pressure Checked?

Having your blood pressure checked is quick, easy, and painless. Your blood pressure is measured with an instrument called a sphygmomanometer (sfig-mo-ma-nom-e-ter).

It works like this: A blood pressure cuff is wrapped around your upper arm and inflated to stop the blood flow in your artery for a few

27

seconds. A valve is opened and air is then released from the cuff and the sounds of your blood rushing through an artery are heard through a stethoscope. The first sound heard and registered on the gauge or mercury column is called the **systolic** blood pressure. It represents the maximum pressure in the artery produced as the heart contracts and the blood begins to flow. The last sound heard as more air is released from the cuff is the **diastolic** blood pressure. It represents the lowest pressure that remains within the artery when the heart is at rest.

What Do the Numbers Mean?

Blood pressure is always expressed in two numbers that represent the systolic and diastolic pressures. These numbers are measurements of millimeters (mm) of mercury (Hg). The measurement is written one above or before the other, with the systolic number on the top and the diastolic number on the bottom. For example, a blood pressure measurement of 120/80 mm Hg is expressed verbally as "120 over 80." See the table below which shows categories for blood pressure levels in adults.

Table 6.1. Categories For Blood Pressure Levels in Adults (Age 18 Years and Older)*

Category	Blood Pressure Level (mm Hg)	
	Systolic	Diastolic
Normal	<130	<85
High Normal	130-139	85-89
High Blood Pressure		
Stage 1	140-159	90-99
Stage 2	160-179	100-109
Stage 3	≥180	≥110

*For those not taking medicine for high blood pressure and not having a short term serious illness. These categories are from the National High Blood Pressure Education Program.

(< means less than; ≥ means greater than or equal to)

If your blood pressure is less than 140/90 mm Hg, it is considered normal. However, a blood pressure below 120/80 mm Hg is even better for your heart and blood vessels. People use to think that low blood pressure (for example, 105/65 mm Hg in an adult) was unhealthy. Except for rare cases, this is not true. High blood pressure or "hypertension" is classified by stages and is more serious as the numbers get higher.

What Causes High Blood Pressure?

For most people, there is no single known cause of high blood pressure. This type of high blood pressure is called "primary" or "essential" hypertension. This type of blood pressure can't be cured, although in most cases it can be controlled. That's why it's so important for everyone to take steps to reduce their chances of developing high blood pressure.

In a few people, high blood pressure can be traced to a known cause like tumors of the adrenal gland, chronic kidney disease, hormone abnormalities, use of birth control pills, or pregnancy. This is called "secondary hypertension." Secondary hypertension is usually cured if its cause passes or is corrected.

Want To Know More?

For more information on either high blood pressure or weight and physical activity, contact:
National Heart, Lung, and Blood Institute Information Center
P.O. Box 30105
Bethesda, MD 20824-0105
(301) 251-1222

Chapter 7

Geriatric Health Screening That Is Clearly Effective

Preventive Medicine

During the past two decades, the population over 65 years has grown twice as quickly as the rest of the U.S. population. By the year 2000, 13% of the population is expected to be over age 65. As the population ages and becomes more impaired, concern for the prevention of disease and promotion of good health increases. In this era of rapid change in the financing and delivery of health services, however, it is essential to determine the effectiveness of specific preventive services and counseling delivered to the elderly. Little information is available, however, regarding the appropriate screening tests and services for older adults. The U.S. Preventive Services Task Force (USPSTF) applied specific criteria to evaluate several services and procedures to a wide age range, although few were specifically targeted to the elderly population.

The older population tends to be a heterogeneous group. Although the elderly can be categorized by age cohorts, there is no consensus which age groups to consider as the "young old" or "old old." Categorization by functional ability, number of comorbidities, and presence of infirmity has also been done. Those with the poorest health status are considered frail or "at risk" elderly. In addition, older adults have

---

This chapter includes "Topics in Geriatrics," "The 'Get Up and Go' Test," "Balance Assessment: A Modified Romberg Test," and "The Functional Reach Test," from Mayo Health Information. Reprinted with permission © 1996-1998 Mayo Foundation for Medical Education and Research.

been stratified according to residence (e.g., community-dwelling or institutionalized) for research purposes.

Most studies evaluating preventive services use reduction of disease specific mortality as an outcome. In the elderly there are clearly additional and more relevant health outcomes to be considered. Health in old age can be said to consist of three related factors:

1. The absence of disease,
2. The maintenance of optimal function; and
3. The presence of an adequate support system.

However, while older adults tend to have a greater burden of disease than younger subjects, individuals may still be considered "healthy". Therefore, the major goals of preventive care in the elderly are delay or reduction of morbidity and prevention of disease, in order to maximize quality of life, satisfaction with life and productivity. These outcomes are more difficult to measure and infrequently done in studies of preventive services.

In this chapter, we have reviewed the current literature regarding geriatric health maintenance and key areas of preventive care. Critical evaluation of the health issues integral to maintaining health in the older adult was performed using established criteria. The objective was to highlight articles pertaining to geriatric health maintenance, allowing the clinician to weigh current evidence for or against screening and/or treatment. The authors took the liberty of making specific recommendation about specific screening tests when the evidence in the literature was convincing. The list of topics is not exhaustive but covers many of the important areas in geriatric health maintenance. The chapter is divided into four major headings; history, physical examination, laboratory and interventions.

Historical Information

Nutrition

A key preventive strategy in caring for older persons is maintaining adequate nutrition. 15% of older outpatients, nearly half of hospitalized elderly, and from 12-85% of aged institutionalized residents have been shown to be malnourished. Under nutrition is clearly linked to prolonged hospital stays, re-admissions, pressure ulcers, and increased mortality. Anorexia and malnutrition can result from poverty, social isolation, depression, dementia, pain, immobility, reflux, constipation, alcoholism, medications, dental problems, altered hunger and thirst recognition, or impaired taste. Dysphagia due to strokes, Parkinsonism, medicines, or dementia has been estimated to affect half of institutionalized elderly. However, no laboratory measures have been validated in screening for malnutrition in the elderly. Nutritional status can be assessed by inquiring about anorexia or weight loss. It is essential to record elderly patients' weights regularly for unrecognized weight loss. Combining historical data about changes in appetite and weight, physical signs of malnutrition (jaundice, cheilosis, glossitis, loss of subcutaneous fat, muscle wasting, edema), and serial weight measurements may be the most useful method to assess nutritional status in the elderly. Additional assessment of any physical, cognitive, or financial barriers to obtaining appropriate nutrition can be approached on an individual basis.

The authors recommend periodic/annual weight measurement in older adults. The USPSTF recommends periodic counseling regarding dietary intake without specific consideration to the elderly patient.

Tobacco

Since 1974 smoking has declined among men aged 65 and older and increased among women aged 65 and older. Attributable risk corresponds to the excess number of deaths that occurred among smokers relative to nonsmokers. The number of deaths attributable to smoking increases after age 65. Within five years of smoking cessation in community-dwelling adults aged 65 and older, the relative risk from all cause mortality was lower than among current smokers. Smokers are more likely to refrain from smoking if their physician recommends it.

The authors agree with the USPSTF recommendations to repeatedly encourage smokers to quit smoking. The nicotine patch may be a useful adjutant in older adults.

Burns

Burn injuries in individuals over 60 years occur more frequently and are associated with higher morbidity and mortality than any other age group. Flame and scald injuries are the predominant mode of burn in the elderly. Fire department statistics have demonstrated a two to three fold increased risk of dying in a house fire in homes without smoke detectors. However, it is unknown if advising patients to install and test smoke detectors results in prevention of fire injury. In addition, some older individuals may be unable to hear or respond to the alarm. The elderly individual should be advised not to smoke in bed, and to reduce water temperatures to 120 degrees Fahrenheit. Once again, the effectiveness of these counseling interventions is unknown.

The authors agree with the USPSTF that it is clinically prudent to provide counseling on measures to reduce the risk of unintentional household injuries.

Continence

Fifteen to thirty percent of community dwelling older adults suffer from urinary incontinence (UI), while nearly 50 percent of older nursing home residents are affected. Twenty-five to 35 percent of those with incontinence have daily or weekly incontinence episodes. The prevalence of UI in elderly women is twice that of elderly men. This increased prevalence in women is related to anatomic differences (e.g., urethral length), pelvic floor dysfunction, and perineal injury. Incontinence in older males tends to be related to prostatic enlargement and sphincter impairment. Additional factors contributing to UI include urinary infections, confusional states, medications, immobility, hyperglycemia, alcohol abuse, congestive heart failure, catheter-induced bladder dysfunction and stool impaction. Patients need to be aware that most UI problems can be evaluated with minimal testing and that most initial treatment options are nonsurgical. These interventions can have significant degrees of success, even among nursing home residents.

The authors recommend periodic nonjudgemental assessment as to the presence of urinary continence in all older adults. This was not reviewed by the USPSTF.

Motor Vehicle Accidents

Drivers over 70 years of age have more accidents, more hospitalizations resulting from accidents, and more driver and pedestrian accidents resulting in fatalities per millions miles driven than middle aged drivers. The decline of visual acuity, hearing, information processing, and psychomotor skills is believed to be related to impairment of driving ability. Patients with dementia may have profound impairments in driving ability, although the degree of cognitive loss at which to recommend cessation of driving is unknown. Dementia of any degree raises significant concerns about driving safety. The specific contribution of dementia to driving accidents is unknown.

Although physicians may advise patients with dementia not to drive, the effectiveness of this advice is unknown. Referral for formal ("behind the wheel") driving assessment by the State Department of Transportation seems prudent and fair. For all ages, seat belts have been shown to decrease morbidity and mortality from motor vehicle accidents. (USPSTF) Randomized control trials have suggested that seat belt use can be increased by office-based interventions. Re-education in driving skills can be helpful, although the effectiveness of this training is unknown. Insurance companies offer reduced rates for older drivers who have completed classes to update driving skills.

The authors recommend advising dementia patients not to drive and referring mildly demented patients to the State Department of Transportation for periodic "behind the wheel" testing. All patients should be advised to wear seatbelts. Periodic hearing and vision testing is advised. The USPTF agrees with advising high-risk individuals to wear seat belts, but does not comment on driving with dementia.

Physical Examination

Blood Pressure

Heart disease and cerebral vascular disease account for the number one and three cause of death in those over 75 years of age. Hypertension is one of the major risk factors for heart disease and cerebrovascular disease. Over the past 25 years, 13 randomized controlled trials have demonstrated a significant reduction in cardiovascular events by pharmacologic control of hypertension in individuals over 60 years of age. A pooling of six large, high-quality trials found only 18 subjects (95% CI, 14 to 25) needed to be treated to prevent one cardiovascular event (cerebrovascular or cardiac).

The authors agree with the USPSTF recommendations that persons thought to be normotensive should receive blood pressure measurements at least once every two years. Elderly found to be hypertensive should be managed with behavioral modification and pharmacotherapy in accordance with the Joint National Committee on Detection, Evaluation and Treatment of High Blood Pressure.

Skin Cancer

Cutaneous cancers are among the most common malignancies. In 1995, an estimated 34,100 new cases of melanoma will be diagnosed and there will be 7,200 deaths. Skin inspection, a simple examination without risk, is the principal screening test to detect skin cancer. Unlike most cancers, 75% of melanomas are diagnosed before age 65. The primary risk factors are a previous history of precancerous lesions, a family history of melanoma, and sun exposure. There is little evidence supporting the effectiveness of physician-performed screening over self-recognition. However, visual impairment (which is common in the elderly) may reduce the ability to self-inspect. No data from experimental studies support the efficacy of routine screening. The sensitivity (30-95%) varies widely across different studies.

The authors recommend annual inspection of patients with a family or previous history of skin cancer precursor lesion and those with increased sun exposure. This recommendation is in agreement with the USPSTF.

Hearing

Hearing loss affects one-third of 65-year-olds, two-thirds of those over age 70, and three-fourths of those 80 years of age and older. Presbycusis is the most common form of hearing loss in the elderly. Older patients may not complain of or even recognize that they are hearing impaired. The impact of hearing loss is poorly appreciated. Depression and social isolation are commonly reported consequences in older patients. Communication can be profoundly impaired, compromising family, worship and entertainment activities as well as social, medical and work relationships. Simple accurate tests of hearing can be performed at low cost. Hearing impairment can be acceptably modified by hearing aides or other amplification devices. Hand-held amplifiers may be useful when a patient's cognitive or physical impairments limit effective device operation and when the cost of a hearing aid is prohibitive.

The authors recommend periodic/annual hearing assessment and otologic examination of all older adults. Formal audiometry need not be performed if the patient is unwilling or unable to use appropriate assistive devices. This is in agreement with the USPSTF.

Vision

Normal aging is accompanied by increasing visual impairment resulting from macular degeneration, cataracts, glaucoma and diabetic retinopathy. Cataracts, the second leading cause of blindness in the United States, are present in over sixty percent of patients over age 75. Open angle glaucoma (OAG), a major cause of blindness in the elderly, increases in prevalence with age, requiring treatment in two to four percent of those over age 75. As a result, more than 90 percent of older adults need eyeglasses. In addition, sixteen percent of those aged 75 to 84, and 27 percent of those older than 85 are blind in both eyes or are unable to read newsprint even with glasses. Yet many older adults are unaware of impaired vision, including losses in peripheral and central acuity. Screening eye examinations performed in geriatric daycare and outpatient settings have revealed that up to one-third of those examined had previously undiagnosed conditions, most of which were treatable. However, there is little evidence available to assess the efficacy of widespread screening for visual impairment in the elderly.

Visual acuity charts are a simple method for assessing visual function. However, a lack of correlation between these test results and daily visual function has been shown. Tonometry and ophthalmoscopy lack specificity in detecting OAG, and fundoscopic findings are apparent in only half of cases of OAG. In addition, the majority of those with intraocular hypertension never develop OAG. Although laser photocoagulation can significantly improve vision in certain types of disciform macular degeneration, there are few data regarding screening the general population for this disorder. A brief globe and fundus examination and simple standard confontrative visual field assessment may focus the content of ophthalmologic referrals. However these can be difficult in the elderly and are of unproven clinical utility as screening tools in the patient who does not complain of visual problems.

At present, the evidence is insufficient to recommend or discourage widespread screening of the elderly population for eye diseases. Nevertheless, periodic interviews regarding problems with near and distance vision and periodic formal ophthalmologic examinations seem prudent. The USPSTF states it may be appropriate to test the visual acuity and it is clinically prudent to test for glaucoma in the elderly.

Dentition

Compared to previous generations, today's elderly are keeping their teeth longer. A controlled oral hygiene trial in individuals greater than 50 years was shown to prevent the progression of periodontal disease and caries in adults. (The intervention consisted of instruction and practice in oral hygiene techniques and oral prophylaxis every 2-3 months.) The optimal frequency for regular dental visits is unknown.

Fluorides are effective in preventing dental caries in adults as well as children. If local water supplies are not fluorinated, self-applied fluorides (available as rinses or gels) are recommended for daily use.

The authors agree with the USPSTF recommendations to encourage all patients to visit the dentist periodically. In addition, all patients should brush their teeth daily with a fluoride-containing toothpaste. Health care providers should assess the geriatric patient's ability to brush his/her own teeth.

Oral Exam

An estimated 28,150 new cases of oral cancer will occur in the United States during 1995 and 8,370 oral cancer deaths. Persons over 65 years of age account for approximately fifty percent of all cases. Risk factors include age greater than 60 years, excessive alcohol consumption and tobacco use. Inspection and palpation of the oral cavity are the screening tests available for oral cancers. There are no data on the sensitivity or specificity of the oral examination, nor on the effectiveness of screening in the elderly.

The authors support the recommendations of the USPSTF to screen only those individuals considered at high risk, which would mean screening all persons over age 60.

Shoulder Function

At least one in four older people have shoulder pain. Nevertheless, nearly half of shoulder complaints go unreported. Thoracic kyphosis, degenerative arthritis, trauma, disuse, and age-related connective tissue changes combine to reduce shoulder strength, integrity, and mobility in the elderly. Older patients may be unaware of shoulder limitations since dysfunction can arise insidiously and without pain. Reduced shoulder range of motion can impair an older person's ability to drive and perform personal cares such as dressing. Long-term limitations in shoulder mobility due to pain or dysfunction may result in muscle weakness, chronic pain, sleep disturbance, and impaired functional ability. Over 70 percent of cases are due to soft tissue lesions responsive to nonsurgical treatments, such as physical therapy, exercise and analgesics. A simple screening measure of shoulder function includes inquiring about the presence of pain and observing range of motion.

The authors recommend periodic/annual assessment of shoulder function in older patients. This was not reviewed by the USPSTF.

Prostate Cancer

During 1995 it is estimated there will be 244,000 new cases of prostate cancer diagnosed and 40,400 deaths due to prostate cancer in the United States. Age is a major factor in the incidence of prostate cancer. Over 80% of all cases of prostate cancer occur in men over the age of 64 years. Autopsy studies have found the incidence of occult tumors ranging from less than 30% at age 50 years to 100% in the 9th decade. Three screening techniques are in clinical use: the digital rectal examination (DRE), transrectal ultrasound and prostate specific antigen. The positive predictive value for the DRE, transrectal ultrasound and prostate specific antigen are 22 to 31%, 17-41%, and 35% respectively. These positive predictive values are too low to be clinically useful.

Early diagnosis through screening would benefit only those men in whom the disease is curable and in whom the tumor will be progressive or lethal. To date there are no randomized control trials with an end point of cure with acceptable quality of life in progress to determine if there is benefit from early diagnosis and treatment of prostate cancer. Possible adverse effects to be considered when screening include: morbidity resulting directly from the tests, morbidity and mortality from unnecessary treatment of those patients identified with incurable disease, detection of clinically insignificant disease, emotional trauma and cost of false positive tests.

The authors agree with the USPSTF recommendation in that there is insufficient evidence to recommend for or against routine digital rectal examination as an effective screening test for prostate cancer in asymptomatic men. Transrectal ultrasound and serum tumor markers are not recommended for routine screening in asymptomatic men.

Ovarian Cancer

In 1995 it is estimated there will be 26,600 new cases of ovarian cancer in the United States. The annual incidence increases with age with the mean age of clinical presentation occurring at 59 years. Currently there are three broad categories of screening techniques available: pelvic examination, ultrasound and other imaging techniques, and carcinoembrionic antigen 125 and other tumor markers. In general, ovarian malignancies have disseminated by the time they are palpable. Studies have suggested that a pelvic examination by a highly skilled examiner may detect early ovarian cancer. Carson et al reviewed all studies evaluating abdominal or transvaginal ultrasound and calculated a summary estimate of the sensitivity of ultrasound for detection of cancer is 85 percent and the specificity is 93.8 percent. Two large screening studies in postmenopausal women found the sensitivity of CA 125 in detecting ovarian cancer to range from 53 percent to 100 percent for a reference level of 35 U/ml. From three community screening studies a specificity of 98.6 percent to 99.4 percent was found for CA 125 utilizing a reference level of 35 U/ml. Unfortunately, whether screening by any technique would result in decreased mortality is unknown.

The authors do not recommend screening of asymptomatic women for ovarian cancer. It is reasonable to examine the ovaries at the time of pelvic examination done for other clinical reasons. In women with the rare hereditary ovarian cancer syndrome, specialist care is recommended. These recommendations are identical to those given by the USPSTF.

Uterine Cancer

The peak incidence of uterine cancer is in women 60 to 74 years of age and the peak mortality is in women 85 years and older. Current screening modalities include bimanual pelvic examination, Papanicolaou smear, endocervical aspiration and endometrial sampling. All four modalities are unreliable and inaccurate "in older women." Most importantly, early detection in asymptomatic women has not been shown to decrease the mortality from uterine cancer.

The authors do not recommend screening asymptomatic women for uterine cancer until there is evidence to support the effectiveness. This area was not reviewed by the USPSTF.

Feet

There is a high prevalence of foot problems in the elderly. A study from England found only 6 of 96 people aged 80 and over had normal, healthy feet. Seventy-seven per cent had difficulty cutting their toenails due to poor vision, inability to reach their toes, or hypertrophied nails. Neglected foot care can lead to discomfort, diminished or impaired ambulation, decreased quality of life, and possible infection or amputation. Physicians can identify foot problems by simply examining the feet and by asking about the presence of pain or individual's ability to perform needed foot care. Impairments in mobility that may prevent independent foot care can be assessed by having the subject touch their toes while seated.

The authors recommend annual assessment of foot care by history and physical examination. The intervention is low effort. The USPSTF did not review this intervention.

Gait and Falls

As a result of aging, illness, pain and disuse, older adults commonly show changes in gait that can result in imbalance and falls. One in five older adults have disorders in gait or transferring ability. Among persons over 75 years of age, 30 percent report difficulty with stairs, 40 percent cannot walk one-half mile and seven percent need assistance to walk at all. Approximately 30 percent of non-institutionalized older adults fall each year. Costs related to care of fall-related fractures approach $10 billion each year. Nonambulatory elderly who are bed or chair bound may become deconditioned and may develop edema, contractures, incontinence, or pressure sores. Such patients are often at risk for falls and nursing home placement.

A number of assessment instruments can accurately screen for gait and balance impairments.

The "Get Up and Go" Test

The subject is seated in a straight-backed high-seat chair. Sitting balance and transfers from sitting to standing are noted. The subject is instructed to rise (without using the armrests, if possible), stand still momentarily, walk forward approximately ten feet and turn around. The subject then walks back to the chair, turns, and sits back down. Certain abnormalities of gait and balance identified in walking tests have been shown to be good predictors of recurrent falls:

- unsafe or incomplete transfers
  1. poor sitting balance
  2. difficulty rising
  3. difficulty or unsafe sitting down
- instability on first standing
- staggering on turns
- short, discontinuous steps
- undue slowness
- hesitancy
- unsafe maneuvers
- excessive truncal sway

- grabbing for support
- stumbling

The subject's gait is considered severely abnormal if the individual appeared at risk for a fall at any time during the test. Although there are no established norms, timing the "Get Up and Go" test allows for serial comparisons. Indeed, self-selected gait speed is the single greatest predictor of self-perceived function and overall physical performance in a wide range of abilities.

Balance Assessment: A Modified Romberg Test

The standing patient performs tasks of increasing difficulty, observing the response to positional stress, loss of visual input and displacement. The patient assumes different standing positions, first with eyes open, then with eyes closed. With each successive maneuver, stability is observed and the patient is asked, "Do you feel steady?" A light nudge to the sternum can be helpful in assessing the response to displacement. This allows a rough estimate of balance and can help identify causative factors (e.g., osteoarthritis, peripheral neuropathy, foot problems, atherosclerosis, weakness, stroke, pain, or contractures).

- Position of Feet for Modified Romberg Test
  1. Feet comfortably apart
  2. Feet together
  3. Feet semi-tandem (heel-to-instep)
  4. Feet tandem (heel-to-toe)

The Functional Reach Test

The Functional Reach test is another simple tool for assessing balance. A patient standing with one shoulder close to a wall is asked to extend the fist along the wall directly frontward. The subject then leans forward, fist extended in front as far as possible without taking a step or losing stability. The patient should be able to move the fist forward a distance of at least six inches; lesser distances indicate a significant risk for falling.

A recent multicenter trial has demonstrated that interventions directed at modification of these gait abnormalities result in a reduction in the risk of falls and injury. Treatment options include: environmental safety changes, gait retraining, strengthening exercises, use of gait aids and treatment of associated pain, medical and podiatric disorders.

The authors recommend inquiring about falls or fear of falling and periodic evaluation of gait and balance in the elderly. This was not reviewed by the USPSTF.

Cognitive Function

The prevalence of dementia in patients over 65 years of age has been reported to be between five and 15 percent, approaching 20 to 50 percent after age 85. A patient's ability to live independently, manage financial affairs, drive, and comply with medication regimens may all be impaired by cognitive decline. Care of the cognitively impaired elder imposes a tremendous psychosocial and economic burden on caregivers. A diagnosis of dementia or mild cognitive impairment would necessarily impact all aspects of an individual's future care (e.g., medications, instructions, consent), reversible conditions may also be identified in some. Without screening tools, early or mild dementia can remain undetected. The Mini-Mental Status Examination is adequate for detecting cognitive impairment, establishing a baseline, and measuring decline over time. However, there is insufficient evidence to determine whether routine screening for cognitive impairment should be included or excluded in the periodic examination of the older adult. Screening cognitive tests are low-yield in the general geriatric population, and are best targeted to persons over age 80, individuals entering RTC, hospital inpatients (e.g. pre-operatively) and in those demonstrating functional decline. Studies do not yet show improvement in various outcomes in those identified with dementia, although this area is not well studied.

The authors recommend periodic evaluation of cognitive status in the higher risk elderly. Although there are no curative medications, management of dementia-related problems can be assisted once the diagnosis is recognized. This was not reviewed by the USPSTF.

Tests

Thyroid Disease

Thyroid dysfunction increases with age, particularly in women over age 50. Hypothyroidism is more common in the elderly, with a prevalence of overt and mild disease in two to three percent of men and six to ten percent of women. Subclinical hypothyroidism affects nine to 16% of those over age 60. The prevalence of unsuspected thyrotoxicosis ranges from two to 20 cases per 1000 persons; the annual incidence of thyrotoxicosis ranges from one to five cases per 10,000 persons. There are few studies on the prevalence of subclinical hyperthyroidism, although it is commonly a result of over-replacement of thyroxine hormone.

Patients with hypothyroidism or thyrotoxicosis can present with signs and symptoms that are subtle, nonspecific, and indistinguishable from complaints common in elderly adults. Constipation, weight loss, dry skin, memory changes, leg edema, tiredness, and cold or exertional intolerance may reflect thyroid disease or conditions frequent in the aged population. The American College of Physicians has recommended against routine screening asymptomatic elderly patients for thyroid disease due to lack of demonstrated efficacy or proven benefit. In addition, monitoring and treatment of subclinical thyroid disease are of uncertain clinical utility and have not been shown to improve outcomes in affected patients. Treatment of subclinical hypothyroidism may risk aggravation of coronary artery disease and osteoporosis.

The USPSTF recommended that it may be clinically prudent to routinely perform thyroid testing on elderly women. With the lack of evidence, however, the authors believe no definitive recommendations can currently be made. These recommendations do not apply to patients who may require surveillance due to prior illnesses or procedures that might affect thyroid function, or to monitor the adequacy of thyroxine replacement.

Lung Cancer

Lung cancer is the leading cause of cancer death in both men and women in the United States. In men, the rate starts to rise at approximately age 40 years and climbs rapidly until it peaks at a rate of about 470 per 100,000 at age 75. In women, the incidence is lower but follows a similar pattern; starting to climb at age 40 and peaking at about 155 per 100,000 at age 70. During the 1970's and 1980's National Cancer Institute Cooperative Early Lung Cancer Detection Program (CELCDP) randomized controlled trial was implemented to determine the screening efficacy of sputum cytology and chest radiography in reducing the morality from lung cancer in a group of asymptomatic male smokers (CELCDP). The Mayo Lung Project evaluated the closest approximation of community-based screening program in the CELCDP. The intervention group were randomized to every four months sputum cytology and chest x-ray. The control group were given the recommendation to obtain once a year chest x-ray and cytology. The death rate from lung cancer between the two groups were identical.

Unfortunately, in the CELCDP only 10 percent of those screened were men over 65 years of age. There are several studies demonstrating a greater likelihood of local stage lung cancer with increasing age. In light of the higher incidence of lung cancer (in those over 65 years) and of more local disease, the results of the Mayo Lung Project possibly shouldn't be extrapolated to those over 65 years of age. There is a need for further investigation in the elderly population.

Until further data are available, the authors do not recommend screening asymptomatic persons (with or without a history of smoking) for lung cancer by performing routine chest radiography or sputum cytology. These recommendations are identical to the USPSTF.

Breast Cancer

In 1995 it is estimated there will be 182,000 new cases of breast cancer diagnosed. In 1991, there were 583 deaths due to breast cancer; 77% of these deaths were in women over age 55 years and 31% were in women over 75 years. Several screening strategies have been recommended for detection of breast cancer, including: breast self examination, clinical breast examination, and mammography. Breast self examination has a low sensitivity—between 20 to 30 percent—which is even lower among elderly women.

Over the past six years, numerous studies on mammographic screening for breast cancer have been published; however, none of the interventional studies included women over 74 years of age and only two included women over 65 years of age. The Two County (Sweden) study which randomized by area of residence and utilized single-view mammography every two and a half years found a 39 percent reduction (Relative Risk [RR] =.61 95%, 95% Confidence Interval [CI] =.44-.84) in cumulative mortality from breast cancer in women 50 to 74 years of age after six years of follow up. The Malmo trial randomized individual subjects and enrolled women ages 45 to 69 years. Single or double view mammography were performed every 18 to 24 months. After an average of 8.8 years of follow-up for women 55 years and older at entry there was a 21 percent reduction in cumulative mortality from breast cancer (RR = 0.79; 95% CI = 0.51-1.24). Therefore, of the two mammography intervention trials, including women over 65 years, both demonstrated a reduction in breast cancer mortality; however, the Malmo trial was not statistically significant. A decision analysis model to determine whether breast cancer screening extends life for women aged 65 years or more with and without comorbid conditions found no inherent reason to impose an upper-age limit for breast cancer screening.

The authors recommend biennial mammography for average risk women over age 65. The upper-age limit to conclude screening should occur when a woman is expected to die within six years from a non-breast cancer cause. The average life expectancy is 12 years for a 75-year-old and 7 years for an 85-year-old. This recommendation is similar to the USPSTF recommendation, with the exception of continued screening beyond age 74 as long as the woman's life expectancy exceeds 6 years.

Cervical Cancer

In spite of the advent of the Papanicolaou (Pap) smear in the 1940's, approximately 15,800 new cervical cancer cases and 4,800 deaths from cervical cancer are expected to occur in the United States during 1995. Surprisingly, 27 percent of new cases of cervical cancer and 41 percent of annual deaths from cervical cancer occur in women who are 65 years of age and older. The National Health Interview Survey estimates that 15 to 20 percent of older white women have never had a Papanicolaou smear. There is no evidence from experimental trials that routinely screened older women, or women of any age, experience reduced morbidity or mortality from cervical cancer. A large body of indirect evidence exists from the United States, Canada, and Europe in the form of correlation studies and case-control studies supporting the effectiveness of the Papanicolaou in reducing the incidence of invasive cervical cancer. Elderly women have often been underscreened. However, for women 65 years and older who have been screened and have had normal Pap tests every three years, continued Pap tests every three years would increase subsequent life expectancy by three days.

There is no consensus among professional organizations regarding screening guidelines in the elderly. The American Cancer Society, National Cancer Institute, the American College of Obstetrics and Gynecology, and the American Medical Association recommend Papanicolaou screening throughout a woman's life. The Canadian Task Force and the United States Preventive Service Task Force recommend discontinuing Papanicolaou smears at ages 70 and 65 years, respectively, if previous Papanicolaou smears have been consistently normal.

The authors recommend discontinuation of Papanicolaou smears at age 65 if previous Papanicolaou smears have been regular and consistently normal. For underscreened elderly women, screening with Papanicolaou smear at least once, if their functional status and medical condition are sufficient to withstand therapy for any lesion discovered, is recommended.

Colorectal Cancer

Colorectal cancer is the second most common cause of cancer mortality. In 1995 an estimated 138,200 new cases will be diagnosed and an estimated 55,300 people will die of the disease in the United States. An individual has a one in twenty life-time risk of developing colorectal cancer. The incidence rate for those under 65 years of age is 19.2 per 100,000, but among those over 65 years of age, it is 337.1 per 100,000. The present tests available for colorectal cancer screening are: digital rectal examination, fecal occult blood test, sigmoidoscopy, barium enema, radiography, and colonoscopy.

There are five controlled trials underway evaluating the effectiveness of the fecal occult blood test. Two of these studies have recently reported a small decrease in mortality from colorectal cancer in the screened group, however, this reduction was not statistically significant. A third study at the University of Minnesota reported a 33 percent decrease in mortality from colorectal cancer from annual fecal occult blood test screening after 13 years of follow up. Fifty-eight percent of the subjects were 60 years or older. The University of Minnesota study is a landmark study in that it demonstrated a reduction in colorectal cancer mortality; however, it is not clear if this is due to the fecal occult blood test screening or to the colonoscopic evaluation of the colon performed in 38 percent of the annual intervention group. In addition, a recent prospective study found the hemoccult to be 26 percent sensitive in a post resection cohort; therefore, the utility of the fecal occult blood test for screening is questionable.

Two case-control studies have found screening sigmoidoscopy to decrease colorectal cancer mortality by 59 to 95 percent. The mean age of the subjects were 66 years in the Selby study and 72% of the subjects were over age 59 in the Newcomb study. In addition, the Selby study found the negative association was as strong when the most recent sigmoidoscopy was nine to ten years before diagnosis as it was when examinations were more recent. This finding calls into question the need for screening sigmoidoscopy less frequently than every three to five years. There are no experimental or observational studies determining the effectiveness of the digital rectal examination and barium enema radiography in reducing mortality from colorectal cancer.

The authors recommend screening average risk individuals over 65 who are expected to live an additional 13 years with flexible sigmoidoscopy every 5 years. Since the average life expectancy at 75 years is twelve years, this would mean discontinuing screening at age 75 years in most elders.

Lipids

Coronary heart disease is the number one cause of death in individuals over 65 years of age. In older adults from 65 to 75 years of age, hypercholesterolemia is estimated to increase coronary heart disease (CHD) death by 30-60%. In the elderly (> 80 years), epidemiologic studies have reported no association between blood cholesterol level and CHD incidence or death. The National Cholesterol Education Program—Adult Treatment Panel II provides an approach to manage adult patients with elevated serum cholesterol levels; however, the guidelines do not distinguish between younger and older adults. There is only one randomized controlled trial of the effectiveness of cholesterol reduction that included older participants utilizing a dietary intervention in middle-aged and elderly male residents of a Veterans Administration domicile. After eight years of follow-up, the study found that cholesterol reduction decreased CHD events (sudden death, MI, cerebral infarction) but increased mortality from cancer and did not affect overall mortality Thus, cholesterol reduction has the potential to prevent CHD events in the elderly, but the balance of health benefits and risks of treatment is untested and uncertain.

A recent study of 997 community-based elderly subjects in the Established Population for the Epidemiologic Study of the Elderly was reported on data collected from 1982 to 1988. These findings rejected the hypothesis that hypercholesterolemia or low HDL-C are important risk factors for all-cause mortality, CHD mortality, or hospitalization (for unstable angina or MI) in this cohort of persons older than 70 years.

The authors recommend screening and treating high blood cholesterol in adults younger than 70 years of age, who already have manifestations of atherosclerotic disease and whose risk factors place them at high risk of CHD death. Elderly people in their late 70s and beyond generally should not be screened or treated for high blood cholesterol. The USPSTF states that periodic measurement of total serum cholesterol in the elderly may be clinically prudent.

Diabetes

Diabetes is the sixth leading cause of mortality in the United States over the age of 75 years in 1991. Non-insulin dependent diabetes mellitus, the more common form of diabetes in the elderly, affects ten percent of subjects over 65 years of age and 25 per cent of adults over 85 years of age. The prevalence is 60 to 100 percent higher among African-Americans. For a firm diagnosis of diabetes, an individual must have a fasting plasma glucose of 140 mg/dL or greater on two occasions. However, no specific glucose level discriminates completely between persons with impaired glucose tolerance or diabetes in the normal population. There is no evidence regarding age, gender, and race adjusted guidelines for the diagnosis of diabetes. Nor is there evidence demonstrating reduction in disease-specific outcomes as a result of screening asymptomatic older adults.

There is evidence for all age groups of increased morbidity and mortality due to hyperglycemia and diabetes mellitus. There are recent data demonstrating that many of the complications of type I diabetes can be reduced or eliminated by strict glycemic control. Whether these results can be extrapolated to older subjects with type II diabetes mellitus is unknown. In the older adult, especially at the extremes of age, significant risks from aggressive therapy may outweigh any benefits. There is a lack of specific therapeutic guidelines for the management of diabetes mellitus in the older patient, and it is unclear whether the asymptomatic older patient benefits from treatment.

The authors agree with USPSTF and recommend periodic/annual fasting plasma glucose measurements in persons over the age of 65 years, especially those who are at high risk for diabetes mellitus such as marked obesity, persons with a family history of diabetes mellitus, or women with a history of gestational diabetes mellitus.

Electrocardiography

The electrocardiogram (ECG) is the principal test for early detection of coronary atherosclerotic disease. However, there are important limitations to the sensitivity and specificity of electrocardiography when used as a screening test. A normal resting ECG does not rule out coronary disease. Conversely, an abnormal ECG does not reliably predict the presence of coronary artery disease. Some advocate obtaining a "baseline" ECG to assist in interpreting subsequent ECG, but studies indicate that in actual practice, most baseline tracings are either unavailable or do not provide information that affects treatment decisions.

The authors do not recommend routine or baseline electrocardiography in asymptomatic elderly patients. Although the USPSTF recommendations did not specifically address the elderly, it was felt to be clinically prudent to obtain a resting ECG for all adults with two or more cardiac risk factors.

Theraputics

Influenza Vaccination

Ninety-five per cent of all influenza deaths occur among people 60 years or older, and they suffer increased morbidity from the disease as compared to younger persons. Studies support a 40-70% effectiveness of the vaccine, which is easily administered at little risk. One randomized double-blinded placebo-controlled trial of the efficacy of influenza vaccination in individuals aged 60 years or older, found a fifty percent reduction in the incidence of serological and clinical influenza. A serial cohort study in individuals aged 65 years or older found reductions in the rate of hospitalizations and deaths from influenza and its complications, as compared with the rates in unvaccinated elderly persons, and vaccination produced direct dollar savings.

The authors agree with the USPSTF recommendation that all persons aged 65 years and older be given influenza vaccines every year during the fall. Priority should be given to residents of long term care facilities.

Tetanus Immunization

Clinical tetanus is rare, and occurs primarily among older adults who are unvaccinated or underimmmunized. During 1989 to 1990, 117 cases were reported in the United States, 25 of which were fatal. All deaths occurred in patients over age 40. Patients over age 60 have accounted for nearly 60% of all tetanus cases. Data from serologic surveys have shown that from one to two-thirds of adults over age 60 lack presumably protective (0.01 IU/mL) levels of tetanus antibody. Data from Sweden, where tetanus boosters are not given after the teen years, indicate that protective antitoxin levels remained in 56 to 80% of older subjects. Women often have lesser immunization rates due to lack of military service (with attendant vaccinations). The Centers for Disease Control and Prevention and the U.S. Preventive Services Task Force have recommended booster doses of Td every ten years. A recent cost-effectiveness analysis reported increasing evidence that decennial tetanus boosters, though effective, are costly, hampered by poor compliance, and often miss at-risk individuals. This study recommended a single booster at age 65, to be coupled with other needed vaccinations. It was felt that diphtheria immunity would not be affected by this regimen.

The authors recommend that elderly patients who have completed a primary tetanus immunization series receive a single booster dose at age 55 to 65 years. Linking this immunization with provision of the pneumococcal vaccine is appropriate and efficient. This differs from the USPSTF, who recommend a tetanus booster once every 10 years following the primary series.

Pneumococcal Vaccination

Pneumococcal disease is a significant cause of morbidity and mortality in the elderly. The vaccine is inexpensive and easy to administer and side effects are relatively rare, especially when given once. The pneumococcal vaccine has been effective in epidemic situations where healthy adults have been involved. Statistical analysis of outpatient studies in subjects older than 45 years indicate vaccine efficacy of about 60%. However, there is little evidence for efficacy in preventing pneumococcal pneumonia in the elderly. Randomized, controlled trials are lacking. It is unclear whether to revaccinate immunocompetent patients due to the waning immunity and reduced efficacy of immunization related to aging. Increased response to vaccination may occur by lowering the age of initial vaccination to 55, although this has not been firmly established. With the increasing problem of antibiotic-resistant strains of pneumococci, it is compelling to provide vaccine prophylaxis.

It is prudent to provide the pneumococcal vaccine at 55 to 65 years of age, however, no concrete recommendations can be made due to the controversy about its efficacy. The USPSTF recommends giving the pneumococcal vaccination to individuals over 65 years. Further research is needed to assess the effectiveness of pneumococcal vaccinations in the elderly and the cost benefit ratio to society.

Advance Directives

Advance Directives include living wills and the durable power of attorney (DPOA) for health care matters. Living wills are explicit value-based declarations used by patients to refuse or accept various life-sustaining medical interventions in case of terminal illness. Alternatively, the durable power of attorney is designated to speak for the patient in medical conditions when the patient cannot make their wishes known. The Patient Self-determination Act is intended to encourage wider use of advance directives. Advance directives can be inexpensive and have universal ethical recognition. They also may facilitate decisions about life-sustaining interventions when patients lack decision-making capacity. Despite enthusiasm for written advance directives, few adults have completed them. A randomized controlled trial from Kaiser Permanente found the mailing of an educational pamphlet and form on the durable power of attorney to patients over 65 years of age significantly increased the completion of the durable power of attorney form. In some states, the living will may be less useful than the DPOA due to restrictions on implementation.

The authors recommend informing patients over 65 years about advance directives either through dialogue or pamphlets, and supplying the patient with the appropriate form. Regulations from the 1987 Omnibus Budget and Reconciliation Act have mandated inquiry concerning advanced directives in hospitalized and institutionalized patients. The USPSTF did not address this intervention.

Aspirin as Primary Prevention of Cardiovascular Disease

Coronary artery disease is the leading cause of death in the United States. The principal risk factors for coronary artery disease are smoking, hypertension, elevated serum cholesterol, diabetes mellitus, age and family history. There are three studies evaluating the effectiveness of aspirin as a prophylactic against myocardial infarction in patients without clinically evident coronary artery disease. The United States Physicians' Aspirin Trial randomized 22,071 male physicians age 40 to 84 without a history of myocardial infarction, stroke or TIA to aspirin 325 mg every other day or placebo. After 5 years of therapy, the incidence of myocardial infarction was 44% lower in the aspirin group. The treatment effect was seen only in those aged 50 years or older. In a similar study, the British Physicians' Study, a group of 5,139 physicians were randomized to aspirin 500 mg per day or no treatment. After 6 years there was no significant reduction in the incidence of myocardial infarction in the aspirin group. The higher dose of aspirin led to side effects that decreased adherence to the treatment protocol.

A non-randomized prospective study of 87,678 U.S. nurses aged 34 to 65 years examined the self-reported aspirin use by nurses without a history of diagnosed coronary artery disease or stroke. Nurses who reported taking one to six aspirin per week had a 32% reduction in fatal and non-fatal myocardial infarction compared with those who did not take aspirin. (p = 0.005). There was no relationship between aspirin use and the incidence of stroke. Once again the treatment effect was seen only in those aged 50 or older. When the results of the U.S. and British study were pooled, the incidence of non-fatal myocardial infarction was reduced by 33 per cent in the aspirin group (p< .0002) and there was a non-statistically significant increase in the incidence of stroke in the aspirin group.

The authors recommend prophylactic low-dose aspirin to reduce the incidence of myocardial infarction in men and women over the age of 65 who are at moderate to high risk for cardiovascular disease. The USPSTF recommend low-dose aspirin therapy in all men over 40 years who are at high risk for cardiovascular disease. However, the USPSTF does not specifically address aspirin therapy for patients over 65 years and women.

Hormone Replacement Therapy (HRT)

It is estimated that approximately one-quarter of all women over age 60 years have spinal compression fractures and about 15% of women sustain hip fractures during their lifetime. Hip fractures are associated with significant pain and disability, loss of independence and high mortality. In the Study of Osteoporotic Fractures, a prospective study of 9,704 women who were 65 years of age or older, current use of estrogen decreased the risk for fracture. There was a greater reduction in risk of fracture if estrogen was administered within 5 years of menopause.

Since 1970, at least 32 epidemiological studies have evaluated the relationship between hormone replacement therapy (HRT) and coronary heart disease (CHD). There is a consistent risk reduction for CHD among estrogen users compared with non-users. Some evidence shows the protective effect of estrogen is stronger in women who have CHD than in healthy women. There is inconsistent evidence of estrogen plus progesterone effect on CHD risk. At least 39 epidemiologic studies of estrogen therapy and breast cancer risk have also been done since 1970. Results of these studies have been mixed. However, a metanalysis based on these studies found no increased risk. From 35 epidemiologic studies since 1970 it is well established that the risk for endometrial cancer increases with estrogen use. However, there is no increased endometrial cancer risk if estrogen is combined with progesterone administration.

The authors recommend the judicious institution of combined estrogen and progesterone replacement in older women who are at risk for or have already developed osteoporosis. In geriatric women who have had hysterectomies who are at risk for coronary artery disease, the institution of unopposed estrogen should be considered. The decision to use HRT is less clear for the woman with an intact uterus at risk for CHD, due to progesterone effects. There are no conclusive data regarding an upper age limit to initiation of estrogen use. Randomized controlled trials in older women are needed to determine the overall reduction in fractures and cardiovascular deaths, and the effect on breast cancer mortality. The USPSTF recommends estrogen therapy consideration for asymptomatic women who are at increased risk for osteoporosis. The USPSTF did not address the use of estrogen replacement therapy in reducing cardiovascular disease.

Is the Screening Test Worthwhile?

Before the clinician makes any decision to seek early diagnosis, the following questions must be answered:

- Is the target disease an important clinical problem?

- Does the burden of disability warrant early detection?

- Is the natural history of the target disease understood?

- Is there a latent or early symptomatic period?

- Is the screening diagnostic strategy effective?

- Is the accuracy of testing (sensitivity and specificity) established?

- Is the test acceptable to patients with low discomfort or risk?

- If the screening test is positive, will patients accept subsequent diagnostic evaluation?

- Is there a known treatment for the target disease?

- Is the treatment effective and available?

- Are there risks of treatment, such as adverse drug effects or adverse outcomes of surgical treatment?

- Is the cost of testing balanced by the benefit of treatment?

Geriatric Health Maintenance Items That Are Clearly Effective in a Screening Program

Historical

- Smoking

Physical Examination

- Blood pressure
- Hearing/vision
- Dentition
- Skin examination for cancer
- Gait and fall assessment

Laboratory

- Mammography
- Papanicolaou smear in under-screened
- Flexible sigmoidoscopy

Interventions

- Aspirin therapy to prevent CAD (Coronary Artery Disease) in men
- Estrogen replacement therapy for osteoporosis prevention in women at risk, and coronary artery disease prevention in women at risk or after hysterectomy

Vaccinations

- Influenza
- Tetanus

Chapter 8

Osteoporosis (Bone Density) Screening

Consider an insidious condition that drains away bone—the hardest, most durable substance in the body. It happens slowly, over years, so that often neither doctor nor patient is aware of weakening bones until one snaps unexpectedly. Unfortunately, this isn't science fiction. It's why osteoporosis is called the silent thief.

And it steals more than bone. It's the primary cause of hip fracture, which can lead to permanent disability, loss of independence, and sometimes even death. Collapsing spinal vertebrae can produce stooped posture and a "dowager's hump." Lives collapse too. The chronic pain and anxiety that accompany a frail frame make people curtail meaningful activities, because the simplest things can cause broken bones; stepping off a curb, a sneeze, bending to pick up something, or a hug. "Don't touch Mom, she might break" is the sad joke in many families.

Osteoporosis leads to 1.5 million fractures, or breaks, per year, mostly in the hip, spine and wrist, and costs $10 billion annually, according to the National Osteoporosis Foundation. It threatens 25 million Americans, mostly older women, but older men get it too. One in three women past 50 will suffer a vertebral fracture, according to the foundation. These numbers are predicted to rise as the population ages.

This chapter includes text from "Boning Up on Osteoporosis" *FDA Consumer*, September 1996, revised August 1997, Publication No. (FDA) 97-1257, and U.S. Department of Health and Human Services *HHS News Release*, "FDA Approves First Ultrasound Device for Diagnosing Osteoporosis," March 13, 1998.

Osteoporosis, which means "porous bones," is a condition of excessive skeletal fragility resulting in bones that break easily. A combination of genetic, dietary, hormonal, age-related, and lifestyle factors all contribute to this condition.

Changing attitudes and improving technology are brightening the outlook for people with osteoporosis. Nowadays, many women live 30 years or more—perhaps a quarter to a third of their lives—after menopause. Improving the quality of those years has become an important health-care goal. Although some bone loss is expected as people age, osteoporosis is no longer viewed as an inevitable consequence of aging. Diagnosis and treatment need no longer wait until bones break.

There is no cure for osteoporosis, and it can't be prevented outright, but the onset can be delayed, and the severity diminished. Most important, early intervention can prevent devastating fractures. The Food and Drug Administration has revised labeling on foods and supplements to provide valuable information about the level of nutrients that help build and maintain strong bones. FDA has also approved a wide variety of products to help diagnose and treat osteoporosis, including several in the last few years.

Bone Life

Bone consists of a matrix of fibers of the tough protein collagen, hardened with calcium, phosphorus and other minerals. Two types of architecture give bones strength. Surrounding every bone is a tough, dense rind of cortical bone. Inside is spongy-looking trabecular bone. Its interconnecting structure provides much of the strength of healthy bone, but is especially vulnerable to osteoporosis.

"We tend to think of the skeleton as an inert erector set that holds us up and doesn't do much else. That's not true," says Karl L. Insogna, M.D., director of the Bone Center at Yale School of Medicine, New Haven, Conn. Every bit as dynamic as other tissues, bone responds to the pull of muscles and gravity, repairs itself, and constantly renews itself.

Besides protecting internal organs and allowing us to move about, bone is also involved in the body's handling of minerals. Of the 2 to 4 pounds of calcium in the body, nearly 99 percent is in the teeth and skeleton. The remainder plays a critical role in blood clotting, nerve transmission, muscle contraction (including heartbeat), and other functions. The body keeps the blood level of calcium within a narrow range. When needed, bones release calcium.

A complex interplay of many hormones balances the activity of the two types of cells—osteoclasts and osteoblasts—responsible for the continuous turnover process called remodeling. Osteoclasts break down bone, and osteoblasts build it. In youth, bone building prevails. Bone mass peaks by about age 30, then bone breakdown outpaces formation, and density declines.

The skeleton is like a retirement account, but in our skeletal "account" we can deposit bone only during our first three decades. After that, all we can do is try to postpone and minimize the steady withdrawals. Osteoporosis is the bankruptcy that occurs when too little bone is formed during youth, or too much is lost later, or both.

"You've got to get as much bone as you can and not lose it," Insogna says. "The most important risk factor for osteoporosis is a low bone mass."

"The upper limit of bone mass that you can acquire is genetically determined," says Mona S. Calvo, Ph.D., in FDA's Office of Special Nutritionals. "But even though you may be programmed for high bone mass, other factors can influence how much bone you end up with," she says. For instance, men tend to build greater bone mass, which is partly why more women face osteoporosis.

But there's another reason. With the decline of the female hormone estrogen at menopause, usually around age 50, bone breakdown markedly increases. For several years, women lose bone two to four times faster than they did before menopause. The rate usually slows down again, but some women may continue to lose bone rapidly. By age 65, some women have lost half their skeletal mass. Because the changes at menopause increase a woman's risk, many physicians feel it's a good time to measure a woman's bone density, especially if she has other risk factors for osteoporosis.

"The best way to gauge a woman's risk for osteoporotic fracture is to measure her bone mass," says Insogna.

Routine x-rays can't detect osteoporosis until it's quite advanced, but other radiological methods can. FDA has approved several kinds of devices that use various methods to estimate bone density. Most require far less radiation than a chest x-ray. Doctors consider a patient's medical history and risk factors in deciding who should have a bone density test. The method used is often determined by the equipment available locally. Readings are compared to a standard for the patient's age, sex and body size. Different parts of the skeleton may be measured, and low density at any site is worrisome.

The Food and Drug Administration has approved an ultrasound device which will help physicians diagnose osteoporosis and assess the risk of bone fracture.

This is the first device for diagnosing osteoporosis which does not involve the use of x-rays. It is intended to be used for women at risk of bone fracture, not as a general screening tool.

The Sahara Clinical Bone Sonometer, manufactured by Hologic, Inc., of Waltham, Mass., estimates bone strength using ultrasound measurements. The portable device transmits high frequency sound waves through the patient's heel for about 10 seconds and automatically analyzes the results.

FDA's approval of the sonometer was based on data from three clinical studies comparing the ultrasound measurements to x-ray bone densitometry measurements: a study of 2,208 healthy women of all ages to establish normal values for the device; a study of 247 women of all ages including groups of women with and without a history of fracture to compare performance of this device to more traditional methods of measuring bone strength; and a study of 212 women which demonstrated the ability of this device to select women at high risk for future fractures.

The ultrasound device was shown to be as good as x-ray bone density measurements for diagnosing osteoporosis and predicting fracture risk.

"Early diagnosis is important," said HHS Secretary Donna E. Shalala. "This new test can be done easily in many doctors' offices. Early diagnosis and treatment will improve the quality of life for millions of Americans who are at risk

Bone density tests are useful for confirming a diagnosis of osteoporosis if a person has already had a suspicious fracture, or for detecting low bone density so that preventative steps can be taken.

"There's a profound relationship between bone mass and risk of fracture," says Robert Recker, M.D., director of the Osteoporosis Research Center at Creighton University, Omaha, Neb.

Readings repeated at intervals of a year or more can determine the rate of bone loss and help monitor treatment effectiveness. However, estimates are not necessarily comparable between machine types because they use different measurement methods, cautions Joseph Arnaudo, in the Center for Devices and Radiological Health. "You always want to go back to the same machine, if you can," he says.

Another test provides an indicator of bone breakdown. FDA approved in 1995 a simple, noninvasive biochemical test that detects in a urine sample a specific component of bone breakdown, called NTx. Clinical labs can get results in about 2 hours. The NTx test, marketed as Osteomark, can help physicians monitor treatment and identify fast losers of bone for more aggressive treatment, but the test may not be used to diagnose osteoporosis.

Brighter Horizons

"A number of new things seem to be in the offing, eventually to come to us, and we're looking forward to getting some additional treatments for osteoporosis," says Troendle.

Uses of existing drugs may be broadened. Early drug trials are often conducted with patients who have severe disease, often after a fracture has occurred or bone loss is quite serious. Some studies under way are testing to see if certain drugs are effective in less severe cases, if they can be started sooner, or used in combination.

The search for bone-building drugs continues. Some naturally occurring bone-specific growth factors have been identified and their use as drugs is being investigated. "The way I visualize the ideal future is that we'll be able to give Drug X that builds up bone to where it's stronger and the risk of fracture is no longer present, then Drug Y maintains it by preventing breakdown," says Stern.

Osteoporosis has been described as an adolescent disease with a geriatric onset, highlighting the importance of beginning to take steps—in exercise and diet—early in life to reduce its disabling impact in later years.

Reducing Your Risk

A host of factors can affect your chances of developing osteoporosis. The good news is that you control some of them. Even though you can't change your genes, you can still lower your risk with attention to certain lifestyle changes. The younger you start, and the longer you keep it up, the better. Here's what you can do for yourself:

- Be sure you get enough calcium and vitamin D.
- Engage in regular physical activity, such as walking.
- Don't smoke.
- If you drink alcohol, do so in moderation.

A sedentary lifestyle, smoking, excessive drinking, and low calcium intake all increase risk. Although coffee has been suspected as a risk factor, studies so far are inconclusive.

Other factors are beyond your control. Being aware of them can provide extra motivation to help yourself in the ways you are able, and aids you and your doctor in health-care decisions. These risk factors are:

- being female: Women have a five times greater risk than men.

- thin, small-boned frame

- broken bones or stooped posture in older family members, especially women, which suggest a family history of osteoporosis

- early estrogen deficiency in women who experience menopause before age 45, either naturally or resulting from surgical removal of the ovaries

- estrogen deficiency due to abnormal absence of menstruation (as may accompany eating disorders)

- ethnic heritage: White and Asian women are at highest risk; African-American and Hispanic women are at lower, but significant, risk.

- advanced age

- prolonged use of some medications, such as excessive thyroid hormone; some antiseizure medications; and glucocorticoids (certain anti-inflammatory medications, such as prednisone, used to treat conditions such as asthma, arthritis and some cancers).

Risk factors may not tell the whole story. You may have none of these factors and still have osteoporosis. Or you may have many of them and not develop the condition. It's best to discuss your specific situation with your doctor.

For More Information

National Osteoporosis Foundation
1150 17th St., N.W., Suite 500
Washington, DC 20036
(202) 223-2226
World Wide Web: http://www.nof.org/

For locations of your nearest bone density testing sites, call: (800) 464-6700.

Osteoporosis and Related Bone Diseases National Resource Center (ORBD-NRC)
(800) 624-BONE
TDD: (202) 223-0344

Older Women's League (OWL)
666 11th St., N.W., Suite 700
Washington, DC 20001
(202) 783-6686

North American Menopause Society
c/o University Hospitals of Cleveland
Department of Obstetrics and Gynecology
11100 Euclid Ave., Suite 7024
Cleveland, OH 44106
(216) 844-8748
World Wide Web: http://www.menopause.org/

American Association of Retired Persons (AARP)
601 E St., N.W.
Washington, DC 20049
(202) 434-2277
World Wide Web: http://www.aarp.org/

— by Carolyn J. Strange

Carolyn J. Strange is a science and medical writer living in Northern California.

Chapter 9

Neurology Tests Your Doctor Might Order

This chapter is a brief introduction of the tests your neurologist might order. Discuss details, side effects, costs, rational, and other concerns with the doctor as appropriate.

Blood Work (Most Frequently Requested)

CBC (Complete Blood Count)

- Hemoglobin/Hematocrit—used to measure the oxygen carrying capacity of the blood and its thickness. Important in many conditions, especially those that impact cerebral circulation.

- WBC (White Blood Cell count) especially important in infections, leukemia, and AIDS.

Electrolytes

- Sodium and Potassium levels are critical for nervous system function.

BUN (Blood Urea Nitrogen)/Creatinine

- A measure of kidney function. Kidney failure leads to confusion, seizures, coma, tremor and other problems.

Reprinted with permission. © Neurologist Online, *Diagnostic Tests*, by Rosario Guarino, M.D.; also reprinted with permission, "Neurologic Diagnostic Tests," by Randall R. Light, M.D., Bryan Neurology Services © 1997.

Glucose

- Too much or too little glucose can cause confusion, seizures, coma. Diabetes is the most common cause of peripheral neuropathy.

Magnesium, Calcium

- Imbalance is important in seizures and muscle problems.

Protime/PTT (protein truncation test)

- Measures of blood clotting, especially important in stroke management.

ESR sed rate (erythrocyte sedimentation rate)

- A general measure of inflammation in the body. Especially important in headaches in elderly patients and collagen vascular diseases.

VDRL (designed by Venereal Disease Research Laboratories)/FTA (fluorescent treponemal antibody)

- Diagnoses syphilis and false positives and helps diagnose collagen vascular disease. Syphilis can cause dementia, nerve and blood vessel damage.

ANA (antinuclear antibody)/RF (rheumatoid factor)

- Helps to diagnose lupus and rheumatoid arthritis which can affect the peripheral nerves and central nervous system.

SPEP/IPEP (erthrocyte protoporphyrin)

- Protein and Immune globulin measurements used to rule out disorders of white blood cells that lead to nerve damage.

Imaging Tests for Neurology Diagnosis

Skull X–Ray

Useful to check for intracranial calcification, midline brain shift, pituitary gland enlargement, and fractures. Largely replaced by CT imaging where available.

Cranial Ultrasound

Used in infants with openings between skull bones to diagnose brain hemorrhage.

CT (Computerized Axial Tomography or CAT Scan)

A computer generated image from x-rays that is excellent for harder tissues, good for most soft tissues, excellent for fresh blood. Newer techniques available for blood vessels. Fast but uses ionizing radiation. Best for trauma and subarachnoid hemorrhage.

MRI (magnetic resonance imaging)

Computer generated image based on alignment of molecules in a magnetic field. Excellent for brain and spinal cord. Excellent for soft tissues and white matter diseases. Best for cervical disks and multiple sclerosis. Gives more detail than CT. Takes longer and claustrophobia a problem with closed units. Pacemakers and some metal in the body, especially in the eye, restrict its use. New techniques can image vessels (MRA) and replace invasive angiography.

Cerebral Angiography

Injection of contrast dye directly into arteries after insertion of a catheter followed by x–ray picture. Best for aneurysm and carotid artery blockage. There is a small risk of stroke. MRA and CT may replace this soon.

EEG (Electroencephalogram)

Measures brain waves with safe scalp surface electrodes. Mainly used for analysis of seizure disorders but also useful with dementia and confused, encephalopathic or comatose patients. Main test for brain death.

SPECT (Single Photon Emission Computed Tomography)

Computer generated image based on brain function at time of test. Image produced based on distribution of radioactive tracers injected into blood and pickup by active brain tissue. Reflects blood flow, glucose uptake, receptor binding locally in brain.

PET (Positron Emission Tomography)

Like SPECT but can check on more than glucose metabolism with various other tracers. Technically more difficult, more expensive, need a particle accelerator on site to make tracers. Promising for certain seizure patients.

MRS (Magnetic Resonance Spectroscopy)

A biochemical measurement of specific brain metabolites with MRI technology that promises to help measure the neuronal number and function. Used in seizure research.

Functional MRI

A new rapid scanning MRI technique that demonstrates alteration in blood oxygenation. Used in seizure research.

Carotid Duplex Ultrasound

A safe test using sonar to generate a picture of carotid arteries in the neck and to estimate blood velocity. Greater than 70% blockage carries a risk of stroke that surgery and/or medicine can reduce.

Transcranial Doppler Ultrasound

A safe test that uses sonar to measure intracranial artery blood velocity. Mainly used to check for spasm after subarachnoid hemorrhage. May be useful for spotting clots to brain and measuring adequacy of collateral cerebral blood flow.

Myelography/CT

A myelogram is a lumbar puncture with contrast dye inserted into the spinal canal followed by x-ray to check for blocks especially from disks or tumors. MRI can do this without needles. Myelography followed by CT is the most accurate test for imaging disk herniation.

Brain Mapping

A computer generated picture of the brain based on EEG activity. Not of proven use clinically at this time.

Additional Tests Used for Neurology Diagnosis

Lumbar Puncture (LP or spinal tap)

Insertion of a long thin needle into the spinal canal and sample fluid and measure opening pressure. A must if infection is suspected. Also needed if ruptured aneurysm is suspected and CT is normal. Helps diagnose multiple sclerosis and other inflammatory diseases of the central nervous system. CT needed first to rule out a brain mass if suspected.

Electromyography (EMG)

Electromyography is a diagnostic test performed in the neurologist's office. An EMG is an evaluation of the muscle's electrical activity. It is performed to look for evidence of damage to a muscle's nerve supply or signs of muscle disease. It is most often used to help diagnose neck, back, or extremity pain, numbness, or weakness.

Based on the history, neurologic exam, x-rays, and available laboratory studies, the EMG is planned and performed by the neurologist at the time of the office visit. Specialized computer based equipment is used to record and analyze the electrical activity recorded from the tip of a small needle inserted into the muscle being evaluated. While there is a slight discomfort associated with the EMG exam, no special medication or preparation is necessary. After the EMG, a patient may resume his usual activities.

Nerve Conduction Velocities (NCV)

A nerve conduction velocity study is a diagnostic test performed in a neurologist's office to evaluate the function of individual nerves. NCV's are performed to help diagnose extremity numbness, weakness, or pain. Based on the history, neurologic exam, x-rays, and available laboratory studies, the NCV is planned and performed by the neurologist at the time of the office visit. A NCV is performed using specialized, computer based equipment to stimulate and record the responses of individual nerves. When the nerve is stimulated, there is brief discomfort. The results are recorded and compared to a set of normal values. After the NCV has been completed, the patient may resume his usual activities.

Evoked Potentials

A measure of nerve conduction time from peripheral to central nervous system from eye, ear, or limbs. Information is gathered about brain and nerve function. Formerly very useful as aid in diagnosing multiple sclerosis, largely replaced by MRI. Still useful for 8th cranial nerve problems by brain stem auditory evoked potential. Sometimes used to monitor brain function under anesthesia.

Tensilon Test

A Tensilon test is a diagnostic test performed by a physician in the office or hospital to help differentiate causes of weakness, double vision, and drooping eye lids. The test is most often performed when myasthenia gravis is suspected. It is performed by injecting Tensilon, a short acting medication, into a vein and evaluating a patient's strength before and after the injection. The medication effect lasts about ten minutes or less. A Tensilon test is considered positive when there is a definite improvement in the patient's strength.

Chapter 10

Tuberculin (TB) Tests, Necessary for Public Health

Tuberculosis (TB), a chronic bacterial infection, causes more deaths worldwide than any other infectious disease. TB is spread through the air and usually infects the lungs, although other organs are sometimes involved. Some 1.7 billion people—one third of the world's population—are infected with the predominant TB organism, *Mycobacterium tuberculosis*.

Most people infected with *M. tuberculosis* never develop active TB. However, in people with weakened immune systems, especially those infected with the human immunodeficiency virus (HIV, the cause of AIDS), TB organisms may overcome the body's defenses, multiply, and cause active disease. Each year, 8 million people worldwide develop active TB and 3 million die.

TB on the Rise in the United States

In the United States, TB has re-emerged as a serious public health problem. In 1993, a total of 25,287 active TB cases, in all 50 states and the District of Columbia, were reported to the Centers for Disease Control and Prevention (CDC), an increase of 14 percent since 1985. Thanks largely to improved public health control measures, this number decreased to 22,860 in 1995. In addition to those with active TB, however, an estimated 15 million people in the United States have

"Tuberculosis" Fact Sheet, National Institute of Allergy and Infectious Diseases (NIAID), NIH, March 1997.

latent TB infections and may develop active TB at some time in their lives.

Minorities are affected disproportionately by TB: 54 percent of active TB cases in 1995 were among African-American and Hispanic people, with an additional 17.5 percent found in Asians. In some sectors of U.S. society, TB rates now surpass those in the world's poorest countries. Among African-American men in New York City aged 35 to 44, for example, 315 out of 100,000 had active TB in 1993, many times the national average of 9.8 cases per 100,000 people.

Drug Resistance a Concern

With appropriate antibiotic therapy, TB usually can be cured. In recent years, however, drug-resistant cases of TB have increased dramatically.

Drug resistance results when patients fail to take their medicine consistently for the six to 12 months necessary to destroy all vestiges of *M. tuberculosis*. In some U.S. cities, more than 50 percent of patients—often homeless people, drug addicts, and others caught in poverty—fail to complete their prescribed course of TB therapy. One reason for this lack of compliance is that TB patients may feel better after only two to four weeks of treatment and stop taking their TB drugs, some of which have unpleasant side effects.

Resistance also may develop when patients are treated with too few drugs or with inadequate doses.

Particularly alarming is the increase in the number of people with multi-drug-resistant TB (MDR-TB), caused by *M. tuberculosis* strains resistant to two or more drugs. Even with treatment, the death rate for MDR-TB patients is 40 to 60 percent, the same as for TB patients who receive no treatment. For people co-infected with HIV and MDR-TB, the death rate may be as high as 80 percent. The time from diagnosis to death for some patients with MDR-TB and HIV may be only months as they are sometimes left with no treatment options.

Of all culture-positive TB cases in New York State in 1995, at least 13 percent were resistant to one or more antibiotic drugs. This figure is similar to that seen in an earlier national survey. At least 39 states reported drug-resistant cases of TB in 1995. In addition, CDC received numerous reports of outbreaks of MDR-TB in hospitals and prisons. During these outbreaks, MDR-TB has sometimes spread to hospital patients, health care workers, prisoners, and prison guards.

What Caused TB's Resurgence?

During the 19th century, TB claimed more lives in the United States than any other disease. Improvements in nutrition, housing, sanitation, and medical care in the first half of the 20th century dramatically reduced the number of cases and deaths. TB's decline hastened in the 1940s and 1950s with the introduction of the first effective antibiotic therapies for TB. By 1985, the number of cases had fallen to 22,201 in the United States, the lowest figure recorded in modern U.S. history.

In 1985, however, the decline ended and the number of active TB cases in the United States began to rise again. Several forces, often interrelated, were behind TB's resurgence:

- The HIV/AIDS epidemic. People with HIV are particularly vulnerable to reactivation of latent TB infections, as well as to disease caused by new TB infections. TB transmission occurs most frequently in crowded environments such as hospitals, prisons, and shelters where HIV-infected individuals make up a growing proportion of the population.

- Increased numbers of immigrants from countries with many cases of TB, many of whom live in crowded housing. Because of language and economic difficulties, many immigrants have limited access to health care and may not receive treatment.

- Increased poverty, injection drug use, and homelessness. TB transmission is rampant in crowded shelters and prisons where people weakened by poor nutrition, drug addiction, and alcoholism are exposed to *M. tuberculosis*. People in poor health, especially those infected with HIV, also are prone to reactivation of latent TB infections.

- Poor compliance with treatment regimens, especially among disadvantaged groups. Some of these people may remain contagious while others develop and pass on resistant strains of *M. tuberculosis* that are difficult to treat.

- Increased numbers of residents in long-term care facilities such as nursing homes. Immune function declines with age, and as patients live longer, many suffer recurrences of latent infections often acquired in early adulthood. As a result, other elderly people, especially those with weak immune systems, become newly infected with TB.

The TB Organism

TB is caused by repeated exposure to airborne droplets contaminated with *M. tuberculosis*, a rod-shaped bacterium. The TB bacterium also is known as the tubercle bacillus. (A small fraction of cases are caused by related bacteria, *M. africanum* and *M. bovis*.)

M. tuberculosis, like other mycobacteria, has an unusual cell wall, a waxy coat comprised of fatty molecules whose structure and functions are not well known. This cell wall appears to allow *M. tuberculosis* to survive in its preferred environment: inside immune cells called macrophages, which ordinarily degrade pathogens with enzymes. The coat of *M. tuberculosis* also renders it impermeable to many common drugs.

Biologists call *M. tuberculosis* and other mycobacteria "acid fast" bacteria because their fatty cell walls prevent the cells from being decolorized by acid solutions after staining during diagnostic tests.

Several factors make *M. tuberculosis* a difficult organism to study in the laboratory, hampering TB research. The bacteria multiply very slowly, only once every 24 hours, and take a month to form a colony. By comparison, other bacteria such as *E. coli* form colonies within eight hours. TB bacilli tend to form clumps, which makes working with them and counting them difficult. Most daunting, *M. tuberculosis*, a dangerous, airborne organism, can be studied only in laboratories that have specialized safety equipment.

Transmission

TB is primarily an airborne disease. The disease is not likely to be transmitted through personal items belonging to those with TB, such as clothing, bedding, or other items they have touched. Adequate ventilation is the most important measure to prevent the transmission of TB.

Because most infected people expel relatively few bacilli, transmission of TB usually occurs only after prolonged exposure to someone with active TB. On average, people have a 50 percent chance of becoming infected with TB if they spend eight hours a day for six months or 24 hours a day for two months working or living with someone with active TB, researchers have estimated.

People are most likely to be contagious when their sputum contains bacilli, when they cough frequently and when the extent of their lung disease, as revealed by a chest x-ray, is great. TB is spread from person to person in microscopic droplets—droplet nuclei—expelled from the lungs when a TB sufferer coughs, sneezes, speaks, sings, or laughs. Only people with active disease are contagious.

Droplet nuclei are tiny and may remain in the air for prolonged periods, ready to be inhaled. They are small enough to bypass the natural defenses of upper respiratory passages, such as hairs in the nose or the hairlike cilia in the bronchial tubes. Infection begins when the bacilli reach the tiny air sacs of the lungs known as alveoli, where they multiply within macrophages.

People who have been treated with appropriate drugs for at least two weeks usually are not infectious.

Infection

The site of initial infection is usually the alveoli—the balloon-like sacs at the ends of the small air passages in the lungs known as bronchioles. In the alveoli, white blood cells called macrophages ingest the inhaled *M. tuberculosis* bacilli.

Some of the bacilli may be killed immediately; others may multiply within the macrophages. Infrequently, but especially in HIV-infected people and in children, the bacilli spread to other sites in the body. This dissemination sometimes results in life-threatening meningitis and other problems.

During the two to eight weeks after initial infection in people with intact immune systems, macrophages present pieces of the bacilli, displayed on their cell surfaces, to another type of white blood cell—the T cell. When stimulated, T cells release an elaborate array of chemical signals. Once this response, called cell-mediated hypersensitivity, is established, a person's T cells usually will respond to the tuberculin skin test (PPD test) and produce a characteristic red welt.

Some of the T-cell signals produce inflammatory reactions; other signals recruit and activate specialized cells to kill bacilli and wall-off infected macrophages in tiny, hard grayish capsules known as tubercles.

From then on the body's immune system maintains a standoff with the infection, sometimes for years. In the tubercles, TB bacilli may persist within macrophages, but further multiplication and spread of *M. tuberculosis* are confined. Most people undergo complete healing of their initial infection, and the tubercles calcify and lose their viability. A positive TB skin test, and in some cases a chest x-ray, may provide the only evidence of the infection.

If, however, the body's resistance is low because of aging, infections such as HIV, malnutrition, or other factors, the bacilli may break out of the tubercles in the alveoli and lead to active disease.

Active Disease

On the average, people infected with *M. tuberculosis* have a 10 percent chance of developing active TB at some time in their lives. The risk of developing active disease is greatest in the first year after infection, but active disease sometimes does not occur until many years later.

Active TB usually results from the spread of bacilli from the alveoli through the bloodstream or lymphatic system to other sites, usually elsewhere in the lungs or local lymph nodes. In 15 percent of cases, the bacilli cause disease in other regions, such as the skin, kidneys, bones, or reproductive and urinary systems.

At the new sites, the body's immune defenses kill many bacilli, but immune cells and local tissue die as well. The dead cells and tissue form granulomas with the consistency of soft cheese, where the bacilli survive but do not flourish. The early symptoms of active TB can include weight loss, fever, night sweats, and loss of appetite, or they may be vague and go unnoticed by the affected individual.

As more lung tissue is destroyed and the granulomas expand, cavities in the lungs develop, and sometimes break into larger airways called bronchi. This allows large numbers of bacilli to spread when patients cough. As the disease progresses, the granulomas may liquefy, perhaps as a result of enzymes secreted by the body's own immune cells. This creates a rich medium in which the bacilli multiply rapidly and spread, creating further lesions and the characteristic chest pain, cough, and, when a blood vessel is eroded, bloody sputum.

Most patients do not suffer shortness of breath until the lungs are extensively damaged by the formation of cavities. Symptoms of TB involving areas other than the lungs vary, depending upon the organ affected.

Diagnosing TB

The tuberculin skin test, also known as the Mantoux test, can identify most people infected with tubercle bacilli six to eight weeks after initial exposure. A substance called purified protein derivative (PPD) is injected under the skin of the forearm and examined about 48 to 72 hours later. If a red welt forms around the injection site, the person may have been infected with *M. tuberculosis*, but doesn't necessarily have active disease. Most people with previous exposure to TB will test positive on the tuberculin test, as will some people exposed to related mycobacteria. An important exception is people with severely weakened immune systems, such as those with HIV.

If a person has a significant reaction to the tuberculin skin test, additional methods can determine if the individual has active TB. This is sometimes difficult because TB can mimic other diseases, such as pneumonia, lung abscesses, tumors, and fungal infections, or occur along with them. In making a diagnosis, doctors rely on symptoms and other physical signs, a person's history of exposure to TB, and x-rays that may show evidence of TB infection, usually in the form of cavities or lesions in the lungs.

The physician also will take sputum and other samples, because a positive bacteriologic culture of *M. tuberculosis* is essential to confirm the diagnosis and determine which drugs will work against the strain of TB the patient carries. Because *M. tuberculosis* grows very slowly, the laboratory diagnosis requires approximately four weeks. An additional two to three weeks usually are needed to determine the drug susceptibility of the organism, making treatment decisions difficult.

Advances in Diagnosis

Recently, researchers supported by the National Institute of Allergy and Infectious Diseases (NIAID) as well as other investigators developed tests that use nucleic acid amplification to speed the diagnosis of TB from four weeks to two days. Another test in development uses luminescent chemicals from the firefly to determine, in 24 to 48 hours, which drugs can kill the TB strain a patient carries.

Treatment of Active Disease

The death rate for untreated TB patients is between 40 and 60 percent. With appropriate antibiotics, however, people with drug-susceptible cases of TB can be cured more than 90 percent of the time.

Successful management of TB depends on close cooperation between the patient and physicians and other health care workers. Patient education is essential, and many doctors opt for supervised, directly observed therapy (DOT). Treatment usually combines the drugs isoniazid (INH) and rifampin, which are given for at least six months, and pyrazinamide, which is used only in the first two months of treatment. This treatment is referred to as short-course chemotherapy. A fourth drug, ethambutol, sometimes is added if a physician suspects that drug-resistant organisms are present.

Therapy for MDR-TB

Treatment for MDR-TB often requires the use of a second line of TB drugs, all of which can produce serious side effects. Therapy for 18 months to two years may be necessary, and patients often receive three drugs, one as an injection, after drug susceptibility testing.

Prevention

TB is largely a preventable disease. In the United States, prevention has focused on identifying infected individuals early—especially those who run the highest risk of developing active disease—and treating them with drugs in a program of directly observed therapy.

INH prevents the disease in most people in close contact with infected people or who are infected with the tubercle bacilli but who do not have active TB. The drug is given daily for six to 12 months and strict patient compliance in taking medication is essential to prevent drug-resistant strains from emerging. Adverse reactions to INH are rare, although a small percentage of patients, especially those older than 35, suffer INH-related hepatitis. Rifampin for one year is recommended for close contacts of patients with INH-resistant TB organisms.

In the United States, people with any of the following risk factors should be considered for preventive therapy, regardless of age, if they have not been previously treated for TB:

- Close contacts of people with newly diagnosed infectious TB; (In addition, children and adolescents who react negatively to the PPD test, but who have been in close contact with infectious people within the past three months should be considered for preventive therapy. Therapy should continue until a second skin test is done 12 weeks after their first contact with an infectious person.)

- People with positive tuberculin skin tests and abnormal chest x-rays compatible with inactive TB (lesions caused by prior disease);

- People whose skin test results have recently converted from negative to positive;

- People with positive skin test reactions who also have special medical conditions known to increase the risk of TB (e.g., HIV

infection, diabetes mellitus) or who are on corticosteroid
therapy;

- HIV-positive people or those suspected to be HIV-infected who
  now have, or had at any time in the past, positive skin test reactions, but who do not have active infection; and

- Injection drug users who have positive skin test reactions.

In addition, people younger than 35 in the following groups should
be considered for preventive therapy if they have positive skin test
reactions:

- Foreign-born people from countries where TB is common;

- People in medically underserved, low-income groups, especially
  African Americans, Hispanics, and Native Americans; and

- Residents of long-term care facilities such as prisons, nursing
  homes, and mental institutions.

Health care workers in frequent contact with TB patients or involved with high-risk procedures such as those that induce coughing
should have a skin test every six months.

Hospitals and clinics caring for high-risk populations can take
precautions to prevent the spread of TB. All patients should be taught
to cover their mouths and noses when coughing or sneezing. Ultraviolet light can be used to sterilize the air, and negative pressure
rooms and special filters are available, as are special respirators and
masks, that filter out the droplet nuclei. Until they are no longer infectious, hospitalized TB patients should be isolated in rooms with
controlled ventilation and airflow.

More Effective Vaccines are Needed

In those parts of the world where the disease is common, a vac-
cine composed of live, attenuated (weakened) mycobacteria from cows
(*M. bovis*, called bacillus Calmette-Guerin [BCG]) is given to infants
as part of the immunization program recommended by the World
Health Organization (WHO). In infants, BCG prevents the spread of
M. tuberculosis within the body, but does not prevent initial infection.

In adults, the effectiveness of BCG has varied widely in large-scale
studies. In addition, positive skin test reactions occur in people who
have received BCG vaccine, thus limiting the effectiveness of the PPD

skin test to identify new infections. As a result, BCG is not recommended for general use in the United States. Because of BCG's limitations, more effective vaccines are needed.

TB and HIV Infection

WHO estimates that 4.4 million people worldwide are co-infected with TB and HIV. By the year 2000, TB will claim 1 million lives annually among the HIV-infected, WHO projects. In the United States, an estimated 100,000 HIV-infected people also carry *M. tuberculosis*, according to CDC.

TB frequently occurs early in the course of HIV infection, often months to years before other opportunistic infections such as *Pneumocystis carinii* pneumonia. TB may be the first indication that a person is HIV-infected, and often occurs in areas outside the lungs, particularly in the later stages of HIV disease.

In the United States, people co-infected with TB and HIV develop active TB at a rate of about 8 percent each **year**. By comparison, otherwise healthy individuals infected with *M. tuberculosis* have a 10 percent **lifetime** risk of developing active TB. People with HIV also are at greater risk of having a new infection progress directly to active disease.

MDR-TB in people co-infected with HIV appears to have a more rapid and deadly disease course than seen in patients with MDR-TB who are otherwise healthy.

Diagnosing TB in HIV-infected people is often difficult. These patients frequently have conditions that produce symptoms similar to those of TB, and may not react to the standard tuberculin skin test because their immune systems are suppressed. Although investigators have hypothesized that a two-stage TB skin test might be more reliable than a single-stage test in HIV-infected individuals, a recently completed NIAID study found this not to be the case.

X-rays, sputum smears and physical exams may also fail to provide an indication of TB infection in the HIV-infected. As a consequence, doctors must often decide to begin anti-TB therapy in HIV-infected people suspected of having active TB while waiting for the results of cultures of sputum or other specimens.

Chapter 11

Allergy Tests

Introduction

Sneezing is not always the symptom of a cold. Sometimes, it is an allergic reaction to something in the air. Experts estimate that 35 million Americans suffer from upper respiratory symptoms that are allergic reactions to airborne pollen. Pollen allergy, commonly called hay fever, is one of the most common chronic diseases in the United States. Worldwide, airborne dust causes the most problems for people with allergies. The respiratory symptoms of asthma, which affects approximately 15 million Americans, are often provoked by airborne allergens (substances that cause an allergic reaction).

Overall, allergic diseases are among the major causes of illness and disability in the United States, affecting as many as 40 to 50 million Americans.

What Is an Allergy?

An allergy is a specific immunologic reaction to a normally harmless substance, one that does not bother most people. People who have allergies often are sensitive to more than one substance. Types of allergens that cause allergic reactions include pollens, dust particles, mold spores, food, latex rubber, insect venom, or medicines.

This chapter includes text from the following National Institute of Allergy and Infectious Diseases (NIAID), NIH documents. *Something in the Air: Airborne Allergens*, February 1998, *Food Allergy and Intolerances*, January 1998, and *Asthma and Allergy Statistics*, June 1996.

Why Are Some People Allergic to These Substances While Others Are Not?

Scientists think that people inherit a tendency to be allergic, meaning an increased likelihood of being allergic to one or more allergens, although they probably do not have an inherited tendency to be allergic to any specific allergens. Children are much more likely to develop allergies if their parents have allergies, even if only one parent is allergic. Exposure to allergens at certain times when the body's defenses are lowered or weakened, such as after a viral infection or during pregnancy, seems to contribute to the development of allergies.

What Is an Allergic Reaction?

Normally, the immune system functions as the body's defense against invading agents such as bacteria and viruses. In most allergic reactions, however, the immune system is responding to a false alarm. When an allergic person first comes into contact with an allergen, the immune system treats the allergen as an invader and mobilizes to attack. The immune system does this by generating large amounts of a type of antibody (a disease-fighting protein) called immunoglobin E, or IgE. Each IgE antibody is specific for one particular allergenic (allergy-producing) substance. In the case of pollen allergy, the antibody is specific for each type of pollen: one type of antibody may be produced to react against oak pollen and another against ragweed pollen, for example.

These IgE molecules are special because IgE is the only class of antibody that attaches tightly to the body's mast cells, which are tissue cells, and to basophils, which are blood cells. When the allergen next encounters its specific IgE, it attaches to the antibody like a key fitting into a lock, signaling the cell to which the IgE is attached to release (and in some cases to produce) powerful inflammatory chemicals like histamine, cytokines, and leukotrienes. These chemicals act on tissues in various parts of the body, such as the respiratory system, and cause the symptoms of allergy.

Some people with allergy develop asthma. The symptoms of asthma include coughing, wheezing, and shortness of breath due to a narrowing of the bronchial passages (airways) in the lungs, and to excess mucus production and inflammation. Asthma can be disabling and sometimes can be fatal. If wheezing and shortness of breath accompany allergy symptoms, it is a signal that the bronchial tubes also have become involved, indicating the need for medical attention.

82

Symptoms of Allergies to Airborne Substances

- Sneezing often accompanied by a runny or clogged nose.

- Coughing and postnasal drip.

- Itching eyes, nose, and throat.

- Allergic shiners (dark circles under the eyes caused by increased blood flow near the sinuses).

- The "allergic salute" (in a child, persistent upward rubbing of the nose that causes a crease mark on the nose).

- Watering eyes.

- Conjunctivitis (an inflammation of the membrane that lines the eyelids, causing red-rimmed, swollen eyes, and crusting of the eyelids).

In people who are not allergic, the mucus in the nasal passages simply moves foreign particles to the throat, where they are swallowed or coughed out. But something different happens to a person who is sensitive to airborne allergens.

As soon as the allergen lands on the mucous membranes lining the inside of the nose, a chain reaction occurs that leads the mast cells in these tissues to release histamine and other chemicals. These powerful chemicals contract certain cells that line some small blood vessels in the nose. This allows fluids to escape, which causes the nasal passages to swell, resulting in nasal congestion.

Histamine also can cause sneezing, itching, irritation, and excess mucus production, which can result in allergic rhinitis (runny nose). Other chemicals made and released by mast cells, including cytokines and leukotrienes, also contribute to allergic symptoms.

Diagnosing Airborne Allergic Diseases

People with allergy symptoms, such as the runny nose of allergic rhinitis, may at first suspect they have a cold—but the "cold" lingers on. It is important to see a doctor about any respiratory illness that lasts longer than a week or two. When it appears that the symptoms are caused by an allergy, the patient should see a physician who understands the diagnosis and treatment of allergies. If the patient's medical history indicates that the symptoms recur at the same time each year, the physician will work under the theory that a seasonal allergen (like pollen) is involved. Properly trained specialists recognize the patterns of potential allergens common during local seasons and the association between these patterns and symptoms. The medical history suggests which allergens are the likely culprits. The doctor also will examine the mucous membranes, which often appear swollen and pale or bluish in persons with allergic conditions.

Skin Tests

Doctors use skin tests to determine whether a patient has IgE antibodies in the skin that react to a specific allergen. The doctor will use diluted extracts from allergens such as dust mites, pollens, or molds commonly found in the local area. The extract of each kind of allergen is injected under the patient's skin or is applied to a tiny scratch or puncture made on the patient's arm or back.

Skin tests are one way of measuring the level of IgE antibody in a patient. With a positive reaction, a small, raised, reddened area (called a wheal) with a surrounding flush (called a flare) will appear at the test site. The size of the wheal can give the physician an important diagnostic clue, but a positive reaction does not prove that a particular pollen is the cause of a patient's symptoms. Although such a reaction indicates that IgE antibody to a specific allergen is present in the skin, respiratory symptoms do not necessarily result.

Blood Tests

Although skin testing is the most sensitive and least costly way to identify allergies in patients, some patients such as those with widespread skin conditions like eczema should not be tested using that method. There are other diagnostic tests that use a blood sample from the patient to detect levels of IgE antibody to a particular allergen. One such blood test is called the RAST (radioallergosorbent test), which can be performed when eczema is present or if a patient has taken medications that interfere with skin testing.

Food Allergy and Intolerance

Food allergies or food intolerances affect the lives of virtually everyone at some point. People often may have an unpleasant reaction to something they ate and wonder if they have a food allergy. Almost one out of three people either say that they themselves have a food allergy or that they modify the family diet because a family member is suspected of having a food allergy. But only about three percent of children have clinically proven allergic reactions to foods. In adults, the prevalence of food allergy drops to about one percent of the total population.

This difference between the clinically proven prevalence of food allergy and the public perception is, in part, due to reactions that are termed "food intolerances" and not food allergies. A food allergy, or hypersensitivity, is an abnormal response to a food that is triggered by the immune system. The immune system is not responsible for the symptoms of a food intolerance, even though these symptoms can resemble those of a food allergy.

It is extremely important for people who have true food allergies to identify them and prevent allergic reactions to food because these reactions can cause devastating illness and, in some cases, be fatal.

Food Allergy Symptoms

There is a wide range of food allergy symptoms. This variability of symptoms stems from the large number of tissues in the body which can be affected by an immune reaction to food.

Frequently the first part of the body to react to food is the gastrointestinal tract. The allergic reaction in this portion of the body can cause vomiting, abdominal pain, and diarrhea. As the immune response to food affects other areas of the body, a person may develop hives (urticaria), swelling, sneezing and a runny nose, asthma or difficulty breathing.

The most severe food allergy reaction is anaphylaxis—a systemic, life-threatening shock that can occur minutes after a person eats a food to which they are allergic. Anaphylactic reactions to food probably result in as many as 50 deaths a year in the United States. One of the characteristic features of this kind of reaction is trouble breathing caused by edema (swelling) of the throat or bronchi; it can also cause severe asthma, hives, a drop in blood pressure and loss of consciousness, and death, if not treated immediately.

Eczema due to food allergy is a different kind of reaction in which the target organ is the skin, which becomes crusty, red, scaly, and itchy. In children, eczema is frequently due to foods, but it can also be a preexisting condition made worse by certain foods. Probably fewer than one in twenty adults with eczema have an associated food allergy.

Common Food Allergies

In adults, the most common foods to cause allergic reactions include: shellfish, such as shrimp, crayfish, lobster, and crab; peanuts, which is one of the chief foods to cause severe anaphylactic reactions; tree nuts, such as walnuts; fish; and egg.

In children, the pattern is somewhat different. The most common food allergens that cause problems in children are egg, milk, and peanuts.

The foods that adults or children react to are those foods they eat often. In Japan, for example, rice allergy is more frequent. In Scandinavia, codfish allergy is common.

Differential Diagnosis

A differential diagnosis means distinguishing food allergy from food intolerance or other illnesses. If a patient goes to the doctor's office and says, "I think I have a food allergy," the doctor has to consider the list of other possibilities that may lead to symptoms that could be confused with food allergy.

One possibility is the contamination of foods with microorganisms, such as bacteria, and their products, such as toxins. Contaminated meat sometimes mimics a food reaction when it is really a type of food poisoning.

There are also natural substances, such as histamine, that can occur in foods and stimulate a reaction similar to an allergic reaction. For example, histamine can reach high levels in cheese, some wines, and in certain kinds of fish, particularly tuna and mackerel. In fish, histamine is believed to stem from bacterial contamination, particularly in fish that hasn't been refrigerated properly. If someone eats one of these foods with a high level of histamine, that person may have a reaction that strongly resembles an allergic reaction to food. This reaction is called histamine toxicity.

Another cause of food intolerance that is often confused with a food allergy is lactase deficiency. This most common food intolerance affects at least one out of ten people. Lactase is an enzyme that is in the lining of the gut. This enzyme degrades lactose, which is in milk. If a person does not have enough lactase, the body cannot digest the lactose in most milk products. Instead, the lactose is used by bacteria, gas is formed, and the person experiences bloating, abdominal pain, and sometimes diarrhea.

Another type of food intolerance is an adverse reaction to certain products that are added to food to enhance taste, provide color, or protect against growth of microorganisms. Compounds that are most frequently tied to adverse reactions that can be confused with food allergy are yellow dye number 5, monosodium glutamate, and sulfites.

Yellow dye number 5 can cause hives, although rarely. Monosodium glutamate (MSG) is a flavor enhancer, and when consumed in large amounts, can cause flushing, sensations of warmth, headache, facial pressure, chest pain or feelings of detachment in some people. These transient reactions occur rapidly after eating large amounts of food to which MSG has been added.

Sulfites can occur naturally in foods or are added to enhance crispness or prevent mold growth. Sulfites in high concentrations sometimes pose problems for people with severe asthma. Sulfites can give off a gas called sulfur dioxide, which the asthmatic inhales while eating the sulfited food. This irritates the lungs and can send an asthmatic into severe bronchospasm, a constriction of the lungs. Such reactions led the U.S. Food and Drug Administration (FDA) to ban sulfites as spray-on preservatives in fresh fruits and vegetables. But they are still used in some foods and are made naturally during the fermentation of wine.

There are a number of other diseases that share symptoms with food allergies including ulcers and cancers of the gastrointestinal tract. These disorders can be associated with vomiting, diarrhea, or cramping abdominal pain exacerbated by eating.

Some people may have a food intolerance that has a psychological trigger. In selected cases, a careful psychiatric evaluation may identify an unpleasant event in that person's life, often during childhood, tied to eating a particular food. The eating of that food years later, even as an adult, is associated with a rush of unpleasant sensations that can resemble an allergic reaction to food.

Diagnosis of Food Allergy

To diagnose food allergy a doctor must first determine if the patient is having an adverse reaction to specific foods. This assessment is made with the help of a detailed patient history, the patient's diet diary, or an elimination diet.

The first of these techniques is the most valuable. The physician sits down with the person suspected of having a food allergy and takes a history to determine if the facts are consistent with a food allergy. The doctor asks such questions as:

- What was the timing of the reaction? Did the reaction come on quickly, usually within an hour after eating the food?

- Was allergy treatment successful? (Antihistamines should relieve hives, for example, if they stem from a food allergy.)

- Is the reaction always associated with a certain food?

- Did anyone else get sick? For example, if the person has eaten fish contaminated with histamine, everyone who ate the fish should be sick. However, in an allergic reaction, only the person allergic to the fish becomes ill.

- How much did the patient eat before experiencing a reaction? The doctor will want to know how much you ate each time and try to relate it to the severity of the reaction.

- How was the food prepared? Some people will have a violent allergic reaction only to raw or undercooked fish. Complete cooking of the fish destroys those allergens in the fish to which they react. If the fish is cooked thoroughly, they can eat it with no allergic reaction.

- Were other foods ingested at the same time of the allergic reaction? Some foods may delay digestion and thus delay the onset of the allergic reaction.

Sometimes a diagnosis cannot be made solely on the basis of history. The doctor may also ask the patient to go back and keep a record of the contents of each meal and whether he or she had a reaction. This gives more detail from which the doctor and the patient can determine if there is consistency in the reactions.

The next step some doctors use is an elimination diet. Under the doctor's direction, the patient does not eat a food suspected of causing the allergy, like eggs, and substitutes another food in this case another source of protein. If the patient removes the food and the symptoms go away, a diagnosis can almost be made. If the patient then eats the food (under the doctor's direction) and the symptoms come back, then the diagnosis is confirmed. This technique cannot be used, however, if the reactions are severe (in which case the patient should not resume eating the food) or infrequent.

If the patient's history, diet diary or elimination diet suggest a specific food allergy is likely, the doctor will then use tests that can more objectively measure an allergic response to food. One of these is a scratch skin test, during which a dilute extract of the food is placed on the skin of the forearm or back. This portion of the skin is then scratched with a needle and observed for swelling or redness that would indicate a local allergic reaction. If the scratch test is positive, the patient has IgE on the skin's mast cells that is specific to the food being tested.

Skin tests are rapid, simple and relatively safe. But a patient can have a positive skin test to a food allergen without experiencing allergic reactions to that food. A diagnosis of food allergy is made only when a patient has a positive skin test to a specific allergen and the history of their reactions also suggests an allergy to the same food.

In some extremely allergic patients who have severe anaphylactic reactions, skin testing can't be used because it could evoke a dangerous reaction. Skin testing also cannot be done on patients with extensive eczema.

For these patients a doctor may use one of two blood tests called RAST and ELISA .These tests measure the presence of food-specific IgE in the blood of patients. These tests may cost more than skin tests and results are not immediately available. As with skin testing, positive tests do not necessarily make the diagnosis.

The final method used to objectively diagnose food allergy is double-blind food challenge. This testing has come into vogue over the last few years as the "gold standard" of allergy testing. For this food challenge, various foods, some of which are suspected of inducing an allergic reaction, are each placed in individual opaque capsules. The patient is asked to swallow a capsule and is then watched to see if a reaction occurs. This process is repeated until all the capsules have been swallowed. In a true double-blind test, the doctor is also "blinded," the capsules having been made up by some other medical person, so that neither the patient nor the doctor knows which capsule contains the allergen.

The one strong advantage of such a challenge is that, if the patient has a reaction only to suspected foods and not to other foods tested, it confirms the diagnosis. However, someone with a history of severe reactions cannot be tested this way. In addition, this testing is expensive because it takes a lot of time to perform. Multiple food allergies are also difficult to evaluate with this procedure.

Consequently, double-blind food challenges are not done often. This type of testing is most commonly used when the doctor believes that the reaction a person is describing is not due to a specific food and wishes to obtain evidence to support this judgment so that additional efforts may be directed at finding the real cause of the reaction.

Controversial Issues

There are several disorders thought by some to be caused by food allergies, but the evidence is currently insufficient or contrary to such claims. It is controversial, for example, whether migraine headaches can be caused by food allergies. There are studies showing that people who are prone to migraines can have their headaches brought on by histamines and other substances in foods. The more difficult issue is whether food allergies actually cause migraines in such people. There is virtually no evidence that rheumatoid arthritis or osteoarthritis can be made worse by foods, despite claims to the contrary. There is also no evidence that food allergies can cause a disorder called the allergic tension fatigue syndrome, in which people are tired, nervous, and may have problems concentrating, or have headaches.

Cerebral allergy is a term that has been applied to people who have trouble concentrating and have headaches, as well as other complaints. This is sometimes attributed to mast cells degranulating in the brain, but no other place in the body. There is no evidence that such a scenario can happen, and cerebral allergy is not currently recognized by allergists.

Another controversial topic is environmental illness. In a seemingly pristine environment, some people have many non-specific complaints such as problems concentrating or depression. Sometimes this is attributed to small amounts of allergens or toxins in the environment. There is no evidence that such problems are due to food allergies.

Some people believe hyperactivity in children is caused by food allergies. But this behavioral disorder has only been suggested to be associated with food additives occasionally in children, and then only when such additives are consumed in large amounts. There is no evidence that a true food allergy can affect a child's activity except for the proviso that if a child itches and sneezes and wheezes a lot, the child may be miserable and therefore more difficult to control. Also, children who are on anti-allergy medicines that can cause drowsiness may get sleepy in school or at home.

Controversial Diagnostic Techniques

Just as there are controversial food allergy syndromes and treatments there are also controversial ways of diagnosing food allergies. One of these is cytotoxicity testing, in which food allergen is added to a patient's blood sample. A technician then examines the sample under the microscope to see if white cells in the blood "die." This technique has been evaluated in a number of studies and has not been found to effectively diagnose food allergy.

Another controversial approach is called sublingual or, if it is injected under the skin, subcutaneous provocative challenge. In this procedure, dilute food allergen is administered under the tongue of the person who may feel that his or her arthritis, for instance, is due to foods. The technician then asks the patient if the food allergen has aggravated the arthritis symptoms. In clinical studies, this procedure has not been shown to effectively diagnose food allergies.

An immune complex assay is sometimes done on patients suspected of having food allergies to see if there are complexes of certain antibodies bound to the food allergen in the bloodstream. It is said that these immune complexes correlate with food allergies. But the formation of such immune complexes is a normal offshoot of food digestion and everyone, if tested with a sensitive enough measurement, has them. To date, no one has conclusively shown that this test correlates with allergies to foods.

Another test is the IgG subclass assay, which looks specifically for certain kinds of IgG antibody. Again, there is no evidence that this diagnoses food allergy.

Food Allergy Summary

Food allergies are caused by immunologic reactions to foods. There actually are several discrete diseases under this category and a number of foods that can cause these problems.

A medical evaluation after one suspects a food allergy is the key to proper management. Treatment is basically avoidance of the other food(s) after they are identified. People with food allergies should become knowledgeable about allergies and how they are treated and should work with their physicians.

Asthma and Allergy Statistics

- From 1990 to 1994, the number of people with **self-reported asthma** in the U.S. increased from 10.4 million to 14.6 million [1,2].

- **Asthma** was the first-listed diagnosis in 468,000 U.S. hospital admissions in 1993 [3].

- **Asthma** affected an estimated 4.8 million **U.S. children** (under age 18) in 1994. Asthmatic youngsters under age 15 underwent 159,000 hospitalizations in 1993, with an average length of stay of 3.4 days [2,3].

- **Asthma** is 26% more prevalent in **black children** than in white children. Black children with asthma experience more

91

severe disability and have more frequent hospitalizations than do white children [4,5].

- Among 5-24 year olds, the **asthma death rate** nearly doubled from 1980 to 1993. In 1993, **blacks** in this age group were 4 to 6 times more likely to die from asthma than whites; and **males** were 1.5 times at greater risk than females [6].

- **Asthma treatment cost** an estimated $6.2 billion in 1990, including direct and indirect expenditures; 43% of that total cost was associated with emergency room use, hospitalization, and death. Loss of school days, alone, caused decreased productivity that cost an estimated $1 billion [7].

- While there are no solid statistics, estimates from a skin test survey suggest that **allergies** affect as many as 40 to 50 million people in the U.S.[8].

- **Allergy testing** was listed as the reason for 1.4 million **office visits to physicians** in 1991 [9].

- **Pollen allergy (hay fever or allergic rhinitis)** affects nearly 9.3% of the people in the U.S., not including those with asthma [2]. Allergic rhinitis was the reason for 7.6 million office visits to physicians in 1992 [9]. The estimated direct and indirect costs of hay fever in the U.S. in 1990 totaled $1.8 billion [10].

- **Allergic dermatitis** (itchy rash) is the most common skin condition in **children** younger than 11 years of age [11]. The percentage of American children diagnosed with it has increased from 3% in the 1960s to 10% in the 1990s [12].

- **Urticaria** (hives; raised areas of reddened skin that become itchy) and **angioedema** (swelling of throat tissues) together affect approximately 15% of the U.S. population every year [12].

- More than 1,000 systemic **allergic reactions to natural rubber latex,** including 15 deaths, were reported to the FDA from 1988 to 1992. Case follow-ups showed that the reactions were caused by residual rubber tree proteins in medical devices such as rubber gloves and catheters. Most (82%) allergic reactions to latex are caused by rubber additives [13].

- **Chronic sinusitis**, most often caused by allergies, affects nearly 35 million people in the U.S. [2].

- **Allergic drug reactions,** commonly caused by antibiotics such as penicillin and cephalosporins, occur in 2 to 3% of hospitalized patients [14].

- Eight percent of **children** younger than 6 years experience **food intolerances.** Of this group, 2 to 4% appear to have reproducible allergic reactions to food. Of **adults,** an estimated 1 to 2% are sensitive to foods or food additives [15].

- A severe allergic reaction known as **anaphylaxis** occurs in 0.5 to 5% of the U.S. population as a result of **insect stings.** At least 40 deaths per year result from insect sting anaphylaxis [16].

References

1. Adams, P.F., Benson, V; Current Estimates from the National Health Interview Survey, National Center for Health Statistics, *Vital Health Statistics*; 10(181), 1991.

2. Centers for Disease Control and Prevention; Vital and Health Statistics, Current Estimates From the National Health Interview Survey, 1994 (U.S. Department of Health and Human Services, Public Health Service, National Center for Health Statistics); *DHHS Publication No. PHS 96-1521*; December 1995.

3. Centers for Disease Control and Prevention; Vital and Health Statistics, National Hospital Discharge Survey: Annual Summary, 1993 (U.S. Department of Health and Human Services, Public Health Service, National Center for Health Statistics); *DHHS Publication No. PHS 95-1782*; August 1995.

4. Taylor, W.R., Newscheck, P.W.; Impact of Childhood Asthma on Health; *Pediatrics*; 90(5):657-662, 1992.

5. Evans, R.; Asthma Among Minority children: A Growing Problem; *Chest*; 101(6):368S-371S, 1992.

6. Centers for Disease Control; Asthma Mortality and Hospitalization Among children and Young Adults, 1980-1993; *MMWR*; 45(17):350-353, May 3, 1996.

7. Weiss, K.B., Gergen, P.J., Hodgson, T.A. An Economic Evaluation of Asthma in the U.S. *NEJM*; 326:862-6, March 26, 1992.

8. Gergen, P.J., Turkeltaub, P.C., Kaovar, M.G.; The Prevalence of Allergic Skin Reactivity to Eight Common Allergens in the US Population: Results from the Second National Health and Nutrition Examination Survey; *J. Allergy Clin. Immunol.*; 800:669-79, 1987.

9. Centers for Disease Control and Prevention; Vital and Health Statistics, National Ambulatory Medical Care Survey: 1991 Summary (U.S. Department of Health and Human Services, Public Health Service, National Center for Health Statistics.); *DHHS Publication No. PHS 94-1777*; May 1994.

10. McMenamin, P. Costs of Hay Fever in the U.S. in 1990. *Annals of Allergy*; 73:35-39, 1994.

11. Lapidus, C.S., Schwarz, D.F., Honig, P.J.; Atopic dermatitis in children: Who cares? Who pays? *Journal of the American Academy of Dermatology*. 28(5):699-703, 1993.

12. Horan, R.F., Schneider, L.C., Sheffer, A.L. Allergic skin disorders and mastocytosis.; *Journal of the American Medical Association*; 268(20):2858-2868, 1992.

13. Sussman, G.L, Beezhold, D.H. Allergy to Latex Rubber. *Ann.Int. Med*; 122:43-46, 1995.

14. Sullivan, T.J., Drug Allergy, in *Allergy, Principles and Practice*, 4th edition; E. Middleton et al., Mosby, St. Louis, p.1726, 1993.

15. Sampson, H.A, Metcalfe, D.D. Food Allergies. *JAMA*; 268:2840-5, 1992.

16. Valentine, M.D., Anaphylaxis and Stinging Insect Hypersensitivity. *JAMA*; 268:2830-2833, 1992.

Chapter 12

Hearing Tests

Audiogram

The basic hearing test or audiogram tests one's ability to hear pure tones in each ear. Best results are obtained by a trained audiologist in a special soundproof testing booth. Simple tests, such as ones done in many schools, may be useful for screening, but a careful audiogram is necessary for accurate diagnosis of most hearing problems.

A complete audiogram will test both the bone conduction (the ability to hear a sound when it is transmitted through bone) and the air conduction (the ability to hear a sound when it is transmitted through air). A comparison between these two types of conduction can be very useful in localizing which part of the hearing mechanism is responsible for the loss. In particular, the test is useful in determining if the loss is due to a problem with the portion of the middle ear that conducts sound from the ear canal to the inner ear (in which case it would be called a "conductive" hearing loss) or if it is due to the inner ear or the nerve that conducts the sound signals to the brain (in which case it would be called a "sensorineural" hearing loss).

The results of audiograms are most often displayed in graph form. This graph shows the amount of hearing loss expressed in units called decibels at different sound frequencies (also called Hertz).

This chapter contains text from "Patient Care–Hearing Tests," by Randall L. Plant, M.D., reprinted with permission © July 1998 University of Washington School of Medicine; and "Hearing Evaluation in Children," by Anne Rouleau Peck, used with permission © 1998 The Nemours Foundation.

High frequencies correspond to high tones, and low frequencies are low tones. Most audiograms go from around 250 hertz to 8000 hertz. A loss up to 20 decibels on this graph is considered "normal". Hearing losses over 20 decibels are considered abnormal.

Tympanogram

The tympanogram is a test that measures how easily the eardrum vibrates back and forth and at what pressure the vibration is the easiest. The middle ear is normally filled with air at a pressure equal to the surrounding atmosphere. If the middle ear is filled with fluid, the eardrum will not vibrate properly and the tympanogram will be flat. If the middle ear is filled with air but at a higher or lower pressure than the surrounding atmosphere, the tympanogram will be shifted in its position.

The tympanogram is a quick and easy test. A special probe is placed up against the ear canal, like an earplug, and the equipment automatically makes the measurements.

Auditory Brain Stem Response (ABR)

The ABR is a special hearing test that can be used to track the nerve signals arising in the inner ear as they travel through the hearing nerve (called the auditory nerve) to the region of the brain responsible for hearing. The test is useful because it can tell us where along that path the hearing loss has occurred. For example, the ABR is often used for individuals with a sensorineural (nerve) loss in just one ear. This loss can sometimes be caused by a benign (non-cancerous) tumor on the auditory nerve. If the ABR is normal along that region of the path, the chances of having this tumor are quite small.

The ABR can also be used on small infants since it requires no conscious response from the person being tested. A small speaker is placed near the ear which produces clicking sound. Special electrodes automatically record the nerve signal; the patient can even be asleep during the test.

Electronystagmogram (ENG)

The ENG is actually not a hearing test but rather a special test of the balance mechanism of the inner ear. The test involves running a cool liquid and then a warm liquid through the ear canal (it is usually done through a small tube so the ear itself remains dry). This change in temperature stimulates the inner ear which in turn causes rapid reflex movements of the eyes. These movements are recorded, and from these it can be determined how well this balance mechanism is functioning.

Hearing Evaluation in Children

Many parents worry about their child's hearing, especially when the child is too young to communicate verbally. Usually there is no need for concern, but it's comforting to know that hearing may be evaluated **at any age**.

Hearing is a critical part of a child's development. Even a mild or partial hearing loss can affect a child's ability to speak and to understand oral language. The earlier hearing loss is detected, the sooner a child may be helped.

The outer ear picks up sounds and passes them to the middle ear through the eardrum. Three small bones (the hammer, anvil, and stirrup bones) vibrate with the sound, passing the vibrations to the inner ear. In the cochlea in the inner ear, the vibrations are changed into electric signals that move along the nerves to the brain.

How Well Does My Child Hear?

Most newborn infants startle or "jump" to sudden loud noises. By three months, a baby usually recognizes a parent's voice. By six months, an infant should turn his or her eyes or head toward a sound. By twelve months, a child should imitate some sounds and produce a few words, such as "Mama" or "bye-bye."

When Is Hearing Evaluation Indicated?

Hearing evaluation may be indicated if a young child has limited, poor, or no speech; seems frequently inattentive; has difficulty learning; or has any signs of hearing loss, such as increasing the television volume.

In conjunction with any behavioral symptoms, hearing assessment also may be necessary if there are certain risk factors for hearing loss, such as childhood hearing loss in family members, severe complications at birth, frequent ear infections, or infections such as meningitis or cytomegalovirus.

What Kinds of Hearing Loss Are There?

Conductive hearing loss is caused by an interference in the transmission of sound to the inner ear. Infants and young children frequently develop conductive hearing loss due to ear infections. This loss is usually mild, temporary, and treatable with medicine or surgery.

Sensorineural hearing loss involves malformation, dysfunction, or damage to the inner ear (cochlea). It usually exists at birth. It may be hereditary or may be caused by a number of medical problems, but often the cause is unknown. This type of hearing loss is usually permanent.

The degree of sensorineural hearing loss can be mild, moderate, severe, or profound. Sometimes the loss is progressive (hearing gradually becomes poorer) and sometimes unilateral (one ear only). Sensorineural hearing loss is generally not medically or surgically treatable, but children with this type of hearing loss can often be helped with hearing aids.

A **mixed hearing loss** occurs when both conductive and sensorineural hearing loss are present at the same time.

A **central hearing loss** involves the hearing areas of the brain, which may show as difficulty "processing" speech and other auditory information.

How Is My Child's Hearing Tested?

There are several methods of testing a child's hearing. The method chosen depends in part on the child's age, development, or medical status.

Behavoral Tests involve careful observation of a patient's behavioral response to sounds like calibrated speech and pure tones. Pure tones are the distinct pitches (frequencies) of sounds. Sometimes other calibrated signals are used to obtain frequency information.

The behavioral response might be an infant's eye movements, a head-turn by a toddler, placement of a game piece by a pre-schooler, or a hand-raise by a grade-schooler. Speech responses may involve picture identification of a word or repeating words at soft or comfortable levels. Very young children are capable of a number of behavioral tests.

Physiologic Tests are not hearing tests but are measures used with very young children that can partially estimate hearing function. It is important that behavioral tests are performed in addition to physiologic tests. Behavioral tests and parental reports should have some agreement with estimated hearing status provided by physiologic tests.

Auditory Brainstem Response (ABR) Test

An infant is sleeping or sedated for the ABR. Tiny earphones are placed in the baby's ear canals. Usually, click-type sounds are introduced through the earphones, and electrodes measure the hearing nerve's response to the sounds. A computer averages these responses and displays waveforms. Since there are characteristic waveforms for normal hearing in portions of the speech range, a normal ABR can predict fairly well that a baby's hearing is normal in that part of the range. An abnormal ABR may be due to hearing loss, but it may also be due to some medical problems or measurement difficulties.

Otoacoustic Emissions (OAE) Test

An infant can be awake but should be fairly quiet for the OAE. In this brief test, a tiny probe is placed in the ear canal. Numerous pulse-type sounds are introduced, and an "echo" response from the inner ear is recorded. These recordings are averaged by a computer. Certain types of recordings are associated with normal inner-ear function.

ABR or OAE tests are often used at hospitals to screen newborn infants. If a baby fails a screening, the test is usually repeated. If the screening is failed again, the baby is referred for full hearing evaluation.

Tympanometry

Tympanometry is not a hearing test but a procedure that can show how well the eardrum moves when a soft sound and air pressure are introduced in the ear canal. It is helpful in identifying middle ear problems, such as fluid collecting behind the eardrum. A tympanogram is a graphic representation of tympanometry. A "flat" line on a tympanogram may indicate that the eardrum is not mobile, while a "peaked" pattern often indicates normal function. An ear inspection should be performed with tympanometry.

Who Should Test My Child's Hearing?

A pediatric audiologist is the professional who specializes in evaluating and assisting children with hearing loss. This person works closely with physicians, educators, and speech/language pathologists. Audiologists have a lot of specialized training. They have masters or doctorate degrees in audiology, have performed internships, and are certified by the American-Speech-Language-Hearing Association or are Fellows of the American Academy of Audiology (F-AAA).

More Information

Ear Canals

Ear canals are the tubular openings that carry sounds from the outside of the body to the eardrum.

The Middle Ear

Deep within the outer ear canal is the eardrum (tympanic membrane). The eardrum is a thin, transparent membrane that vibrates in response to sound waves. The middle ear is a small, air-containing cavity that sits behind the eardrum. When the eardrum vibrates, tiny bones within the middle ear transmit the sound signals to the inner ear. Here nerves are stimulated to relay the sound signals to the brain. A tiny passageway, the eustachian tube, connects the middle ear to the nose. The eustachian tube normally serves to ventilate and equalize pressure to the middle ear. When you child's ears "pop" when yawning or swallowing, the eustachian tube is adjusting the air pressure in the middle ear.

Chapter 13

Vision Tests

Introduction

This chapter is designed to help people with eye diseases including glaucoma, age-related macular degeneration, and diabetic retinopathy better understand these diseases. It describes the causes, symptoms, tests, and diagnosis of these eye diseases. The vision tests described for glaucoma are typical of all basic vision exams.

Glaucoma

Glaucoma is a group of diseases that can lead to damage to the eye's optic nerve and result in blindness.

Open-angle glaucoma, the most common form of glaucoma, affects about 3 million Americans—half of whom don't know they have it. It has no symptoms at first. But over the years it can steal your sight. With early treatment, you can often protect your eyes against serious vision loss and blindness.

What Is the Optic Nerve?

The **optic nerve** is a bundle of more than 1 million nerve fibers. It connects the **retina,** the light-sensitive layer of tissue at the back of the eye, with the brain. A healthy optic nerve is necessary for good vision.

This chapter includes text from the following National Eye Institute (NEI), 1996 NIH Publications: "Glaucoma," Publication No. 96-651, "Age-Related Macular Degeneration," Publication No. 96-2294, and "Diabetic Retinopathy," Publication No. 96-2171.

How Does Glaucoma Damage the Optic Nerve?

In many people, increased pressure inside the eye causes glaucoma. In the front of the eye is a space called the **anterior chamber.** A clear fluid flows continuously in and out of this space and nourishes nearby tissues.

The fluid leaves the anterior chamber at the **angle** where the **cornea** and **iris** meet. When the fluid reaches the angle, it flows through a spongy meshwork, like a drain, and leaves the eye.

Open-angle glaucoma gets its name because the angle that allows fluid to drain out of the anterior chamber is *open.* However, for unknown reasons, the fluid passes too slowly through the meshwork drain. As the fluid builds up, the pressure inside the eye rises. Unless the pressure at the front of the eye is controlled, it can damage the optic nerve and cause vision loss.

Who Is at Risk?

Although anyone can get glaucoma, some people are at higher risk than others. They include:

- Blacks over age 40.
- Everyone over age 60.
- People with a family history of glaucoma.

What Are the Symptoms of Glaucoma?

At first, open-angle glaucoma has no symptoms. Vision stays normal, and there is no pain. As glaucoma remains untreated, people may notice that although they see things clearly in front of them, they miss objects to the side and out of the corner of their eye.

Without treatment, people with glaucoma may find that they suddenly have no side vision. It may seem as though they are looking through a tunnel. Over time, the remaining forward vision may decrease until there is no vision left.

How Is Glaucoma Detected?

Most people think that they have glaucoma if the pressure in their eye is increased. This is not always true. High pressure puts you at risk for glaucoma. It may not mean that you have the disease.

Whether or not you get glaucoma depends on the level of pressure that your optic nerve can tolerate without being damaged. This level is different for each person.

Although normal pressure is usually between 12-21 mm Hg, a person might have glaucoma even if the pressure is in this range. That is why an eye examination is very important.

To detect glaucoma, your eye care professional will do the following tests:

- **Visual acuity:** This eye chart test measures how well you see at various distances.

- **Tonometry:** This standard test determines the fluid pressure inside the eye. There are many types of tonometry. One type uses a purple light to measure pressure. Another type is the "air puff" test, which measures the resistance of the eye to a puff of air.

- **Pupil dilation:** This examination provides your eye care professional with a better view of the optic nerve to check for signs of damage. To do this, your eye care professional places drops into the eye to dilate (widen) the pupil. After the examination, your close-up vision may remain blurred for several hours.

- **Visual Field:** This test measures your side (peripheral) vision. It helps your eye care professional find out if you have lost side vision, a sign of glaucoma.

Can Glaucoma Be Treated?

Yes. Although you will never be cured of glaucoma, treatment often can control it. This makes early diagnosis and treatment important to protect your sight. Most doctors use medications for newly diagnosed glaucoma; however, new research findings show that laser surgery is a safe and effective alternative.

What Are Some Other Forms of Glaucoma?

Although open-angle glaucoma is the most common form, some people have other forms of the disease.

In **low-tension or normal-tension glaucoma,** optic nerve damage and narrowed side vision occur unexpectedly in people with normal eye pressure. People with this form of the disease have the same types of treatment as open-angle glaucoma.

In **closed-angle glaucoma,** the fluid at the front of the eye cannot reach the angle and leave the eye because the angle gets blocked by part of the iris. People with this type of glaucoma have a sudden increase in pressure. Symptoms include severe pain and nausea as well as redness of the eye and blurred vision. **This is a medical emergency.** The patient needs immediate treatment to improve the flow of fluid. Without treatment, the eye can become blind in as little as one or two days. Usually, prompt laser surgery can clear the blockage and protect sight.

In **congenital glaucoma,** children are born with defects in the angle of the eye that slow the normal drainage of fluid. Children with this problem usually have obvious symptoms such as cloudy eyes, sensitivity to light, and excessive tearing. Surgery is usually the suggested treatment, because medicines may have unknown effects in infants and be difficult to give to them. The surgery is safe and effective. If surgery is done promptly, these children usually have an excellent chance of having good vision.

Secondary glaucomas can develop as a complication of other medical conditions. They are sometimes associated with eye surgery or advanced cataracts, eye injuries, certain eye tumors, or uveitis (eye inflammation). One type, known as pigmentary glaucoma, occurs when pigment from the iris flakes off and blocks the meshwork, slowing fluid drainage. A severe form, called neovascular glaucoma, is linked to diabetes. Also, corticosteroid drugs—used to treat eye inflammations and other diseases—can trigger glaucoma in a few people. Treatment is with medicines, laser surgery, or conventional surgery.

What Can You Do to Protect Your Vision?

If you are being treated for glaucoma, be sure to take your glaucoma medicine every day and see your eye care professional regularly.

You can also help protect the vision of family members and friends who may be at high risk for glaucoma—Blacks over age 40 and everyone over age 60. Encourage them to have an eye examination through dilated pupils every two years.

Age-Related Macular Degeneration

Age-related macular degeneration (AMD) is a disease that affects your central vision. It is a common cause of vision loss among people over age of 60. Because only the center of your vision is usually affected, people rarely go blind from the disease. However, AMD can sometimes make it difficult to read, drive, or perform other daily activities that require fine, central vision.

What Is the Macula?

The macula is in the center of the **retina,** the light-sensitive layer of tissue at the back of the eye. As you read, light is focused onto your macula. There, millions of cells change the light into nerve signals that tell the brain what you are seeing. This is called your **central vision.** With it, you are able to read, drive, and perform other activities that require fine, sharp, straight-ahead vision.

How Does AMD Damage Vision?

AMD occurs in two forms:

- **Dry AMD** affects about 90 percent of those with the disease. Its cause is unknown. Slowly, the light sensitive cells in the macula break down. With less of the macula working, you may start to lose central vision in the affected eye as the years go by. Dry AMD often occurs in just one eye at first. You may get the disease later in the other eye. Doctors have no way of knowing if or when both eyes may be affected.

- **Wet AMD**—Although only 10 percent of all people with AMD have this type, it accounts for 90 percent of all blindness from the disease. It occurs when new blood vessels behind the retina start to grow toward the macula. Because these new blood vessels tend to be very fragile, they will often leak blood and fluid under the macula. This causes rapid damage to the macula that can lead to the loss of central vision in a short period of time.

Who Is at Risk for AMD?

Although AMD can occur during middle age, the risk increases as a person gets older. Results of a large study show that people in their 50s have about a 2 percent chance of getting AMD. This risk rises to nearly 30 percent in those over age 75. Besides age, other AMD risk factors include:

- **Gender**—Women may be at greater risk than men, according to some studies.

- **Smoking**—Smoking may increase the risk of AMD.

- **Family History**—People with a family history of AMD may be at higher risk of getting the disease.

- **Cholesterol**—People with elevated levels of blood cholesterol may be at higher risk for wet AMD.

What Are the Symptoms of AMD?

Neither dry nor wet AMD causes any pain. The most common symptom of dry AMD is slightly blurred vision. You may need more light for reading and other tasks. Also, you may find it hard to recognize faces until you are very close to them. As dry AMD gets worse, you may see a blurred spot in the center of your vision. This spot occurs because a group of cells in the macula have stopped working. Over time, the blurred spot may get bigger and denser, taking more of your central vision.

People with dry AMD in one eye often do not notice any changes in their vision. With one eye seeing clearly, they can still drive, read, and see fine details. Some people may notice changes in their vision only if AMD affects both of their eyes.

An early symptom of wet AMD is that straight lines appear wavy. This happens because the newly formed blood vessels leak fluid under the macula. The fluid raises the macula from its normal place at the back of the eye and distorts your vision. Another sign that you may have wet AMD is rapid loss of your central vision. This is different from dry AMD in which loss of central vision occurs slowly. As in dry AMD, you may also notice a blind spot.

How Is AMD Detected?

Eye care professionals detect AMD during an eye examination that includes:

- **Visual acuity test:** This eye chart test measures how well you see at various distances.

- **Pupil dilation:** This examination enables your eye care professional to see more of the retina and look for signs of AMD. To do this, drops are placed into the eye to dilate (widen) the pupil. After the examination, your vision may remain blurred for several hours.

- **Tonometry:** This is a standard test that determines the fluid pressure inside the eye. Increased pressure is a possible sign of glaucoma, another common eye problem in people over age 60.

One of the most common early signs of AMD is the presence of **drusen**. Drusen are tiny yellow deposits in the retina. Your eye care professional can see them during an eye examination. The presence of drusen alone does not indicate a disease, but it might mean that the eye is at risk for developing more severe AMD.

While conducting the examination, your eye care professional may ask you to look at an **Amsler grid.** This grid is a pattern that resembles a checkerboard. You will be asked to cover one eye and stare at a black dot in the center of the grid. While staring at the dot, you may notice that the straight lines in the pattern appear wavy to you. This may be a sign of wet AMD. (See **Amsler Grid** below.)

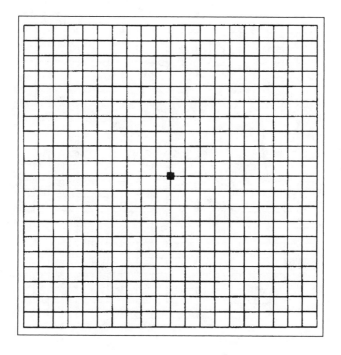

Figure 13.1. *An Amsler Grid Through Normal Eyes*

If your eye care professional suspects you have wet AMD, you may need to have a test called **fluorescein angiography.** In this test, a special dye is injected into a vein in your arm. Pictures are then taken as the dye passes through the blood vessels in the retina. The photos help your eye care professional evaluate leaking blood vessels to determine whether they can be treated.

What Can You Do to Protect Your Vision?

- **Dry AMD.** If you have dry AMD, you should have your eyes examined through dilated pupils at least once a year. This will allow your eye care professional to monitor your condition and check for other eye diseases as well.

You should also obtain an Amsler grid from an eye care professional to use at home. This will provide you with a quick and inexpensive

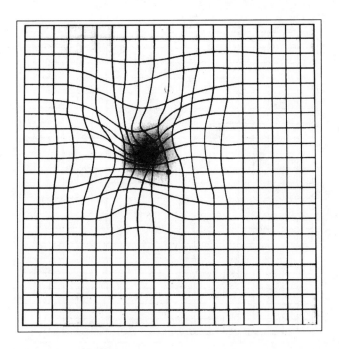

Figure 13.2. An Amsler Grid Through the Eyes of Someone with AMD.

test to evaluate your vision each day for signs of wet AMD. It works best for people who still have good central vision. You should check each eye separately—cover one eye and look at the grid, then cover your other eye and look at the grid. You also may want to check your vision by reading the newspaper, watching television, and just looking at people's faces. If you detect any changes, you should have an eye exam.

- **Wet AMD.** If you have wet AMD, it is important not to delay laser surgery if your eye care professional advises you to have it. After surgery, you will need to have frequent eye examinations to detect any recurrence of leaking blood vessels. Studies show that people who smoke have a greater risk of recurrence than those who don't. In addition, you should continue to check your vision (at home with the Amsler grid or other methods) as described under dry AMD and schedule an eye exam immediately if you detect any changes.

Diabetic Retinopathy

Diabetic retinopathy is a potentially blinding complication of diabetes that damages the eye's retina. It affects half of the 14 million Americans with diabetes.

At first, you may notice no changes in your vision. But don't let diabetic retinopathy fool you. It could get worse over the years and threaten your good vision. With timely treatment, 90 percent of those with advanced diabetic retinopathy can be saved from going blind.

The National Eye Institute (NEI) is the Federal government's lead agency for vision research. The NEI urges all people with diabetes to have an eye examination through dilated pupils at least once a year.

What Is the Retina?

The retina is a light-sensitive tissue at the back of the eye. When light enters the eye, the retina changes the light into nerve signals. The retina then sends these signals along the optic nerve to the brain. Without a retina, the eye cannot communicate with the brain, making vision impossible.

How Does Diabetic Retinopathy Damage the Retina?

Diabetic retinopathy occurs when diabetes damages the tiny blood vessels in the retina. At this point, most people do not notice any changes in their vision.

Some people develop a condition called macular edema. It occurs when the damaged blood vessels leak fluid and lipids onto the macula, the part of the retina that lets us see detail. The fluid makes the macula swell, blurring vision.

As the disease progresses, it enters its advanced, or proliferative, stage. Fragile, new blood vessels grow along the retina and in the clear, gel-like vitreous that fills the inside of the eye. Without timely treatment, these new blood vessels can bleed, cloud vision, and destroy the retina.

Who Is At Risk for this Disease?

All people with diabetes are at risk—those with Type I diabetes (juvenile onset) and those with Type II diabetes (adult onset).

During pregnancy, diabetic retinopathy may also be a problem for women with diabetes. It is recommended that all pregnant women with diabetes have dilated eye examinations each trimester to protect their vision.

What Are Its Symptoms?

Diabetic retinopathy often has no early warning signs. At some point, though, you may have macular edema. It blurs vision, making it hard to do things like read and drive. In some cases, your vision will get better or worse during the day.

As new blood vessels form at the back of the eye, they can bleed (hemorrhage) and blur vision. The first time this happens it may not be very severe. In most cases, it will leave just a few specks of blood, or spots, floating in your vision. They often go away after a few hours.

These spots are often followed within a few days or weeks by a much greater leakage of blood. The blood will blur your vision. In extreme cases, a person will only be able to tell light from dark in that eye. It may take the blood anywhere from a few days to months or even years to clear from inside of your eye. In some cases, the blood will not clear. You should be aware that large hemorrhages tend to happen more than once, often during sleep.

How Is Diabetic Retinopathy Detected?

Diabetic retinopathy is detected during an eye examination that includes:

- **Visual acuity test:** This eye chart test measures how well you see at various distances.

- **Pupil dilation:** The eye care professional places drops into the eye to widen the pupil. This allows him or her to see more of the retina and look for signs of diabetic retinopathy. After the examination, close-up vision may remain blurred for several hours.

- **Ophthalmoscopy:** This is an examination of the retina in which the eye care professional: (1) looks through a device with a special magnifying lens that provides a narrow view of the retina, or (2) wearing a headset with a bright light, looks through a special magnifying glass and gains a wide view of the retina.

- **Tonometry:** A standard test that determines the fluid pressure inside the eye. Elevated pressure is a possible sign of glaucoma, another common eye problem in people with diabetes.

Your eye care professional will look at your retina for early signs of the disease, such as: (1) leaking blood vessels, (2) retinal swelling, such as macular edema, (3) pale, fatty deposits on the retina—signs of leaking blood vessels, (4) damaged nerve tissue, and (5) any changes in the blood vessels.

- **Fluorescein Angiography:** A test that helps the doctor determine if you need treatment for macular edema.

In this test, a special dye is injected into your arm. Pictures are then taken as the dye passes through the blood vessels in the retina. This test allows your doctor to find the leaking blood vessels.

Where to Get More Information

Groups and agencies that offer information about counseling, training, and other special services are available. You may also want to contact a nearby school of medicine or optometry as well as a local agency devoted to helping the visually impaired.

American Academy of Ophthalmology
655 Beach Street, P.O. Box 7424
San Francisco, CA 94109-7424
415-561-8500
Fax: 415-561-8533
E-mail: lmckinstry@aao.org
http://www.eyenet.org

American Diabetes Association
1660 Duke Street
Alexandria, VA 22314
703-549-1500
800-342-2383
E-mail: customerservice@diabetes.org
http://www.diabetes.org

American Foundation for the Blind
11 Penn Plaza, Suite 300
New York, NY 10001
800-232-5463
212-502-7600
E-mail: afbinfo@afb.org
http://www.afb.org

American Optometric Association
243 Lindbergh Boulevard
St. Louis, MO 63141
314-991-4100
314-991-4101
http://www.aoanet.org

Association for Macular Diseases
210 E. 64th Street
New York, NY 10021
212-605-3719
http://www.macula.org/assoc.htm

Council of Citizens with Low Vision International
1859 North Washington Avenue, Suite 2000
Clearwater, FL 33755-1862
800-733-2258
E-mail: jim@tbaynet.com
http://www.cclvi.org

(The) Foundation Fighting Blindness
Executive Plaza 1, Suite 800
11350 McCormick Road
Hunt Valley, MD 21031-1014
888-349-3937
410-785-1414
TDD 800-683-5551
http://www.blindness.org

(The) Glaucoma Foundation
33 Maiden Lane
New York, NY 10038
800-452-8266
Fax: 212-504-1933
E-mail: glaucomafdn@mindspring.com
http://www.glaucoma-foundation.org/info

Glaucoma Research Foundation
200 Pine Street, Suite 200
San Francisco, CA 94104
800-826-6693
415-986-3162
Fax: 415-986-3763
E-mail: gleams@glaucoma.org
http://www.glaucoma.org

Juvenile Diabetes Foundation International
120 Wall Street
New York, NY 10005
212-785-9500
212-785-9595
E-mail: info@jdcure.org
http://www.jdfcure.com

Lighthouse International
111 E. 59th Street
New York, NY 10022
800-829-0500
212-281-9707
212-821-9713 TTY
Fax: 212-821-9713
E-mail: info@lighthouse.org
http://www.lighthouse.org

Macular Degeneration International
2968 West Ina Road, #106
Tucson, AZ 85741
800-393-7634
520-797-2525
http://www.medhelp.org/agsg/agsg1071.htm

National Diabetes Information Clearinghouse of the National Institute of Diabetes and Digestive and Kidney Diseases
1 Information Way
Bethesda, MD 20892-3560
E-mail: ndic@info.niddk.nih.gov
http://www.niddk.nih.gov/health/diabetes/ndic.htm

National Eye Institute
2020 Vision Place
Bethesda, MD 20892-3655
301-496-5248
http://www.nei.nih.gov

National Federation of the Blind
1800 Johnson Street
Baltimore, MD 21230
401-659-9314
E-mail: epc@roudley.com
http://www.nfb.org

Prevent Blindness America
500 East Remington Road
Schamburg, IL 60173
800-331-2020
847-843-2020
E-mail: info@preventblindness.org
http://www.prevent-blindness.org

Chapter 14

Diabetes Diagnosis and Control

Diagnosing Diabetes

A doctor can diagnose diabetes by checking for symptoms such as excessive thirst and frequent urination and by testing for glucose in blood or urine. When blood glucose rises above a certain point, the kidneys pass the extra glucose in the urine. However, a urine test alone is not sufficient to diagnose diabetes.

A second method for testing glucose is a blood test usually done in the morning before breakfast (fasting glucose test) or after a meal (postprandial glucose test).

Points to Remember

A doctor will diagnose diabetes by looking for four kinds of evidence:

- risk factors like exercise weight and a family history of diabetes
- symptoms such as thirst and frequent urination
- complications like heart trouble
- signs of excess glucose or sugar in blood and urine tests.

National Institutes of Health (NIH), Publication No. 97-241, February 10, 1997; and "Clearer Names and a Lower Number for Diagnosis," National Diabetes Information Clearing House. e-text last updated: 9 February 1998; also, Reprinted with permission © 1996 "Exam/Test Chart" from *Managing Type II Diabetes: Your Invitation to a Healthier Lifestyle*, by Arlene Monk, Jan Pearson, Priscilla Hollander, and Richard M. Bergenstal, IDC Publishing, Minneapolis, International Diabetes Center.

The oral glucose tolerance test is a second type of blood test used to check for diabetes. Sometimes it can detect diabetes when a simple blood test does not. In this test, blood glucose is measured before and after a person has consumed a thick, sweet drink of glucose and other sugars. Normally, the glucose in a person's blood rises quickly after the drink and then falls gradually again as insulin signals the body to metabolize the glucose. In someone with diabetes, blood glucose rises and remains high after consumption of the liquid.

A doctor can decide, based on these tests and a physical exam, whether someone has diabetes. If a blood test is borderline abnormal, the doctor may want to monitor the person's blood glucose regularly. If a person is overweight, he or she probably will be advised to lose weight. The doctor also may monitor the patient's heart, since diabetes increases the risk of heart disease.

Diabetes: Clearer Names and a Lower Number for Diagnosis

An international expert committee recently recommended a change in the names of the two main types of diabetes because the former names caused confusion. The type of diabetes that was known as Type I, juvenile-onset diabetes, or insulin-dependent diabetes (IDDM) is now type 1 diabetes. The type of diabetes that was known as Type II, noninsulin-dependent diabetes (NIDDM), or adult-onset diabetes, is now type 2 diabetes. The new names reflect an effort to move away from basing the names on the treatment or age of onset.

The expert committee recommended a lower fasting plasma glucose (FPG) number to diagnose diabetes. The new FPG number is greater than or equal to 126 milligrams per deciliter (mg/dl), rather than greater than or equal to 140 mg/dl. This recommendation was based on a 2-year review of more than 15 years of research. This research showed that when blood glucose was consistently over 126 mg/dl the prevalence of diabetes complications, such as heart disease and loss of eyesight, increased dramatically and developed before the diagnosis of diabetes. The experts believe the earlier diagnosis and treatment can prevent or delay the costly and burdensome complications of diabetes.

For the first time, these experts suggest that adults age 45 and older be tested for diabetes. If their blood glucose is normal at the first test, they should be tested at 3-year intervals. People under 45 should be tested if they are at high risk for diabetes. Risk factors include:

- Being more than 20 percent above ideal body weight or having a body mass index (BMI) of greater than or equal to 27 kgm/m.

- Having a first-degree relative with diabetes (mother, father, or sibling).

- Being a member of a high-risk ethnic group (African American, Hispanic, Asian, or Native American).

- Delivering a baby weighing more than 9 pounds or having diabetes during a pregnancy.

- Having blood pressure at or above 140/90 mm/Hg.

- Having abnormal blood fat levels, such as high density lipoproteins (HDL) less than or equal to 35 mg/dl or triglycerides greater than or equal to 250 mg/dl.

- Having impaired glucose tolerance when previously tested for diabetes.

The committee states a diagnosis of diabetes is warranted for any of three positive tests, with a second positive test on a different day:

- A fasting plasma glucose of greater than or equal to 126 mg/dl.

- A casual plasma glucose (taken any time of day) of greater than or equal to 200 mg/dl with the symptoms of diabetes.

- 'An oral glucose tolerance test (OGTT) value of greater than or equal to 200 mg/dl in the blood measured at the 2-hour interval. (The OGTT is given over a 3-hour time span and administered by a physician or medical laboratory. The person comes in fasting and a blood sample is taken. He or she drinks a glucose syrup. Then a blood sample is taken from the person to measure glucose once an hour for 3 hours.)

The committee recommended that the fasting plasma glucose is preferable to OGTT because it is less expensive, easier to administer, and more acceptable to the person being tested.

A new category for glucose intolerance or impaired fasting glucose (IFG) was defined as having a fasting plasma glucose value of greater than or equal to 110 mg/dl but less than 126 mg/dl. The existing category, impaired glucose intolerance (IGT), is now defined as results of an OGTT greater than or equal to 140 mg/dl but less than 200 mg/dl in the 2-hour sample.

Table 14.1. Diabetes Exam Chart

Test/Exam	Target	Every 3 Months	Every 6 Months	Every 9 Months	Every Year
Height/Weight		X	X	X	X
Blood Pressure	Under 130/85mm Hg	X	X	X	X
HbA1c	Within 1.5 percentage points of lab normal	X	X	X	X
Total Cholesterol	Under 200 mg/dL				X
LDL-Cholesterol	Under 130 mg/dL				X
HDL-Cholesterol (Men)	35 mg/dL or higher				X
HDL-Cholesterol (Women)	45 mg/dL or higher				X
Cholesterol/ HDL Ratio	4.5 or under				X
Triglycerides	Under 200 mg/dL				X
Urine Protein					X
EKG (electro-cardiogram)	Normal				X
Thyroid Function	T4 4.5-12.5 g/dL, TSH 0.2-5.50 IU/mL			X	
Dental Exam			X		X
Foot Exam		X	X	X	X
Eye Exam					X
Meter Check			X		X
Observe Injection (if taking insulin)			X		X

Testing for Diabetes During Pregnancy

The expert panel also suggested a change in the testing for diabetes during pregnancy, stating that women at low risk for gestational diabetes do not need to be tested. This group includes women who are

- Younger than 25 years of age.
- At normal body weight.
- Without family history of diabetes.
- Not members of a high-risk ethnic group.

All women who do not fall into the low-risk category should continue to be tested for gestational diabetes during the 24th to 28th weeks of pregnancy.

Keeping Diabetes Under Control

Tests

Keeping diabetes under control includes taking a series of tests to monitor your treatment and your health. This chart provides information on more than a dozen tests and exams, why they're needed and the target range for the test results.

This chart shows which exams you need and how often they need to be done. Bear in mind that target ranges may vary based on your age and your health, so be sure to talk with your diabetes care team about your personal targets.

For More Information:

The National Diabetes Information Clearinghouse (NDIC) has more free information on diabetes. To learn whether you have diabetes and what type of diabetes you have, ask your health care provider.

National Diabetes Information Clearinghouse
1 Information Way
Bethesda, MD 20892-3560
Fax: (301) 907-8906
E-mail: "mailto:ndic@info.niddk.nih.gov"

The National Diabetes Information Clearinghouse (NDIC) is a service of the National Institute of Diabetes and Digestive and Kidney Diseases (NIDDK). NIDDK is part of the National Institutes of Health under the U.S. Public Health Service. Established in 1978, the clearinghouse provides information about diabetes to people with diabetes and their families, health care professionals, and the public. NDIC answers inquiries; develops, reviews, and distributes publications; and works closely with professional and patient organizations and government agencies to coordinate resources about diabetes.

Chapter 15

Some Tests May Be Unnecessary

Many Medical Screening Tests May Be Unnecessary

Doctors can face an ethical dilemma when patients request screening tests, such as those for breast cancer and prostate cancer, that may be ill-advised under certain circumstances.

University of Michigan physician David J. Doukas and three co-authors explored that predicament in an article entitled "Ethical Considerations in the Provision of Controversial Screening Tests," in the October 1997 Archives of Family Medicine.

Physicians may face this quandary when patients claim entitlement to such tests under their insurance plans, when health advocacy and professional groups recommend their use, or when media attention heightens interest in the latest screening breakthrough, the article noted.

These claims, however, may not be supported by scientific evidence demonstrating that the screening tests meet a minimum criteria of effectiveness.

For example, the article pointed out that there is considerable disagreement in the medical community over the routine use of

---

This chapter includes text from "Many Medical Screening Tests May Be Unnecessary," by Sandra W. Key and Michelle Marble, *Cancer Weekly Plus*, November 3, 1997 © Charles W. Henderson 1997, reprinted with permissions; and "Tests You Need ... Tests You Don't Need," *Getting the Most for Your Medical Dollar*, November 1996, Vol. 5, No. 4, © reprinted with permission of People's Medical Society.

mammograms in women under the age of 50 and prostate specific antigen tests in men. The ethical issue becomes more complicated when doctors provide controversial screening tests because they fear a future lawsuit by a patient who later develops a disease.

Doukas et al. Described several potential risks of screening tests with controversial benefits including:

- Reliance on screening tests before their effectiveness has been corroborated by adequate research.

- Creating the impression that such exams can reduce a patient's risk to zero—possibly leading them to make uninformed medical decisions.

- Inaccurate, false positive results which can cause profound anxiety and require additional testing that can be increasingly invasive and costly.

- Depleting society's limited medical resources.

The authors asserted that physicians have a responsibility to inform patients of the limitations and risks of screening tests, and to refuse to order tests that would violate their medical and ethical judgment. Physicians can counsel patients about the lack of scientific evidence regarding a test's benefits and the fact that no test can assure zero-risk of disease.

Physicians also may choose to administer a test if initial scientific evidence supports a claim of benefit and the patient is aware of the risks. Alternatively, the physician has the option to refuse to provide the test, or refer that patient to another doctor who will provide it.

This education and negotiation process is intended to apprise the patient about which screening tests have been proven to be beneficial and which have not. Such a discussion can result in patients making informed and learned health care decisions.

"For most diseases for which there is a potential screening test, the effectiveness of screening is controversial," wrote Doukas et al. "Physicians can use a 'preventive ethics' approach to explain that tests with controversial benefits are unlikely to be helpful."

Unnecessary Testing

Millions of medical tests are performed annually, and Americans and insurers spend billions of dollars for them. Yet many millions of these medical tests are not necessary, say some experts. And many of these tests aren't very accurate. Others have serious risks and iffy benefits. So, you may well wonder—should you have that test? Does your malady really require two or three tests to determine a diagnosis?

If you feel healthy and don't seem to have any problems, should you spend the money every year to have certain medical tests done? For instance, how effective or essential is the annual physical starting at about $100 a visit?

The entire issue comes down to this: The specter of excessive and unnecessary testing lurks in every corner of the doctor's office. A notion that has insinuated itself into the core of medical-practice habits is, "If testing is good, a lot of it is even better." And as Edward R. Pinckney, M.D., former editor of the Journal of the American Medical Association is quoted as saying in the Wall Street Journal: "Most medical tests—and by that I mean well over half—do not really contribute to a patient's diagnosis or therapy."

You can take charge, however, and minimize the risks and costs of overtesting in your doctor's office.

- Ask why you need the test. In their comprehensive guide to more than 200 diagnostic and home medical tests, *The People's Book of Medical Tests* (New York: Summit Books, 1985), David S. Sobel, M.D., and Tom Ferguson, M.D., recommend that before you agree to any test, you ask your doctor what will be done if the test results are abnormal and what will be done if the test results are normal. They advise you that you may not need the test if the doctor's answers are the same for both questions. Also be sure to demand additional information or clarification if you don't understand something.

- Ask how reliable the test is, what the chance is of a false-positive or a false-negative indication and how risks of either can be minimized. (A false-positive result means that the test shows up positive or abnormal, but no disease is actually present. A false-negative result means that the test shows up negative, or normal, but you actually have the disease.) No test is 100 percent accurate, but you should be told the usefulness and the limits of tests if you are to make an informed decision and get your money's worth. False—or even misread results, for that matter—can direct your doctor to perform inappropriate actions.

- Ask where the test will be processed, whether in the office or an outside commercial lab. If the test is scheduled to go outside, ask if the commercial lab is accredited by the College of American Pathologists. As for tests processed in the doctor's in-office lab, you should know that evidence points to some inaccuracy problems.

- Find out what alternatives you have if you refuse the test.

- Ask how much the test will cost. And check with your insurance company prior to undergoing an expensive test to see if it will cover the total cost.

- Talk to you doctor. While this advice sounds facetious, it really isn't. Admittedly, doctors don't always listen to their patients' explanations and questions or even ask the right questions themselves. And certainly there can be an economic incentive for doctors to order many tests—too many tests, to be sure. But consumers do share in the responsibility of communicating well, and too often they don't mention all symptoms, or they downplay them. Keep notes of everything you feel, every disturbance, every symptom, and bring the notes to your appointment. Give your doctor as much information as you can, and demand the same in return.

Nipping Family Diseases in the Bud

If a certain disease or condition runs in your family, you may want to consider the associated screening tests listed below. They can help detect the disease as early as possible.

Cancers: Breast Cancer

- Mammograms each year beginning at age 30.
- Self-examination for lumps.
- CEA and CA15-3 blood tests.

Cancers: Cervical and Vaginal

- Annual Pap smear and pelvic exam commencing at age 20.

Cancers: Colon Cancer

- Test annually for blood in the stool, starting at age 30.
- CEA blood test for carcinoembryonic antigen.
- Periodic colonoscopy.

- Annual proctosigmoidoscopy beginning at age 46.
- Rigid proctoscopy.

Cancers: Leukemia

- Complete blood count.
- Chromosome analysis.
- Bone marrow biopsy.

Cancers: Lung Cancer

- Annual chest x-ray and sputum exam beginning at age 50.
- NSE blood test.

Cancers: Oral Cancer

- Annual dental examination.
- Biopsy.

Cancers: Ovarian Cancer, Cysts, and Tumors

- Annual pelvic exam.
- Ultrasound.
- CA-125 blood test.

Cancers: Pancreatic Cancer

- CA-19-9 blood test

Cancers: Prostate Cancer

- Digital rectal exam annually after age 40.
- PSA blood test.

Cancers: Stomach Cancer

- Periodic endoscopic examination, particularly if Barrett's syndrome is present.

Cancers: Testicular Cancer

- AFP blood test.
- Regular self-examination.
- Ultrasound

Cancers: Uterine Cancer

- Endometrial biopsy

Cystic Fibrosis

- Regular tests of lung function, stool and perspiration salinity.

Diabetes

- Blood sugar test.
- Urinalysis

Glaucoma

- Glaucoma exam at age 40

Heart Attack, Heart Disease, Atherosclerosis, Stroke

- Regular blood pressure.
- Serum cholesterol and triglyceride tests.
- Electrocardiogram.
- Exercise-tolerance test

Mood Disorders

- Psychiatric evaluation when symptoms—chronic depression, major mood swings—first present themselves.

Osteoporosis

- Bone-density assessment before menopause

Polycystic Kidney Disease, Kidney Tumors

- Urinalysis.
- Ultrasound.
- CAT scan

Schizophrenia

- Psychiatric evaluation when symptoms—delusions, hallucinations, incoherence—first present themselves.

Part Two

Screening Tests You Can Do at Home

Chapter 16

In-Home Tests Make Health Care Easier

When it comes to helping people stay healthy, in-home medical tests may be useful. Blood pressure monitors and the blood cholesterol test, for instance, may play a role in thwarting heart and blood vessel disease. A positive result from a pregnancy test might prompt a woman to go to her doctor sooner, so she gets prenatal care earlier in her pregnancy.

Another device, the home meter for testing blood glucose (sugar) levels can, within seconds, electronically analyze a blood drop from a finger prick, so a person with diabetes knows whether to adjust medicine, exercise or diet. "By creating the potential for tight control of diabetes, the blood glucose meter has revolutionized this area of medical practice," says the Food and Drug Administration's Steven Gutman, M.D. "It's a cornerstone of modern diabetic therapy." Gutman is acting director of FDA's division of clinical laboratory devices, Center for Devices and Radiological Health, responsible for reviewing many in-home test devices.

More Benefits

Generally, in-home tests provide easy access to medical knowledge about one's health. In some cases, such as monitoring high blood pressure, home testing reduces the number of times a patient must visit a doctor's office or laboratory, thereby reducing medical costs. People also may feel an increased sense of control over their health.

FDA Consumer, December 1994.

An over-the-counter (OTC) test performs at least one of three functions:

- doctor-recommended monitoring (e.g., blood pressure, for hypertension; blood glucose, for diabetes control; ovulation, for infertility).

- detecting markers for possible health conditions when there are no physical signs or symptoms (blood cholesterol level, for high cholesterol; hidden [occult] blood in stool, for colon or rectal cancer).

- detecting markers for specific conditions when there are physical signs or symptoms (a specific female hormone in urine after a missed period, for pregnancy).

For any in-home test, the manufacturer must convince the agency not only that the test has value (results will benefit consumers), but also that consumers have the knowledge necessary to decide whether testing themselves is appropriate, says Jur Strobos, M.D. J.D., director of FDA's Policy Research Staff. "If the firm does not show that consumers can make this judgment," he says, "we assume the test is for screening without pre-selecting patients. Then, we ask ourselves, is it appropriate for this use?"

Not all tests on the OTC market are equally useful, however, says Philip Phillips, deputy director of FDA's Office of Device Evaluation.

"Some OTC tests that have been marketed for many years," he says, "may not be as useful or acceptable as many consumers believe."

Eye charts, Phillips notes for example, have been sold for decades and are still around in some drugstores, "but you shouldn't rely on them if you think you need eyeglasses or have not had a recent examination." People having eye problems should be examined by a licensed eye-care professional, he says.

Incorrect Results

The more recently approved in-home tests are as reliable as professional tests. Still, all tests can generate false positives (indicating someone has a condition that in fact the person does not) or false negatives (a result that does not identify a condition that is in fact present)—particularly if the user doesn't follow directions.

Instead of signifying colon or rectal cancer, a positive result on a test for hidden blood in stool could reflect such factors as bleeding gums or last night's T-bone steak. Or an untrained person may perform the test incorrectly, causing hidden blood in stool to go undetected.

A false negative can occur with a pregnancy test. When a urine sample has a certain level of human chorionic gonadotropin hormone, the test device indicates a probable pregnancy. But pregnant women don't always produce the hormone at the same rate, so a woman could be pregnant but not yet producing enough hormone to prompt the signal from that particular test. Also, levels needed to trigger the signal vary among the different brands of the device. Thus, a test might indicate no pregnancy in a woman who, in fact, is pregnant. If the woman continued certain practices potentially harmful to the fetus, such as smoking, drinking excessively, or taking certain medicines, she might risk her baby's health.

After a negative pregnancy test, therefore, a woman should wait the number of days suggested in the instructions and test again—making sure she's following the instructions properly. If the second test is negative and she's still not menstruating, she should promptly consult her doctor.

In other words, it can be risky for consumers to consider test results as a definite diagnosis. Professional follow-up is needed.

A doctor's diagnosis involves evaluation of the patient's medical history and physical examination, often other tests, and sometimes consultation with other medical experts. Further, unlike home testing, professional laboratories must meet quality standards, which provide additional reliability and uniformity to test results.

While no test—OTC or professional—is 100 percent accurate, in a medical setting, Gutman says, "professional, trained people would be expected to interpret test results in a broader context."

Preventing Problems

A number of tests unavailable over the counter at pharmacies can be bought from medical supply firms without a prescription. "Consumers should be wary about buying these tests on their own," Gutman says. "Many such products, though nonprescription, are intended for use by trained professionals, or for home use only with medical guidance."

However, interpreting results of the newer OTC tests on pharmacy shelves should not be a problem for consumers. Before FDA will approve OTC sales today, test sponsors must prove that consumers can accurately interpret results.

OTC tests also must be labeled with appropriate warnings. For instance, if a test is not for use by people with diabetes, a large-type warning must state so.

To use in-home tests as safely and effectively as possible, consumers should carefully read the instructions, which the FDA makes sure are user-friendly. As Gutman puts it: "Instructions tell how a test works, when it works, when it doesn't, and what to do when it doesn't."

Term Translations

Accuracy is the ability of a test to give consistent results. FDA requires in-home tests to show the same accuracy as professional tests.

False positive is a test result indicating someone has a condition that in fact the person does not.

False negative is a test result that does not identify a condition that is in fact present.

Using Tests Wisely

To use an in-home test as safely and effectively as possible, take these precautions:

- Check the expiration date. If the date is past, don't buy the product. Chemicals in an outdated test may no longer work properly, so the results may not be valid. Don't use a previously purchased test with an expired date.

- Don't leave a temperature-sensitive product in the car trunk or by a sunny car window in hot weather on the trip home from the store. Don't leave it in the car if you go elsewhere.

- Follow the package directions on where to store the product at home.

- Learn what the test is intended to do and what its limitations are. Remember: No test is 100 percent accurate.

- Read the insert to learn how to use the product. Review the instructions and pictures until you fully understand each step.

- Don't guess if something is unclear. Consult a pharmacist or other health professional, or check the instructions for an "800" number.

- Note special precautions, such as avoiding physical activity or certain foods and drugs before testing.

- Follow instructions exactly, including any specimen collection process. Sequence is important. Don't skip a step. If a step to check the test or calibrate an instrument is included, do it.

- When collecting a urine specimen with a container not from a kit, wash the container thoroughly, and rinse out all soap traces, preferably with distilled water, which generally is purer than other bottled or tap water.

- When a step is timed, be precise. Use a stopwatch or a watch that counts seconds.

- Note what to do if the results are positive, negative or unclear.

- Keep accurate records of results.

- If the test depends on color for a step, and you're colorblind, be sure someone who sees color interprets the results.

- If you have questions about the test results or their implications for your health, consult your doctor or other qualified health professional.

- Keep tests containing chemicals, which may be poisonous, or sharp instruments out of the reach of children. Promptly discard used materials as directed.

—by Dixie Farley

Dixie Farley is a staff writer for *FDA Consumer*.

Chapter 17

Colocare Fecal Occult Blood Test

ChemTrak, Inc., Chicago, Illinois, reported that its Colocare home test clearly outperformed the other fecal occult blood screening tests (FOBT) in an independent research study conducted by a nationally recognized physician researcher.

Of the four test kits used by 85 patients over a two-year period, only the "throw-in-the-bowl" method incorporated in the Colocare product detected the presence of precancerous polyps. The three other FOBT kits used during the study had no correlation with positive results. The study also noted that ColoCare showed the highest positive predictive value for the detection of all types of polyps. Colocare is manufactured by Helena Laboratories and marketed over-the-counter to consumers by ChemTrak.

The results were presented by John I. Hughes, MD, FACP, FACG, associate medical director, Kelsey-Seybold Medical Group, medical director of the Vercellino Gastrointestinal Cancer Institute, and clinical associate professor at Baylor College of Medicine, in a poster presentation at the Annual Meeting of the American College of Gastroenterology.

"These encouraging results indicate that the Colocare product is not only convenient, but extremely accurate in detecting the early signs of colorectal disease," said Niquette Hunt, ChemTrak. "The wide availability of this product, its low price, instant results, and ease of

"Colocare Found Superior to Other Tests In Detecting Cancer," *Cancer Weekly Plus,* November 17, 1997, reprinted with permission © 1997 Charles W. Henderson.

use, should help more people feel comfortable about using a home test—and contacting their doctors sooner about any signs of colorectal disease."

Colorectal cancer currently trails only lung cancer as the nation's leading cancer killer. Some 55,000 Americans die each year from colorectal cancer. One of the major factors in the high mortality rate is late detection. If colorectal cancer is detected early, the five-year survival rate can exceed 80 percent. In cases when cancer is detected later, however, half the patients die within five years.

The latest Clinical Guidelines for Colorectal Cancer Screening, funded by the American College of Gastroenterology, The American Gastroenterological Association, and four other major medical groups, note that FOBT, with positive indications followed promptly by a doctor's appointment, could cut the death rate from colorectal cancer by one-third. The widely endorsed guidelines recommend annual fecal blood testing for all adults more than 50-years-old.

Dr. Hughes conducted a study involving a controlled sample of 85 patients ranging in age from 38 to 78. The patients used four different test kits—three products that involve direct sampling and handling of fecal matter, and a drop-in-the-bowl pad that changes color in the presence of fecal blood. Only the throw-in-the-bowl test—marketed to consumers as ChemTrak's ColoCare—produced positive indications of colorectal polyps.

"Our preliminary view of this throw-in-the-bowl technique is that it may significantly improve the usually low compliance observed up until now with the traditional fecal occult blood tests," Dr. Hughes said. "The $30 million currently being spent each year on these tests is not producing an acceptable return. This different method appears to offer the promise of swifter medical intervention and better prospects for patients."

Sandra W. Key, News Editor, with Michelle Marble

Chapter 18

Diabetic Home Tests

Checking Blood Glucose Levels

When a person's body is operating normally, it automatically checks the level of glucose in blood. If the level is too high or too low, the body will adjust the sugar level to return it to normal. This system operates in much the same way that cruise control adjusts the speed of a car. With diabetes, the body doesn't do the job of controlling blood glucose automatically. To make up for this, someone with diabetes has to check blood sugar regularly and adjust treatment accordingly.

Remember:

- Testing blood glucose levels regularly can show whether treatment is working.

A doctor can measure blood glucose during an office visit. However, levels change from hour to hour and someone who visits the doctor

This chapter contains text from "Checking Blood Glucose Levels," National Institute of Diabetes and Digestive and Kidney Diseases (NIDDK), NIH Publication No. 97-241, September 1992, updated February 1997; and, "How Accurate Are Home Glucose Readings?," from *Health After 50*, July 1997, reprinted with permission from The Johns Hopkins Medical Letter Health After 50. © MedLetter Associates, 1998. To order a one year subscription, call 800-829-9170. Also included is, "Better Test Your Feet—Your Doctor Probably Won't," reprinted with permission from *Diabetes Forecast*, Vol. 51, Issue 6, June 1998 p. 59, © 1998 American Diabetes Association.

only every few weeks won't know what his or her blood glucose is daily. Do-it-yourself tests enable people with diabetes to check their blood sugar daily.

The easiest test someone can do at home is a urine test. When the level of glucose in blood rises above normal, the kidneys eliminate the excess glucose in urine. Glucose in urine, therefore, reflects an excess of glucose in blood.

Urine testing is easy. Tablets or paper strips are dipped in urine. The color change that occurs indicates whether blood glucose is too high. However, urine testing is not completely accurate because the reading reflects the level of blood glucose a few hours earlier. In addition, not everyone's kidneys are the same. Even when the amount of glucose in two people's urine is the same, their sugar levels may be different. Certain drugs and vitamin C also can affect the accuracy of urine tests.

It's more accurate to measure blood glucose directly. Kits are available that allow people with diabetes to test their blood glucose at home. The test involves pricking a finger to draw a drop of blood. A spring-operated "lancet" does this automatically. The drop of blood is placed on a strip of specially coated plastic or into a small machine that "reads" how much glucose is in the blood. A doctor may suggest that someone test his or her blood glucose several times a day. Self blood glucose monitoring can show how the body responds to meals, exercise, stress, and diabetes treatment.

Another test that measures the effectiveness of treatment is a "glycosylated hemoglobin" test. It measures the glucose that has become attached to hemoglobin, the molecule in red blood cells that gives blood its red color. Over time, hemoglobin absorbs glucose, according to its concentration in blood. Once glucose is absorbed by hemoglobin it remains there until the blood cells die and new ones replace them. With the "glycosylated hemoglobin" test, a doctor can tell whether blood glucose has been very high over the last few months.

How Accurate Are Home Glucose Readings?

Using a home meter to monitor blood glucose levels can help reduce the risk of long-term diabetes complications such as nerve damage, declining kidney function, and vision loss. But home values are generally 10 to 15% less accurate than laboratory ones—largely because of human error. Studies show that patients generally produce the best readings soon after completing a diabetes education program. But as time passes, poor habits develop, and accuracy tends to slip.

To address this problem, the American Diabetes Association has asked manufacturers to introduce new meters that further reduce the possibility of human error. The goal is to achieve values that differ from laboratory standards by no more than 5%. But that doesn't mean you need to rush out and purchase a new meter. Because most inaccuracies are caused by poor testing techniques, you can probably improve the quality of home monitoring simply by being more careful about how you maintain your equipment and process your samples.

Home meters measure the amount of glucose in whole blood at the moment the blood sample is obtained. In contrast, laboratory testing often measures the glucose in plasma (a component of the blood). Other useful laboratory tests include fasting blood glucose (which is usually done after an overnight fast) and glycosylated hemoglobin (a blood test that indicates how well glucose has been controlled during the previous four to six weeks.

How To Use a Meter

Home monitoring requires the patient to prick a finger, obtain a drop of blood, and place it on a test strip treated with an enzyme that causes a color change when exposed to glucose. The amount of glucose present is determined by inserting the strip into a meter, which provides a digital readout of the value. The process takes between 15 seconds and two minutes, depending on the meter used. An older method, in which the color change is visually compared to a chart, is far less accurate.

The frequency and timing of monitoring depend on the type of diabetes, how tightly blood-glucose is controlled, and general health. Many patients with type I diabetes, which usually develops in children and young adults, need to monitor themselves several times each day. However, those with very stable type II diabetes, which usually develops after age 40, can sometimes test themselves as little as once a day—or even less. Others who are very elderly, or have problems such as severe arthritis that can make home monitoring difficult, might opt for stepped up laboratory testing.

Home glucose meters come with many features. Factors to consider are the readability of the digital display; how easy or difficult the meter is to use; size and portability; the ongoing cost of test strips; maintenance; and whether the unit automatically keeps a record of values. Maintaining a log, either manually or automatically, is extremely important so that glucose values can be tracked over time. Treatment with some combination of insulin, oral medication, and diet and exercise can be adjusted accordingly. Prices vary widely, ranging from a low of about $30. To a high of around $370. Check with your insurance company to find out about reimbursement possibilities for both the meter and the strips, keeping in mind that over time the strips will cost more than the meter itself.

Action Steps for Accurate Home Readings

Accurate home monitoring requires patience, consistency, and attention to detail. The following simple precautions will eliminate as much error as possible:

- **Test the meter**. At least once a month, check the unit according to the manufacturer's instructions using the specified control solution. Follow this procedure more frequently if test strips have been exposed to unusual conditions, such as extremes of temperature or humidity.

- **Recalibrate the meter**. Whenever you open a new packet of strips, follow the manufacturer's instructions for readjusting the unit. Some meters recalibrate automatically, while others require manual adjustment.

- **Use fresh strips**. Don't use strips after the expiration date; after they've changed color; or if the package is open and they've been exposed to light or air.

- **Keep the meter clean.** Wipe away blood, dust, and lint after each use.

- **Use proper technique**. Follow the manufacturer's directions regarding the amount of blood needed and the material to be used for blotting or wiping. Don't add more blood once the sample is on the strip.

- **Check the meter against lab findings.** Periodically take your meter to your doctor, take a reading, and compare the value to a laboratory finding. If the results differ by more than 15%, follow the above steps and do another comparison. If the discrepancy persists, you need to review your technique with a professional. A new meter may be required.

Testing Your Feet

Your doctor ought to check your feet for nerve damage. Ought to but probably won't. Studies show that many doctors don't do foot exams, let alone sensory testing.

Maybe you ought to do sensory testing yourself. A new study shows that most people find it easy to do, and that they can get accurate results.

Simple Filament

About half the people with diabetes have damage to the nerves in their feet. One result is "loss of protective sensation." If you have lost protective sensation, you don't feel common irritations, such as a blister forming, a tiny stone in your shoe, or a sliver of glass in your skin. The problem starts out small, but if it's not taken care of, it can lead to a foot ulcer and amputation.

If you knew you had lost protective sensation, you'd know to be extra careful about your feet. You'd know to wear appropriate shoes, to check your feet every day for red spots or small cuts, to avoid going barefoot.

Your doctor can do a very simple test to see whether you've lost protective sensation. He or she touches certain spots on your foot with a nylon filament. The filament bends when a 10-gram force is applied. If you can't feel the touches in one or more spots, you've lost protective sensation. According to the American Diabetes Association, filament testing should be part of a comprehensive foot exam, and you should have a foot exam by a health care professional at least once a year.

Researchers at the Gillis W. Long Hansen's Disease Center in Carville, La., know that most health care professionals don't do this sensory testing. So they set out to evaluate whether people could do the testing themselves.

Sensory Kits

For the study, 196 people with diabetes who were scheduled for follow-up appointments at nine diabetes centers in different states were sent "self-testing sensory kits." A kit included a filament, instructions, and a questionnaire about the testing kit. Subjects were asked to do the sensory testing before their follow-up appointments. At their follow-up appointments, participants' feet were retested by their health care professionals.

Of the people who received kits, 145 did the testing, completed the survey, and kept their follow-up appointments. Results:

- 97 percent reported that the filament was easy to use.

- 69 percent reported that they did the filament testing themselves; 31 percent had someone else help.

- 53 people (35 percent) found a loss of sensation; 34 people reported that they had not known about this loss of sensation before the test.

In 87 percent of the cases, the results of the retests by health care professionals agreed with the results the patients got. Patients who got the same result as their health care professionals were younger (average age 56) than those who got different results (average age 65). There were 10 false-negatives—that is, 10 people reported that they did feel the filament; when retested by their providers, they did not feel the filament. This indicates that it would be best for people to have their results confirmed by health car professionals.

Bob Rolfsen, director of the Lower Extremity Amputation Prevention (LEAP) Program, Carville, La., and co-author of the study, says, "For years, patients have taken responsibility for their diabetes: They give themselves insulin, check their blood glucose. They have assumed responsibility for lowering their risk of diabetes complications. There is no reason not to test themselves for loss of sensation."

For More Information

American Diabetes Association
1660 Duke St.
Alexandria, VA 22314
703-549-1500; 800-342-2383
E-mail: customerservice@diabetes.org
www.diabetes.org

LEAP Program (Filament Information)
GWL Hansen's Disease Center
5445 Point Clair Road
Carville, LA 70721
225-642-4714; 225-642-4710 Fax
E-mail: bob.rolfsen@access.gov
http://158.72.105.163/LEAP/

Chapter 19

Testing Yourself for Human Immunodeficiency Virus (HIV-1)

AIDS is a serious disease that can be fatal. You can determine if you are infected with the Human Immunodeficiency Virus-1 (HIV-1), the virus that causes AIDS, by taking a test for the presence of antibodies to the virus. A sample for testing can now be collected in your own home.

There are a number of different HIV home collection test systems and kits that have appeared on the market, available through the Internet and through magazine or newspaper promotions. However, only one HIV-1 Home Collection Test System is currently approved by the United States Food and Drug Administration (FDA):

Home Access Express HIV-1 Test System manufactured by Home Access Health Corporation.

The other HIV-1 home test kits being advertised have not been approved by the FDA for use and marketing in the United States. These unapproved HIV home test kits claim to detect antibodies to HIV-1, the virus that causes AIDS, in blood or saliva, providing results in the home in fifteen minutes or less.

Are All HIV-1 Home Tests the Same?

A few simple questions and answers might help to explain how they differ, and how to select a test that you can trust.

Center for Biologics Evaluation and Research, FDA, Number: D0409, May 1997, Updated July 1997.

How Many Different Kits Are Available, and How Do They Work?

There are more than a dozen different HIV home test kits being advertised on the market today. Only the Home Access test system is FDA approved and legally marketed in the United States.

Because the Home Access test consists of multiple components, including materials for specimen collection, a mailing envelope to send the specimen to a laboratory for analysis, and includes pre- and post-test counseling, it is considered a testing system.

This approved system uses a simple finger prick process for home blood collection which results in dried blood spots on special paper. The dried blood spots are mailed to a laboratory with a confidential and anonymous personal identification number (PIN), and analyzed by trained clinicians in a certified medical laboratory using the same procedures that are used for samples taken in a doctor's office. The results are obtained by the purchaser through a toll free telephone number using the PIN, and post-test counseling is provided by telephone when results are obtained.

The advertisers of the unapproved HIV home test kits claim that the presence of a visual indicator, such as a red dot, within 5 to 15 minutes of taking the test shows a positive result for HIV infection. These unapproved test kits use a simple finger prick process for home blood collection or a special sponge device for saliva collection. The blood or saliva sample is then added to a plastic testing device containing a special type of paper. A developing solution is added to determine if the sample is positive for HIV. The samples are not sent to a laboratory for professional analysis. Although this approach may seem faster and simpler, it may provide a less accurate result than can be achieved using an approved test, which is analyzed under more controlled conditions than is possible in the home.

How Reliable Are the Unapproved HIV Home Test Kits?

Diagnostic testing depends on precise science. Unapproved HIV home test kits do not come with any guarantee of the accuracy of the test, or the sensitivity of the reagents used in the analysis. Nor do they have a documented history of delivering dependable results. Proper training to interpret results is not provided with the kits, and they do not have a validated record of precision. This means that they may not be as accurate and that they may yield inconsistent results. Users can get a positive result when they are, in fact, not infected (called a false positive), or the test may indicate that a person is not infected with the virus, when, in fact, they are (called a false negative). Both of these outcomes can have grave consequences in terms of mental anguish, access to proper medical treatment, and on future transmission of the disease.

None of the unapproved tests have undergone the intense scrutiny and validation required for FDA marketing approval. Although unapproved tests might be promoted as sensitive and reliable, the consumer has no guarantee that the results produced by the test are, in fact, accurate. Even if they have been tested by independent laboratories, they have not been analyzed and validated by the FDA to assure that the test results were correct and reliable.

FDA is unaware of any data to confirm the reliability or accuracy of the process used in the unapproved HIV home test kits.

How Reliable Are Approved HIV Test Systems?

Approved HIV test systems, on the other hand, have undergone extensive study and review by the manufacturer of the product to ensure that they work, that the results they provide are specific, meaning that they will accurately detect antibodies to the HIV-1 virus that causes AIDS, and that they are sensitive, meaning that they can detect even low levels of these antibodies, indicating that someone has been exposed to HIV-1.

Clinical studies have shown that the approved HIV test system is able to correctly identify 100% of known positive blood samples, and 99.5% of HIV-1 negative blood samples.

In addition, manufacturer's tests on the approved HIV test system have been carefully reviewed by the FDA to assure that the tests conducted were themselves adequate to demonstrate that the system is capable of yielding accurate, dependable results. FDA review also assures that the system contains adequate directions for proper use, and that the quality standards will be monitored to ensure that each kit is as consistently accurate and sensitive.

What about Counseling?

The unapproved HIV home test kits do not provide direct counseling to help the user understand results, answer questions about the test or about HIV infection, or to discuss available options.

The approved HIV test system has a built in mechanism for pre- and post-test counseling provided by the manufacturer. Counseling is an important part of HIV testing. It is anonymous and confidential.

Counseling, which uses both printed material, and telephone interaction, not only provides the user with an interpretation of what positive or negative results really mean, but provides information on how to keep from getting infected if you are negative, and how to prevent transmission of disease if you find you are infected. Counseling also provides you with information about treatment options if you are infected, and can even provide referrals to doctors that treat HIV-infected individuals in your area.

Are Approved HIV Test Systems Really Confidential?

The approved HIV home test system is anonymous. It can be purchased anonymously at pharmacies, or by mail order from the manufacturers. The mail-in system uses a confidential code number that is unrelated to the identity of the buyer or user.

Although some states require that new cases of HIV infection be reported to the health department, only the number of cases detected with home test systems can be reported. The identity of the user remains anonymous.

The number of cases reported allows local or state public health officials to assess the extent of infection to properly budget, plan and administer programs for people with HIV.

The lack of reporting of the number of new cases in a geographic area also means that adequate services for people with HIV infection may not be available in your area.

Is One Test Better than Another?

Since the approved HIV home test system has been independently tested, validated, and approved by the FDA for marketing, the consumer can feel confident that the approved HIV test system will provide the most accurate results available from an HIV-1 home test. In addition, the user is provided with counseling and referrals if needed. Use of an approved HIV test system also assures that accurate numbers of infection are reported to public health departments so that adequate services can be provided.

Are There Other Ways I Can Be Tested for Infection with HIV-1?

There are several kinds of tests available through your doctor to determine if you are infected with HIV-1, the virus that causes AIDS.

In addition to blood tests, there is a test that uses oral fluid, collected from between the cheek and gum of the mouth, and a urine test. All of these tests have been thoroughly tested and reviewed, and provide the highest possible level of confidence in determining HIV infection. All are collected in the doctor's office, and analyzed in a medical laboratory. Only a doctor or clinic can administer these tests.

What Is the Best Choice for You:

1. An HIV home test system that has been approved by the FDA for marketing after extensive review and in which you can feel confident about the results? OR

2. An HIV home test kit that has not even been reviewed by the FDA and may not provide accurate results about whether you are HIV positive or negative?

Is it worth your time, money, mental anguish and your life to gamble on an unapproved HIV home test kit? Only you can answer that question.

For Questions about HIV Home Test Kits

HIV/AIDS Program of the FDA
Office of Special Health Issues
Food and Drug Administration
5600 Fishers Lane, HF-12
Rockville, MD 20857
301-827-4460
Fax: 301-443-4555
E-mail: OSHI@oc.fda.gov
http://www.fda.gov/oashi/aids/klein.html

Chapter 20

Over the Counter Drug Tests—Urine and Hair Analysis

Is America losing the battle against teen drug abuse? The 1996-97 PRIDE (Parents' Resource for Drug Education) survey of more than 140,000 students shows that drug use among 11-14 year olds is on the rise, with 11.4 percent of junior-high students reporting monthly use of marijuana, cocaine, and other illicit drugs. A study last year at Columbia University found that drugs are more readily available and used by younger people than ever before.

Parents who anguish over their child's possible drug abuse are now taking responsibility for, and control of, their teenagers by administering in-home drug tests. There are two types of over-the-counter drug tests—urine and hair analysis. The former is the most widely used method, but the latter is gaining popularity and support. A principal difference between the two tests is that urinalysis typically reveals drug use during the previous three to four days. Hair analysis, on the other hand, can detect usage for the previous 90 days.

The Boston-based Psychemedics Corporation began offering its in-home hair sample collection product, PDT-90, for personal use. For the test, an inch-and-a-half snippet of about 50 hairs is collected, put in a plastic bag, and sent to the company's lab to confirm if marijuana, cocaine, opiates (including heroin), methamphetamine, or PCP have been used during the past three months. Parents access the confidential

"Friendly Drug Test Uses Hair Instead of Urine" *Medical Update*, April 1998, Vol. 21, No. 10. Reprinted with permission from Medical Update: A Monthly Medical Newsletter © 1998 Medical Education and Research Foundation.

and anonymous test results only through code numbers: names are never used.

For most parents and teenagers, hair analysis is less intrusive and embarrassing than urinalysis. "It's probably the friendliest drug test a person will ever take," says one business executive, who plans to use the test in his own family.

Chapter 21

Pregnancy Tests

Many women use home pregnancy tests if they suspect they're pregnant. Regulated by the Food and Drug Administration, pregnancy tests have come far since the early to mid-1900s when toads, rats, and rabbits were used in testing. Now, over-the-counter home pregnancy kits provide privacy and fast results, and can detect pregnancy as early as six days after conception, or one day after a missed menstrual period. This gives an early advantage for vital prenatal care.

All pregnancy tests are based on the presence of a hormone, human chorionic gonadotropin (HCG), that the pregnant woman produces after conception. The first self tests of the 1970s used ring, or "tube agglutination," tests consisting of prepackaged red blood cells to detect HCG in urine. A ring at the bottom of the tube indicated a positive result. Sensitive to movement and human error, ring tests are now rarely used.

Today's brands, such as e.p.t. and First Response, contain monoclonal antibodies that detect minute traces of HCG. These antibodies are molecules coated with a substance that bonds to the pregnancy hormone, if it's present, to produce either a positive or negative result. (Each test manufacturer uses a different "trade secret" chemical formula for the bonding substance.) The user collects urine and combines it with the antibodies provided in the package. The test is timed, and a color change indicates the result.

Excerpts from "The Perplexities of Pregnancy," *FDA Consumer*, November 1990.

151

Although most manufacturers claim 99 percent accuracy in laboratory tests, inaccurate results may be more frequent in actual use, due to such factors as improper use of the test, using a product past its expiration date, exposure of the test to the sun, and cancers. The procedures outlined in the instructions must be followed exactly for results to be accurate.

Whitehall Laboratories markets the one-step brand, Clearblue Easy. It gives results in three minutes and informs the user when the test hasn't been done properly. This testing method, called rapid assay delivery system, combines a biochemical process with monoclonal antibodies in one pen-like instrument.

Whatever the result or the brand used, most manufacturers recommend repeating the process a few days later to confirm the results. After conception, a woman produces a minimal amount of HCG. The strength of each test varies, and although a woman may be pregnant, the test may not pick up the amount of HCG hormone present the first time.

—Lisa Iannucci

Lisa Iannucci is a freelance writer in Yonkers, N.Y.

Chapter 22

Cholesterol Test

The Food and Drug Administration has cleared for marketing the first cholesterol test available for home use by consumers without a prescription. Previously, cholesterol tests, which are used to help determine the risk of heart disease, were available only for use by medical professionals.

The test—the Accumeter Cholesterol Self-Test, made by Chem Trak Inc. of Sunnyvale, Calif.—comes in a kit and allows the user to find the level of cholesterol in the blood in about 15 minutes. "This test can help give consumers greater opportunity to monitor their health and take steps to prevent disease," said Health and Human Services Secretary Donna E. Shalala. "Making it more convenient to check on cholesterol can help ensure that people are aware of the level so they can see a doctor before serious problems develop."

High cholesterol is only one factor that leads to heart disease. Others include high blood pressure, smoking, obesity, and family history of heart disease before age 55. An estimated 17.6 million Americans have heart disease, which claims some 734,000 lives in the United States annually. The agency's decision to allow the test to be sold over-the-counter is based on results of a multi-center clinical trial involving nearly 500 adults. The firm's study showed the test to be as accurate as cholesterol tests used by doctors and medical laboratories.

"Accuracy is crucial," said David A. Kessler, M.D., Commissioner of Food and Drugs. "It is also important, as the study showed, that

FDA Press Release March 2, 1993.

participants were able to read and understand the instructions and perform the test without assistance," he noted.

To perform the test, the user pricks his finger, squeezes blood into a cassette that contains a test strip and then waits 10 to 15 minutes for results. The strip changes color as the cholesterol rises on it. When the time is up, the user compares the height of color shown on the cassette with an accompanying conversion chart to get the cholesterol reading.

The test measures total cholesterol. It does not measure individual components, such as LDL or HDL cholesterol. A reading of less than 200 is desirable; 200 to 239 is borderline high; and 240 or above is high, meaning the user may be at a greater risk for heart disease. People whose cholesterol is borderline or high should see a doctor.

The National Institutes of Health's National Cholesterol Education Program recommends that people with a reading in the desirable range have their cholesterol checked once every five years, and that those whose cholesterol is borderline or high follow the recommendation of their doctor for frequency of testing.

The home test should not be used by hemophiliacs or by people who take medicine to thin blood because of the possibility of the finger prick. Those individuals should have their cholesterol checked by their doctors.

The package labeling for the test includes detailed instructions for proper use and a discussion of the test's limits. It also includes information on cholesterol, heart disease, diet and exercise and lists a toll-free number consumers can call for additional information.

Part Three

Findings of the
U.S. Preventive Services
Task Force

Chapter 23

The Periodic Health Exam

Introduction

The periodic health visit is an important opportunity for the delivery of clinical preventive services. Identification of specific preventive services that are appropriate for inclusion in the periodic health examination has been one of the principal objectives of the U.S. Preventive Services Task Force project. This chapter introduces the services that were evaluated by the Task Force and are recommended as part of the periodic health examination of the asymptomatic individual. Tables listing specific preventive services that are recommended for patients in different age groups are presented in Chapters 24–27.

The Task Force judged it especially important to emphasize those preventive services that have been proven to be effective in properly conducted studies, and to tailor the content of the periodic health examination to the individual needs of the patient. This approach is based on the recognition that the limited time afforded to patient encounters may be most constructively used if the clinician focuses on interventions of proven efficacy. The clinician can then choose from among these effective interventions for each patient according to the likeliest causes of illness and injury based on that individual's age, sex, and other risk factors. Thus, the two most important factors to consider are the potential effectiveness of clinical interventions in

This chapter contains text from the *Guide to Clinical Preventive Services*, U.S. Preventive Services Task Force, 1996.

improving clinical outcomes and the leading causes of mortality and morbidity.

Clinical efforts directed toward promoting health and preventing disease are of limited value if the preventive intervention does not improve outcome. Thus, the major consideration in setting priorities is effectiveness of the intervention. Although suicide and homicide are important causes of death among adolescents, for example, the effectiveness of efforts by primary care clinicians to prevent deaths from intentional injuries has not been established. On the other hand, there are effective measures to reduce the risk of motor vehicle injuries, a leading cause of death in this age group. The busy clinician seeing adolescent patients is best advised to direct attention to the use of safety belts and the dangers of driving while under the influence of alcohol, rather than to interventions of unproven effectiveness.

It is also important to consider the leading causes of morbidity and mortality for patients when establishing priorities for the periodic health examination. Leading causes of death by age group are provided.

While more difficult to measure than mortality, leading causes of morbidity also should guide the use of preventive services

Individual risk factors are also important to consider in designing the periodic health examination. The leading causes of morbidity and mortality may differ considerably for persons in special high-risk groups as compared to individuals of the same age and sex in the general population. The differences in priorities among individuals in different age groups and risk categories and the varying effectiveness of some preventive services in different populations make it impossible to recommend a uniform periodic health examination for all persons.

Many of the preventive services appearing in Chapters 24–27 are recommended only for members of high-risk groups. These are listed separately in and are grouped by general patient characteristics that broadly define high-risk populations. This organization will help the clinician to identify patients who might be eligible for one or more of the interventions listed. It is crucial, however, to then read the specific high-risk definition indicated by an annotated high-risk (HR) code after each intervention, because patients may share characteristics of the general high-risk grouping without actually meeting the individual high-risk definitions for every intervention within that group. For example, a 23-year-old woman whose high-risk sexual behavior is limited to having two recent sexual partners should be screened for gonorrhea and chlamydia infection, but she may not require screening for syphilis or a hepatitis A vaccine. To avoid providing unnecessary preventive services, clinicians must evaluate carefully whether patients who are potentially at risk meet the specific high-risk definitions for each potential intervention. While nonstandardized historical questions were not evaluated by the Task Force and therefore are not included in the recommendations, the history and physical examination can be used to identify high-risk individuals who would benefit from targeted interventions.

Age Chart Introduction

The preventive services examined in this report and appearing in Chapters 24–27 include only those preventive services that might be performed by primary care clinicians on asymptomatic persons in the context of *routine* health care. Preventive measures involving persons with signs or symptoms and those performed outside the clinical setting are not within the scope of this report or its recommendations. While the Task Force did not evaluate all components of the physical examination, several specific screening maneuvers that might be performed as part of the physical examination are included if they were considered. The recommendations are not intended as a complete list of all that should occur during the periodic health examination. Rather, these recommendations encompass those preventive services that have been examined by the Task Force and that have been shown to have satisfactory evidence of clinical effectiveness.

At the same time, the preventive interventions listed are not exhaustive. The periodic health examination performed by most pediatricians, for example, includes a number of maneuvers that were not examined by the Task Force, such as screening for developmental disorders and anticipatory guidance.

Preventive services listed are not necessarily recommended at every periodic visit. For example, although sigmoidoscopy is recommended for persons age 50 and over, it is not recommended annually even though periodic visits in this age group may occur once a year. Where a specific periodicity has been proven effective (e.g., annual fecal occult blood testing in persons 50 years of age and over), this information is included in the notes. The Task Force has not attempted to design a periodicity schedule for health supervision visits because for many interventions, evidence of an optimal periodicity is lacking. In addition, periodicity for certain interventions varies with patient characteristics (age, gender, and risk factors).

Although the preventive services listed in Chapters 24–27 can serve as the basis for designing periodic checkups devoted entirely to health promotion and disease prevention, they may also be performed during visits for other reasons (e.g., illness visits, chronic disease checkups) when indicated. Health maintenance needs to be considered at every visit. For patients with limited access to care, the illness visit may provide the only realistic opportunity to discuss prevention. It is recognized that busy clinicians may not be able to perform all recommended preventive services during a single clinical encounter. Indeed, it is not clear that such a grouping is either necessary or clinically effective. If a sparser, evidence-based protocol is used, health maintenance can frequently be done during acute visits. Patients suffering from an acute illness or injury, however, may not be receptive to some preventive interventions. The clinician must therefore use discretion in selecting appropriate preventive services from these recommendations and may wish to give special emphasis to those effective interventions aimed at the leading causes of illness and disability in the age group. Recommended preventive services that cannot be performed by the clinician at the current visit should be scheduled for a later health visit.

Immunizations appearing in Chapters 24–27 are those recommended on a routine basis and do not apply to persons with special exposures to infected individuals. Chapters 24–27 do not include interventions for which the Task Force found insufficient evidence on which to base recommendations for or against inclusion in the periodic health examination. The Task Force recognizes that there may be other grounds on which to base a recommendation for or against an intervention when scientific evidence is not available, including patient preference, costs associated with the procedure, the likelihood of benefit or harms from the procedure, and the burden of suffering from the condition. Consideration of these other grounds can guide the clinician in making decisions about the appropriate use of these interventions. For many important causes of morbidity and mortality, evidence of effective preventive interventions is lacking. There is a great need for well-controlled, randomized studies with adequate sample sizes to evaluate the effectiveness of preventive interventions for many conditions. Such topics merit attention in the planning of future research agendas.

—*Ann O'Malley, MD, MPH, and Carolyn DiGuiseppi, MD, MPH.*

Chapter 24

Birth to 10 Years Screening Recommendations

Leading Causes of Death

- Conditions originating in perinatal period
- Congenital anomalies
- Sudden infant death syndrome (SIDS)
- Unintentional injuries (non-motor vehicle)
- Motor vehicle injuries

Interventions for the General Population

Interventions considered and recommended for the periodic health examination of children from birth through 10 years of age.

Screening

- Height and weight
- Blood pressure
- Vision screen (ages 3-4)
- Hemoglobinopathy screen (birth) [1]
- Phenylalanine livel (birth) [2]
- T4 and/or TSH (birth) [3]

This chapter contains text from the *Guide to Clinical Preventive Services*, U.S. Preventive Services Task Force, 1996.

Counseling

- Injury prevention
- Child safety car seats (age <5 yr)
- Lap-shoulder belts (age ≥5 yr)
- Bicycle helmet, avoid bicycling near traffic
- Smoke detector, flame retardant sleepwear
- Hot water heater temperature <120-130 degrees Fahrenheit
- Window/stair guards, pool fence
- Safe storage of drugs, toxic substances, firearms, and matches
- Syrup of ipecac, poison control phone number
- CPR training for parents/caretakers
- Diet and exercise
- Breast-feeding, iron-enriched formula and foods (infants and toddlers)
- Limit fat and cholesterol, maintain caloric balance, emphasize grains, fruits, vegetables (age ≥2 yr)
- Regular physical activity*

Substance Use

- Effects of passive smoking*
- Anti-tobacco message*

Dental Health

- Regular visits to dental care provider
- Floss, brush with fluoride toothpaste daily
- Advice about baby bottle tooth decay*

Immunizations

- Diphtheria-tetanus-pertussis (DPT) [4]
- Oral poliovirus (OPV) [5]
- Measles-mumps-rubella (MMR) [6]
- H. influenzae type b (Hib) conjugate [7]
- Hepatitis B [8]
- Varicella [9]

Chemoprophylaxis

- Ocular prophylaxis (birth)

Table 24.1. Interventions for High-Risk Populations Birth to 10 Years

Population	Potential Interventions
Preterm or low birth weight	Hemoglobin/hematocrit (HR1)
Infants of mothers at risk for HIV	HIV testing (HR2)
Low income; immigrants	Hemoglobin/hematocrit (HR1); PPD (HR3)
TB contacts	PPD (HR3)
Native American/Alaska Native	Hemoglobin/hematocrit (HR1); PPD (HR3); hepatitis A vaccine (HR4); pneumococcal vaccine (HR5)
Travelers to developing countries	Hepatitis A vaccine (HR4)
Residents of long-term care facilities	PPD (HR3); hepatitis A vaccine (HR4); influenza vaccine (HR6)
Certain chronic medical conditions	PPD (HR3); pneumococcal vaccine (HR5); influenza vaccine (HR6)
Increased individual or community lead exposure	Blood lead level (HR7)
Inadequate water fluoridation	Daily fluoride supplement (HR8)
Family history of skin cancer; fair skin, eyes, hair	Avoid excess/midday sun (HR9)

Notes and References

[1] Whether screening should be universal or targeted to high-risk groups will depend on the proportion of high-risk individuals in the screening area, and other considerations.

[2] If done during first 24 hr of life, repeat by age 2 wk.

[3] Optimally between day 2 and 6, but in all cases before newborn nursery discharge.

[4] 2, 4, 6, and 12-18 mos.; once between ages 4-6 yr. (DTP may be used at 15 mos. and older).

[5] 2, 4, 6-18 mos.; once between ages 4-6 yr.

[6] 12-15 mos. and 4-6 yr.

[7] 2, 4, 6 and 12-15 mos.; no dose needed at 6 mos. if PRP-OMP vaccine is used for first 2 doses.

[8] Birth, 1 mo., 6 mos.; or, 0-2 mos., 1-2 mos. later, and 6-18 mos. If not done in infancy: current visit, and 1 and 6 mos. later.

[9] 12-18 mos.; or older child without history of chickenpox or previous immunization. Include information on risk in adulthood, duration of immunity, and potential need for booster doses.

[*] The ability of clinician counseling to influence this behavior is unproven.

HR1 (high risk)

Infants age 6-12 mos. who are: living in poverty, black, Native American or Alaska Native, immigrants from developing countries, preterm or low birth weight infants, or infants whose principal dietary intake is unfortified cow's milk.

HR2

Infants born to high-risk mothers whose HIV status is unknown. Women at high risk include: past or present injection drug use; persons who exchange sex for money or drugs, and their sex partners; injection drug-using, bisexual, or HIV-positive sex partners currently or in past; persons seeking treatment for STDs; blood transfusion during 1978-1985.

HR3

Persons infected with HIV, close contacts of persons with known or suspected TB, persons with medical risk factors associated with TB, immigrants from countries with high TB prevalence, medically underserved low-income populations (including homeless), residents of long-term care facilities for indications for BCG vaccine.

HR4

Persons ≥2 yrs. living in or traveling to areas where the disease is endemic and where periodic outbreaks occur (e.g., countries with high or intermediate endemicity; certain Alaska Native, Pacific Island, Native American, and religious communities). Consider for institutionalized children aged ≥2 yrs. Clinicians should also consider local epidemiology

HR5

Immunocompetent persons ≥2 yrs. with certain medical conditions, including chronic cardiac or pulmonary disease, diabetes mellitus, and anatomic asplenia. Immunocompetent persons ≥2 yrs. living in high-risk environments or social settings (e.g., certain Native American and Alaska Native populations).

HR6

Annual vaccination of children ≥6 mos. who are residents of chronic care facilities or who have chronic cardiopulmonary disorders, metabolic diseases (including diabetes mellitus), hemoglobinopathies, immunosuppression, or renal dysfunction for indications for amantadine/rimantadine prophylaxis.

HR7

Children about age 12 mos. Who:

1. live in communities in which the prevalence of lead levels requiring individual intervention, including residential lead hazard control or chelation, is high or undefined;

2. live in or frequently visit a home built before 1950 with dilapidated paint or with recent or ongoing renovation or remodeling;

3. have close contact with a person who has an elevated lead level;

4. live near lead industry or heavy traffic;

5. live with someone whose job or hobby involves lead exposure;

6. use lead-based pottery; or

7. take traditional ethnic remedies that contain lead.

HR8

Children living in areas with inadequate water fluoridation (<0.6 ppm).

HR9

Persons with a family history of skin cancer, a large number of moles, atypical moles, poor tanning ability, or light skin, hair, and eye color.

Chapter 25

Ages 11–24 Years Screening Recommendations

Leading Causes of Death

- Motor vehicle/other unintentional injuries
- Homicide
- Suicide
- Malignant neoplasms
- Heart diseases

Interventions for the General Population

Interventions considered and recommended for the periodic health examination of individuals ages 11 to 24.

Screening

- Height and weight
- Blood pressure [1]
- Papanicolaou (Pap) test (females) [2]
- Chlamydia screen (females <20 yr) [3]
- Rubella serology or vaccination history (females >12 yr) [4]
- Assess for problem drinking

This chapter contains text from the *Guide to Clinical Preventive Services*, U.S. Preventive Services Task Force, 1996.

Counseling

Injury Prevention

- Lap/shoulder belts
- Bicycle/motorcycle/ATV helmets [*]
- Smoke detector [*]
- Safe storage/removal of firearms [*]

Substance Use

- Avoid tobacco use
- Avoid underage drinking and illicit drug use [*]
- Avoid alcohol/drug use while driving, swimming, boating, etc. [*]

Sexual Behavior

- STD prevention: abstinence; avoid high-risk behavior, condoms/ female barrier with spermicide [*]
- Unintended pregnancy: contraception
- Diet and exercise
- Limit fat and cholesterol; maintain caloric balance, emphasize grains, fruits, vegetables
- Adequate calcium intake (females)
- Regular physical activity [*]

Dental Health

- Regular visits to dental care provider
- Floss, brush with fluoride toothpaste daily

Immunizations

- Tetanus-diphtheria (Td) boosters (11-16 yr)
- Hepatitis B [5]
- MMR (11-12 yr) [6]
- Varicella (11-12 yr) [7]
- Rubella (females >12 yr) [4]

Chemoprophylaxis

- Multivitamin with folic acid (females planning/capable of pregnancy)

Table 25.1. Interventions for High-Risk Individuals Ages 11-24.

Population	Potential Interventions
High-risk sexual behavior	RPR/VDRL (HR1); screen for gonorrhea (female) (HR2); HIV (HR3); chlamydia (female) (HR4); hepatitis A vaccine (HR5)
Injection or street drug use	RPR/VDRL (HR1); HIV screen (HR3); hepatitis A vaccine (HR5); PPD (HR6); advice to reduce infection risk (HR7)
TB contacts; immigrants; low income	PPD (HR6)
Native Americans/Alaska Natives	Hepatitis A vaccine (HR5); PPD (HR6); pneumococcal vaccine (HR8)
Travelers to developing countries	Hepatitis A vaccine (HR5)
Certain chronic medical conditions	PPD (HR6); pneumococcal vaccine (HR8); influenza vaccine (HR9)
Settings where adolescents and young adults congregate	second MMR (HR10)
Susceptible to varicella, measles, mumps	Varicella vaccine (HR11); MMR (HR12)
Blood transfusion between 1978-1985	HIV screen (HR3)
Institutionalized persons; health care/lab workers	Hepatitis A vaccine (HR5); PPD (HR6); influenza vaccine (HR9)
Family history of skin cancer; abnormal moles; fair skin, eyes, hair	Avoid excess/midday sun, use protective clothing * (HR13)
Prior pregnancy with neural tube defect	Folic acid 4.0 (HR14)
Inadequate water fluoridation	Daily fluoride supplement (HR15)

Notes and References

[1] Periodic Blood pressure for persons aged ≥21 yr.

[2] If sexually active at present or in the past: q ≤ 3 yr. If sexual history is unreliable, begin Pap tests at age 18 yr.

[3] If sexually active.

[4] Serologic testing, documented vaccination history, and routine vaccination against rubella (preferably with MMR) are equally acceptable alternatives.

[5] If not previously immunized: current visit, 1 and 6 mos. later.

[6] If no previous second dose of MMR.

[7] If susceptible to chickenpox.

[*] The ability of clinician counseling to influence this behavior is unproven.

HR1

Persons who exchange sex for money or drugs, and their sex partners; persons with other STDs (including HIV); and sexual contacts of persons with active syphilis. Clinicians should also consider local epidemiology.

HR2

Females who have: two or more sex partners in the last year; a sex partner with multiple sexual contacts; exchanged sex for money or drugs; or a history of repeated episodes of gonorrhea. Clinicians should also consider local epidemiology.

HR3

Males who had sex with males after 1975; past or present injection drug use; persons who exchange sex for money or drugs, and their sex partners; injection drug-using, bisexual, or HIV-positive sex partner currently or in the past; blood transfusion during 1978-1985; persons seeking treatment for STDs. Clinicians should also consider local epidemiology.

HR4

Sexually active females with multiple risk factors including: history of prior STD; new or multiple sex partners; age under 25; nonuse or inconsistent use of barrier contraceptives; cervical ectopy. Clinicians should consider local epidemiology of the disease in identifying other high-risk groups.

HR5

Persons living in, traveling to, or working in areas where the disease is endemic and where periodic outbreaks occur (e.g., countries with high or intermediate endemicity; certain Alaska Native, Pacific Island, Native American, and religious communities); men who have sex with men; injection or street drug users. Vaccine may be considered for institutionalized persons and workers in these institutions, military personnel, and day-care, hospital, and laboratory workers. Clinicians should also consider local epidemiology.

HR6

HIV positive, close contacts of persons with known or suspected TB, health care workers, persons with medical risk factors associated with TB, immigrants from countries with high TB prevalence, medically underserved low-income populations (including homeless), alcoholics, injection drug users, and residents of long-term care facilities for indications for BCG vaccine.

HR7

Persons who continue to inject drugs.

HR8

Immunocompetent persons with certain medical conditions, including chronic cardiac or pulmonary disease, diabetes mellitus, and anatomic asplenia. Immunocompetent persons who live in high-risk environments or social settings (e.g., certain Native American and Alaska Native populations).

HR9

Annual vaccination of: residents of chronic care facilities; persons with chronic cardiopulmonary disorders, metabolic diseases (including diabetes mellitus), hemoglobinopathies, immunosuppression, or renal dysfunction; and health care providers for high-risk patients for indications for amantadine/rimantadine prophylaxis.

HR10

Adolescents and young adults in settings where such individuals congregate (e.g., high schools and colleges), if they have not previously received a second dose.

HR11

Healthy persons aged ≥13 yr without a history of chickenpox or previous immunization. Consider serologic testing for presumed susceptible persons aged ≥13 yr.

HR12

Persons born after 1956 who lack evidence of immunity to measles or mumps (e.g., documented receipt of live vaccine on or after the first birthday, laboratory evidence of immunity, or a history of physician-diagnosed measles or mumps).

HR13

Persons with a family or personal history of skin cancer, a large number of moles, atypical moles, poor tanning ability, or light skin, hair, and eye color.

HR14

Women with prior pregnancy affected by neural tube defect who are planning pregnancy.

HR15

Persons aged <17 yr living in areas with inadequate water fluoridation (<0.6 ppm).

Chapter 26

Ages 25–64 Years Screening Recommendations

Leading Causes of Death

- Malignant neoplasms
- Heart diseases
- Motor vehicle and other unintentional injuries
- Human immunodeficiency virus (HIV) infection
- Suicide and homicide

Interventions for the General Population

Interventions considered and recommended for the periodic health examination of individuals ages 25 to 65.

Screening

- Blood pressure
- Height and weight
- Total blood cholesterol (men ages 35-65, women ages 45-65)
- Papanicolaou (Pap) test (women) [1]
- Fecal occult blood test [2] and/or sigmoidoscopy (≥50 yr)
- Mammogram ± clinical breast exam (women 50-69 yr) [3]
- Assess for problem drinking
- Rubella serology or vaccination history (women of childbearing age [4]

This chapter contains text from the *Guide to Clinical Preventive Services*, U.S. Preventive Services Task Force, 1996.

Counseling

Substance Use

- Tobacco cessation
- Avoid alcohol/drug use while driving, swimming, boating, etc.

Diet and Exercise

- Limit fat and cholesterol; maintain caloric balance; emphasize grains, fruits, vegetables
- Adequate calcium intake (women)
- Regular physical activity [*]

Injury Prevention

- Lap/shoulder belts
- Motorcycle/bicycle/ATV helmets
- Smoke detector [*]
- Safe storage/removal of firearms [*]

Sexual Behavior

- STD prevention: avoid high-risk behavior*; condoms/female barrier with spermicide*
- Unintended pregnancy: contraception

Dental Health

- Regular visits to dental care provider
- Floss, brush with fluoride toothpaste daily

Immunizations

- Tetanus-diphtheria (Td) boosters
- Rubella (women of childbearing age) [4]

Chemoprophylaxis

- Multivitamin with folic acid (women planning or capable of pregnancy)
- Discuss hormone prophylaxis (peri- and postmenopausal women)

Table 26.1. Interventions for High-Risk Populations

Population	Potential Interventions
High-risk sexual behavior	RPR/VDRL (HR1); screen for gonorrhea (female) (HR2); HIV (HR3); chlamydia (female (HR4); hepatitis B vaccine (HR5); hepatitis A vaccine (HR6)
Injection or street drug use	RPR/VDRL (HR1); HIV screen (HR3); hepatitis B vaccine (HR5); hepatitis A vaccine (HR6); PPD (HR7); advice to reduce infection risk (HR8)
Low income; TB contacts; immigrants; alcoholics	PPD (HR7)
Native Americans/Alaska Natives	Hepatitis A vaccine (HR6); PPD (HR7); pneumococcal vaccine (HR9)
Travelers to developing countries	Hepatitis B vaccine (HR5); hepatitis A vaccine (HR6)
Certain chronic medical conditions	PPD (HR7); pneumococcal vaccine (HR9); influenza vaccine (HR10)
Blood product recipients	HIV screen (HR3); hepatitis B vaccine (HR5)
Susceptible to measles, mumps, or varicella	MMR (HR11); varicella vaccine (HR12)
Institutionalized persons	Hepatitis A vaccine (HR6); PPD (HR7); pneumococcal vaccine (HR9); influenza vaccine (HR10)
Health care/lab workers	Hepatitis B vaccine (HR5); hepatitis A vaccine (HR6); PPD (HR7); influenza vaccine (HR10)
Family history of skin cancer; fair skin, eyes, hair	Avoid excess/midday sun, use protective clothing [*] (HR13)
Previous pregnancy with neural tube defect	Folic acid 4.0 mg (HR14)

Notes and References

[1] Women who are or have been sexually active and who have a cervix: q ≤ 3 yr.

[2] Annually.

[3] Mammogram every 1–2 yr, or mammogram every 1–2 yr with annual clinical breast examination.

[4] Serologic testing, documented vaccination history, and routine vaccination (preferably with MMR) are equally acceptable alternatives.

[*] The ability of clinician counseling to influence this behavior is unproven.

HR1

Persons who exchange sex for money or drugs, and their sex partners; persons with other STDs (including HIV); and sexual contacts of persons with active syphilis. Clinicians should also consider local epidemiology.

HR2

Women who exchange sex for money or drugs, or who have had repeated episodes of gonorrhea. Clinicians should also consider local epidemiology.

HR3

Men who had sex with men after 1975; past or present injection drug use; persons who exchange sex for money or drugs, and their sex partners; injection drug-using, bisexual, or HIV-positive sex partner currently or in the past; blood transfusion during 1978-1985; persons seeking treatment for STDs. Clinicians should also consider local epidemiology.

HR4

Sexually active women with multiple risk factors including: history of STD; new or multiple sex partners; nonuse or inconsistent use of barrier contraceptives; cervical ectopy. Clinicians should also consider local epidemiology.

HR5

Blood product recipients (including hemodialysis patients), persons with frequent occupational exposure to blood or blood products, men who have sex with men, injection drug users and their sex partners, persons with multiple recent sex partners, persons with other STDs (including HIV), travelers to countries with endemic hepatitis B.

HR6

Persons living in, traveling to, or working in areas where the disease is endemic and where periodic outbreaks occur (e.g., countries with high or intermediate endemicity; certain Alaska Native, Pacific Island, Native American, and religious communities); men who have sex with men; injection or street drug users. Consider for institutionalized persons and workers in these institutions, military personnel, and day-care, hospital, and laboratory workers. Clinicians should also consider local epidemiology.

HR7

HIV positive, close contacts of persons with known or suspected TB, health care workers, persons with medical risk factors associated with TB, immigrants from countries with high TB prevalence, medically underserved low-income populations (including homeless), alcoholics, injection drug users, and residents of long-term care facilities for indications for BCG vaccine.

HR8

Persons who continue to inject drugs.

HR9

Immunocompetent institutionalized persons aged ≥50 yr and immunocompetent persons with certain medical conditions, including chronic cardiac or pulmonary disease, diabetes mellitus, and anatomic asplenia. Immunocompetent persons who live in high-risk environments or social settings (e.g., certain Native American and Alaska Native populations).

HR10

Annual vaccination of residents of chronic care facilities; persons with chronic cardiopulmonary disorders, metabolic diseases (including diabetes mellitus), hemoglobinopathies, immunosuppression, or renal dysfunction; and health care providers for high-risk patients for indications for amantadine/rimantadine prophylaxis.

HR11

Persons born after 1956 who lack evidence of immunity to measles or mumps (e.g., documented receipt of live vaccine on or after the first birthday, laboratory evidence of immunity, or a history of physician-diagnosed measles or mumps).

HR12

Healthy adults without a history of chickenpox or previous immunization. Consider serologic testing for presumed susceptible adults.

HR13

Persons with a family or personal history of skin cancer, a large number of moles, atypical moles, poor tanning ability, or light skin, hair, and eye color.

HR14

Women with previous pregnancy affected by neural tube defect who are planning pregnancy.

Chapter 27

Age 65 Year and Older Screening Recommendations

Leading Causes of Death

- Heart diseases
- Malignant neoplasms (lung, colorectal, breast)
- Cerebrovascular disease
- Chronic obstructive pulmonary disease
- Pneumonia and influenza

Interventions for the General Population

Interventions considered and recommended for the periodic health examination for individuals age 65 and older.

Screening

- Blood pressure
- Height and weight
- Fecal occult blood test [1] and/or sigmoidoscopy
- Mammogram ± clinical breast exam (women   69 yr) [2]
- Papanicolaou (Pap) test (women
- Vision screening
- Assess for hearing impairment
- Assess for problem drinking

This chapter contains text from the *Guide to Clinical Preventive Services,* U.S. Preventive Services Task Force, 1996.

Counseling

Substance Use

- Tobacco cessation
- Avoid alcohol/drug use while driving, swimming, boating, etc. [*]

Diet and Exercise

- Limit fat and cholesterol; maintain caloric balance; emphasize grains, fruits, vegetables
- Adequate calcium intake (women)
- Regular physical activity [*]

Injury Prevention

- Lap/shoulder belts
- Motorcycle and bicycle helmets
- Fall prevention [*], Safe storage/removal of firearms [*]
- Smoke detector [*]
- Set hot water heater to <120–130 degrees Fahrenheit degrees
- CPR training for household members

Dental Health

- Regular visits to dental care provider [*]
- Floss, brush with fluoride toothpaste daily [*]

Sexual Behavior

- STD prevention: avoid high-risk sexual behavior [*]; use condoms [*]

Immunizations

- Pneumococcal vaccine
- Influenza [1]
- Tetanus-diphtheria (Td) boosters

Chemoprophylaxis

- Discuss hormone prophylaxis (women)

Table 27.1. Interventions for High-Risk Individuals Age 65 and Older

Population	Potential Interventions
Institutionalized persons	PPD (HR1); hepatitis A vaccine (HR2); amantadine/rimantadine (HR4)
Chronic medical conditions; TB contacts; low income; immigrants; alcoholics	PPD (HR1)
Persons ≥75 yr, or ≥70 yr with risk factors for falls	Fall prevention intervention (HR5)
Cardiovascular disease risk factors	Consider cholesterol screening (HR6)
Family history of skin cancer; abnormal moles; fair skin, eyes, hair	Avoid excess/midday sun, use protective clothing [*] (HR7)
Native Americans/Alaska Natives	PPD (HR1); hepatitis A vaccine (HR2)
Travelers to developing countries	Hepatitis A vaccine (HR2); hepatitis B vaccine (HR8)
Blood product recipients	HIV screen (HR3); hepatitis B vaccine (HR8)
High-risk sexual behavior	Hepatitis A vaccine (HR2); HIV screen (HR3); hepatitis B vaccine (HR8); RPR/VDRL (HR9)
Injection or street drug use	PPD (HR1); hepatitis A vaccine (HR2); HIV screen (HR3); hepatitis B vaccine (HR8); RPR/VDRL (HR9); advice to reduce infection risk (HR10)
Health care/lab workers	PPD (HR1); hepatitis A vaccine (HR2); amantadine/rimantadine (HR4); hepatitis B vaccine (HR8)
Persons susceptible to varicella	Varicella vaccine (HR11)

Notes and References

[1] Annually.

[2] Mammogram every 1–2 yr, or mammogram every 1–2 yr with annual clinical breast exam.

[3] All women who are or have been sexually active and who have a cervix: q 3 yr. Consider discontinuation of testing after age 65 yrs if previous regular screening with consistently normal results.

[*] The ability of clinician counseling to influence this behavior is unproven.

HR1

HIV positive, close contacts of persons with known or suspected TB, health care workers, persons with medical risk factors associated with TB, immigrants from countries with high TB prevalence, medically underserved low-income populations (including homeless) or living in a shelter, alcoholics, injection drug users, and residents of long-term care facilities for indications for BCG vaccine.

HR2

Persons living in, traveling to, or working in areas where the disease is endemic and where periodic outbreaks occur (e.g., countries with high or intermediate endemicity; certain Alaska Native, Pacific Island, Native American, and religious communities); men who have sex with men; injection or street drug users. Consider for institutionalized persons and workers in these institutions, and hospital and laboratory workers. Clinicians should also consider local epidemiology.

HR3

Men who had sex with men after 1975; past or present injection drug use; persons who exchange sex for money or drugs, and their sex partners; injection drug-using, bisexual, or HIV-positive sex partner currently or in the past; blood transfusion during 1978-1985; persons seeking treatment for STDs. Clinicians should consider local epidemiology.

HR4

Consider for persons who have not received the vaccine or are vaccinated late; when the vaccine may be ineffective due to major antigenic changes in the virus; for unvaccinated persons who provide home care for high-risk persons; to supplement protection provided by vaccine in persons who are expected to have a poor antibody response; and for high-risk persons in whom the vaccine is contraindicated.

HR5

Persons aged 75 years and older; or aged 70-74 with one or more additional risk factors including: use of certain psychoactive and cardiac medications (e.g., benzodiazepines, antihypertensives); use of 4 or more prescription medications; impaired cognition, strength, balance, or gait. Intensive individualized home-based multifactorial fall prevention intervention is recommended in settings where adequate resources are available to deliver such services.

HR6

Although evidence is insufficient to recommend routine screening in elderly persons, clinicians should consider cholesterol screening on a case-by-case basis for persons ages 65-75 with additional risk factors (e.g., smoking, diabetes, or hypertension).

HR7

Persons with a family or personal history of skin cancer, a large number of moles, atypical moles, poor tanning ability, or light skin, hair, and eye color.

HR8

Blood products recipients (including hemodialysis patients), persons with frequent occupational exposure to blood or to blood products, men who have sex with men, injection drug users and their sex partners, persons with multiple recent sex partners persons with other STDs (including HIV), travelers to countries with endemic hepatitis B.

HR9

Persons who exchange sex for money or drugs and their sex partners; persons with other STDs (including HIV); and sexual contacts of persons with active syphilis. Clinicians should also consider.

HR10

Persons who continue to inject drugs

HR11

Healthy adults without a history of chickenpox or previous immunization. Consider serologic testing may be considered for presumed susceptible adults.

Part Four

X-ray and Radiology Tests

Chapter 28

Patient Preparation for Radiologic Exams

Many radiologic exams require specific patient preparation prior to the exam in order to ensure that the study is performed in the safest and most accurate manner possible. If you are scheduled for one of the following studies, follow the instructions exactly as written. If you have any questions, or feel that you can't comply with the instructions, be sure to call the site where the exam is scheduled.

The Following Exams Require Patient Preparation

- Computed Tomography (CAT Scan, CT Scan)
- Upper GI Series (UGI, Stomach Exam) with or without Small Bowel
- Barium Enema (BE, Lower GI Series, Colon Exam)
- Intravenous Pyelogram (IVP, Kidney Exam)
- Gall Bladder X-Ray (Oral Cholecystogram, OCG)
- Mammogram (Breast X-Ray)
- Pelvic Ultrasound (GYN or Obstetrical)
- Abdominal Ultrasound (Ultrasound of Gallbladder)
- Nuclear Medicine

The Following Exams Usually Require No Patient Preparation

- Other Ultrasound (kidneys, breast, thyroid, scrotum, extremity, aorta)

- General X-rays (chest, spine, bone, sinus, skull)

- Magnetic Resonance Imaging (MRI)

- Arthrogram

- Sialogram

Following are common preparations for the listed exams. This listing is for consumer knowledge only. Follow your doctor's specific directions for any test you require.

Computed Tomography

- Nothing to eat (except medicines) four hours before exam.

- Nothing to drink (except medicines) two hours before the exam.

- CT of abdomen or pelvis: You will need to drink a contrast liquid before this exam. Your doctor or clinic will give you directions.

- Allow 1 hour for the exam.

Upper Gastrointestinal (GI) Series

- Nothing to eat or drink after midnight the night before the exam.

- If barium enema done the day before, take 8 ounce bottle of Citrate of Magnesium following the barium enema at 5:00 p.m.

- *Allow 30 minutes for the exam. Allow 1 to 3 hours for small bowel*

Barium Enema

- Check the specific instructions for the site where your exam is scheduled.

Intravenous Pyelogram

The evening before the exam:

- Your doctor will specify if you should take Citrate of Magnesium.
- Nothing to eat for 4 hours prior to the exam.
- Nothing to drink (except medicines) for 2 hours prior to the exam.
- *Allow 1 hour for the exam.*

Oral Cholecystogram

The day before exam:

- High fat lunch, fat free dinner.
- At 7:00 p.m., take 6 contrast tablets. Patients weighing over 150 lbs. should take 9 tablets.
- After taking tablets, water only until midnight.
- Nothing by mouth after midnight.
- *Allow 30 minutes for the exam.*

Mammogram

- On the day of the exam, do not use any perfume or powder on underarm area or breasts.
- Bring previous mammograms or arrange to have them sent ot your doctor's office.
- Wear 2-piece clothing if possible.
- Allow 30 minutes for the exam.

Pelvic or Obstetrical Ultrasound

- Empty bladder 90 minutes prior to exam time.
- Drink 1 quart (32 ounces) of liquid within 15 minutes of emptying bladder. Do not void (empty bladder) until exam is completed.
- Allow 30 minutes for the exam.

Abdominal or Gallbladder Ultrasound

- No fatty foods or dairy products the day before the exam.
- Nothing to eat or drink after midnight.
- Do not give enemas.
- Allow 30 minutes for the exam.

—Dr. Steven Brick

Chapter 29

X-ray

Contents

Section 29.1

Diagnostic Imaging History

Excerpts from "The Picture of Health," *FDA Consumer*,
January/February 1999.

It's What's Inside that Counts with X-rays, Other Imaging Methods

Within a year of German scientist Wilhelm Roentgen's discovery of x-rays in 1895, people throughout the world knew about Roentgen's work and had seen his first x-ray picture—his wife Bertha's hand, showing her bones, wedding ring, and all. Even before Roentgen was awarded the first Nobel Prize in physics in 1901 for his discovery, x-ray studios were popping up that sold bone portraits for display in the home.

As their popularity grew, some publications contained inflated claims about x-rays—they could restore vision to the blind, they could raise the dead. Other people expressed a far more skeptical view: "I can see no future in the field," the head of one x-ray clinic reportedly proclaimed. "All the bones of the body and foreign bodies have been demonstrated."

But x-ray was far from a dead-end technology. Instead, it marked the start of a revolution in medical diagnosis. Like other medical imaging technologies that followed, including ultrasound, computed tomography (or CT) scanning, and magnetic resonance imaging (or MRI), x-ray can help doctors narrow down the causes of a patient's symptoms without surgery and sometimes diagnose an illness before symptoms even appear. While it can't help a blind person see again, used appropriately, medical imaging can be a useful first step in treating a range of problems, from a simple broken bone to a cancerous tumor.

Using medical imaging *appropriately*, explains William Sacks, M.D., a medical officer in the Food and Drug Administration's radiology branch, means always considering the risks from a device along with its benefits. X-rays and some other imaging tests use radiation, after all, which can have serious health consequences if used improperly. FDA looks at both the risk and benefit sides of the equation to decide whether to allow marketing of a device, Sacks says. And doctors judge the risks versus the benefits in deciding if a test is medically necessary.

FDA, the U.S. Environmental Protection Agency, and other federal and state agencies share the responsibility for protecting the public from unnecessary radiation. For its part, FDA regulates x-ray equipment and all other electronic radiation-emitting products (including nonmedical consumer products, such as microwave ovens) under the Radiation Control for Health and Safety Act. For all electronic imaging devices, the agency develops and enforces standards to ensure that only safe and effective devices are allowed to be marketed.

"Nothing is entirely safe, of course, including walking down the sidewalk," Sacks says. "The question to ask is, 'In balance, do the benefits of x-ray outweigh the safety concerns?' The benefit of making bone portraits for display, like they did at the beginning of the century, is near zero. Now that we know the health risks from certain doses of radiation, we don't order x-rays willy-nilly, but only if there is a health reason to find out something imaging is capable of telling us."

Beyond the Conventional

Unlike conventional x-rays, which take a single picture of a part of the body, an updated version of the technology called computed tomography generates hundreds of x-ray images in a single examination. Despite the large number of images, the total amount of radiation can be less from a 30 to 45 minute CT scan than from some conventional x-ray procedures.

The patient lies still on an examination table that slides into a circular opening in the CT scanner. The x-ray tube that surrounds the patient takes the pictures from many different directions, and then a computer takes the images and constructs them into two-dimensional cross sections of the body, which can be viewed on a television screen.

"There was nothing uncomfortable about the test, nothing to be afraid of," says Wanda Diak, the managing director of a support network called CancerHope, who underwent several CT scans in 1996 and 1997 to track the status of her ovarian cancer.

Computed tomography produces detailed images that can sometimes reveal abnormalities an ordinary x-ray would not pick up. CT scanning can be useful in checking the brain for tumors, aneurysms, bleeding, or other abnormalities. Also, it can unveil tumors, cysts, or other problems in the liver, spleen, pancreas, lungs, kidneys, pelvis, lymph glands, and other body parts.

It was a CT scan that first revealed an abnormality last September (1998) in the colon of Yankees outfielder Darryl Strawberry. Because of the baseball player's prolonged stomach cramps and other symptoms, doctors performed the CT scan and followed up with a procedure called colonoscopy. Based on the tests, doctors reportedly removed a tumor and part of Strawberry's large intestine. Strawberry will undergo six months of chemotherapy, also.

Doctors have expressed optimism about a full recovery for the athlete. Strawberry himself told his fans at an appearance last October, "My chances are great. Don't worry, I'm gonna live."

Powerful Magnet

First cleared for marketing in 1984, magnetic resonance imaging, like x-ray and CT scanning, provides a look inside the body without surgery. MRI differs in a basic respect from its predecessor technologies, however: MRI uses a strong magnetic field, not x-rays, to create a picture of the internal body structure being studied.

Typically, during MRI, the patient lies on a table that slides into a tubular scanner for the 30 to 90 minute test. Patients are often given earphones to wear while inside the tunnel to block out the loud clanking noises the machine makes.

Inside the tube, a large, donut-shaped magnet creates a magnetic field. Pulse radio waves are directed into the magnetic field and absorbed by hydrogen atoms in the body. The machine's computers create an image of the body's internal structure by measuring the emission of energy from the movement of hydrogen atoms within the patient's body.

MRI is especially useful in studying the brain and spinal cord, the soft tissues of the body, and the joints. Because this technique shows distinct contrast between normal and abnormal tissues, it is sometimes superior to CT scanning and other imaging methods in evaluating tumors, tissue damage, and blood flow.

MRI scanning has no known long-term risks. No jewelry or other metal can be carried or worn during the exam, though, because of the very strong magnetic field. Most importantly, the health professional overseeing the treatment must be told if a patient has a pacemaker, hearing aid, any metal implants such as artificial joints, plates, or screws, or other metal implants or electrical devices. The magnet could interfere with these devices and cause serious injury, even death in the case of a pacemaker.

While MRI is a painless procedure, people who tend to feel claustrophobic may be uncomfortable inside the tunnel. For those people, anti-anxiety medicines are available, or they may choose a hospital or clinic that offers the less confining "open MRI" machine.

Sound Study

Ultrasound scanning isn't just for viewing a developing fetus, anymore. Originally used for this purpose, ultrasound today substitutes for conventional x-rays in the diagnosis of many conditions, commonly those involving the kidneys, bladder and uterus, the heart (called echocardiography), and the spleen, gallbladder and pancreas. However, ultrasound does not produce clear images of the lungs and other organs filled with gas or air.

With an ultrasound exam, a gel is spread over the skin covering the area of interest, and a "transducer" is moved back and forth to gather data. The transducer sends out high-frequency sound waves, far above the range of human hearing. When the waves hit the body part being studied, some are absorbed by tissues, and some are echoed back to a transducer. The machine measures the amount of sound reflected back, and displays an image called a sonogram on a monitor or on videotape or graph paper.

An ultrasound exam can take anywhere from 15 minutes to an hour.

While ultrasound is considered risk-free, FDA's Sacks says it still should be used only when medically warranted because, "There's no point in taking a chance for anything but a medical reason."

Helicopter or Zamboni

So, which diagnostic imaging technique is best? "Best for what? It really depends what you're looking for," says board-certified diagnostic radiologist Mark E. Klein, M.D. He likens the question to asking which mode of transportation is best: "In the mountains, you'd want a helicopter or four-wheel drive. On ice, you'd want a Zamboni." For example, he says, a skull x-ray to look for a brain lesion is useless, so the best choice might be a CT scan or MRI. For a broken arm, an x-ray would do the job and is preferred over an MRI.

X-ray, CT scanning, MRI, and ultrasound are among the most common noninvasive procedures (or minimally invasive, in some cases when a contrast agent is used), but the diagnostic options don't end there. Nuclear scanning, including two techniques called positron emission tomography (PET) and single photon emission computed tomography (SPECT), use radioactive substances introduced into the body to discern abnormal from normal body structures or evaluate the body's functioning. Other, sometimes riskier procedures require the insertion of tubes or instruments into the body.

A patient should know why the doctor is choosing a certain imaging technique, Sacks says. "The patient ought to feel secure about what's being done and understand the doctor's reasoning: 'What information does the doctor expect to get from this test?'"

During the test, too, the technician or radiologist can help the patient feel more secure. Julie (who asked that her last name not be used) says she didn't feel upset or panicky during her MRIs in 1997 to follow her uterine cancer. "The technicians were very careful to help me understand what to expect and what I would feel–10 seconds of this, a minute of that, hold still for this length of time. I felt thoroughly prepared for it."

Her last MRI confirmed that she was "all clean" of cancer. "Even if the tests revealed bad news, I'm very thrilled they were there to give doctors a good view of my situation."

Wanda Diak's ovarian cancer has not been evident for almost three years. During her follow-up exams, she says, her doctor sometimes taps on her stomach to check for signs of recurrence. The method seemed primitive to Diak, but her doctor pointed out that before CT scans and other imaging, different sounds were all doctors had to clue them in to an abnormality.

"I think about someone tapping on your stomach rather than having this image that essentially slices you in half so you can see inside," Diak says. "It's like the caveman to the year 2000."

—by Tamar Nordenberg

Tamar Nordenberg is a staff writer for FDA Consumer.

Section 29.2

What Is an X-ray?

"The Picture of Health," *FDA Consumer*, January/February 1999.

Black-and-White Photo

Roentgen labeled the rays he discovered with the scientific symbol "X," meaning unknown, because he didn't understand their makeup at first. X-rays are actually electromagnetic waves. When they are passed through a patient's body to a photographic film on the other side, they create a picture of internal body structures called a radiograph.

Chest radiographs, which are among the most common imaging tests, can reveal abnormalities of the lungs (such as pneumonia, tumor or fluid), heart (such as congestive heart failure or enlarged heart), and rib cage (such as broken or abnormal bones).

Other common types of x-ray examinations include dental studies to detect cavities and other tooth and gum problems; abdominal studies, which can reveal abnormalities of not just the abdomen, but also the liver, spleen, gallbladder, and kidneys; gastrointestinal studies of the upper or lower GI tract; studies of the joints to assess things like arthritis and sports injuries; and mammograms, which can help detect breast cancer with the use of special x-ray equipment.

Getting a radiograph takes only a few minutes, at a doctor's office or a radiology unit of a hospital or separate location. After positioning the patient with the body part to be examined between the unit that emits the rays and an x-ray film cassette, the doctor or technician steps away from the area and presses a button or otherwise activates the x-ray machine to take the picture.

The less dense a structure of the body is, the more radiation passes through it and reaches the film. The x-rays expose the film, changing its color after it is developed to gray or black, much like light would darken photographic film.

Bones, as well as tumors, are more dense than soft tissues. They appear white or light on the x-ray film because they absorb much of the radiation, leaving the film only slightly exposed. Structures that are less solid than bone, such as skin, fat, muscles, blood vessels, and the lungs, intestines, and other organs, appear darker on the film because they let more of the x-rays pass through. Likewise, a break in a bone allows the x-ray beams to pass through, so the break appears as a dark line in the otherwise white bone.

To make certain organs stand out more clearly, a "contrast medium"—a substance that blocks x-rays rather than transmitting any—can be introduced into the body, in the form of a drink or injection. Barium sulfate is commonly used to study the gastrointestinal tract, while iodine-containing dyes are often used to provide information about the gallbladder, kidneys, blood vessels (using a technique called angiography), or the cavities of the heart.

FDA regulates these contrast agent drugs to make sure they are safe for patients and helpful in diagnosing their medical condition.

Section 29.3

How Safe Are X-ray and Imaging Tests

This section contains text from "What We Know About Radiation," Radiation Safety Branch of the Office of the Director, NIH, July 1996 and "The Picture of Health," *FDA Consumer*, January/February 1999.

What Is Radiation?

We live in a sea of radiation. There are many different types of radiation, some of which are visible light, ultraviolet rays from the sun, infrared from a heat lamp, microwaves, radio waves and ionizing radiation. Radiation is said to be ionizing if it has sufficient energy to displace one or more of the electrons that are part of an atom. This creates an electrically charged atom known as an ion. Common examples of ionizing radiation are x-rays, which are generated by machines, and gamma rays, which are emitted by radioactive materials. Others include alpha and beta rays, which are also emitted from radioactive materials, and neutrons, which are emitted during the splitting (fission) of atoms in a nuclear reactor.

When Do We Encounter Ionizing Radiation in Our Daily Lives?

Everyone who lives on this planet is constantly exposed to naturally occurring ionizing radiation (background radiation). This has been true since the dawn of time. The average effective dose equivalent of radiation to which a person in the United States is exposed annually is estimated to be about 350 millirem. (A millirem is a unit that estimates the biological impact of a particular type of radiation absorbed in the body.)

Sources of background radiation include cosmic rays from the sun and stars; naturally occurring radioactive materials in rocks and soil; radionuclides (unstable radioactive counterparts to naturally stable atoms) normally incorporated into our body's tissues; and radon and its products, which we inhale. Radon exists as a gas and is present in soil from which it seeps into the air. Radon gets trapped inside buildings, especially if the ventilation is poor. Levels of environmental radiation depend upon geology, how we construct our dwellings, and altitude. For example, radiation levels from cosmic rays are greater for people on airplanes and those living on the Colorado plateau. This low-level background radiation is a part of the earth's natural environment and any degree of risk associated with it has not been demonstrated to date.

We are also exposed to ionizing radiation from man-made sources, mostly through medical procedures. On the average, doses from a diagnostic x-ray are much lower, in dose effective terms, than natural background radiation. Radiation therapy, however, can reach levels many times higher than background radiation but this is usually targeted only to the affected tissues. Besides extremely small amounts of ionizing radiation from color televisions and smoke detectors, there are small amounts of ionizing radiation in many building materials and mining and agricultural products, such as granite, coal, and potassium salt. People who smoke receive additional radiation from radionuclides in tobacco smoke.

What Are Some of the Beneficial Ways in which Ionizing Radiation Is Used in Medicine and in Medical Research?

The discovery of x-rays in 1895 was a major turning point in diagnosing diseases because physicians finally had an easy way to "see" inside the body without having to operate. Newer x-ray technologies such as CT (computerized tomography) scans have revolutionized the diagnosis and treatment of diseases affecting almost every part of the body. Other sophisticated techniques have provided physicians with low-risk ways to diagnose. For example, doctors can now pinpoint cholesterol deposits that are narrowing or blocking coronary arteries, information essential for bypassing or unclogging them.

Every major hospital in the United States has a nuclear medicine department in which radionuclides are used to diagnose and treat a wide variety of diseases more effectively and safely by "seeing" how the disease process alters the normal function of an organ. To obtain this information a patient swallows, inhales, or receives an injection of a tiny amount of a radionuclide. Special cameras reveal where the radioactivity accumulates briefly in the body, providing, for example, an image of the heart that shows normal and malfunctioning tissue. Radionuclides are also used in laboratory tests to measure important substances in the body, such as thyroid hormone. Radionuclides are used to effectively treat patients with thyroid diseases, including Graves disease—one of the most common forms of hyperthyroidism—and thyroid cancer.

The use of ionizing radiation has led to major improvements in the diagnosis and treatment of patients with cancer. These innovations have resulted in increased survival rates and improved quality of life. Mammography can detect breast cancer at an early stage when it may be curable. Needle biopsies are more safe, accurate, and informative when guided by x-ray or other imaging techniques. Radiation is used in monitoring the response of tumors to treatment and in distinguishing malignant tumors from benign ones. Bone and liver scans can detect cancers that have spread.

Half of all people with cancer are treated with radiation, and the number of those who have been cured continues to rise. There are now tens of thousands of individuals alive and cured from various cancers as a result of radiotherapy. In addition, there are many patients who have had their disease temporarily halted by radiotherapy. Radionuclides are also being used to decrease or eliminate the pain associated with cancer—such as that of the prostate or breast—that has spread to the bone.

Radionuclides are a technological backbone for much of the biomedical research being done today. They are used in identifying and learning how genes work. Much of the research on is dependent upon the use of radionuclides. Scientists are also "arming" monoclonal antibodies—that are produced in the laboratory and engineered to bind to a specific protein on a patient's tumor cells—with radionuclides. When such "armed" antibodies are injected into a patient, they bind to the tumor cells, which are then killed by the attached radioactivity, but the nearby normal cells are spared. So far, this approach has produced encouraging success in treating patients with leukemia. Most new drugs, before they are approved by the, have undergone animal studies that use radionuclides to learn how the body metabolizes them.

Another clinical and research tool, PET scanning (positron emission tomography), involves injecting radioactive material into a person to "see" the metabolic activity and circulation in a living brain. PET studies have enabled scientists to pinpoint the site of brain tumors or the source of epileptic activity, and to better understand many neurologic diseases. For example, researchers were able to learn how dopamine—the chemical messenger (neurotransmitter) that's involved in Parkinson's disease—is used by the brain.

What Are the Adverse Effects of Ionizing Radiation?

Ionizing radiation can cause important changes in our cells by breaking the electron bonds that hold molecules together. For example, radiation can damage our genetic material (deoxy-ribonucleic acid or DNA) either directly by displacing electrons from the DNA molecule, or indirectly by displacing electrons from some other molecule in the cell that then interacts with the DNA. A cell can be destroyed quickly or its growth or function may be altered through a change (or mutation) that may not be evident for many years. However, the possibility of this inducing a clinically significant illness or other problem is quite remote at small radiation doses.

Our cells, however, have several mechanisms to repair the damage done to DNA by radiation. The efficiency of these repair mechanisms differs among cells and depends on several things, including the type and dose of radiation. There also are biological factors that can greatly modify the cancer-causing effects of large doses of radiation.

The severity of radiation's effects depends on many other factors such as the magnitude and duration of the dose; the area of the body exposed to it; and a person's sex, age, and physical condition. A very large dose of radiation to the whole body at one time can result in death. Exposure to large doses of radiation can increase the risk of developing cancer. Because a radiation-induced cancer is indistinguishable from cancer caused by other factors, it is very difficult to pinpoint radiation as the cause of cancer in a particular individual.

Other effects of large doses of radiation include suppression of the immune system and cataracts. Certain tissues of a fetus, particularly the brain, are especially sensitive to radiation at specific stages of development.

It is very difficult to detect biologic effects in animals or people who are exposed to small doses of radiation. Based on studies in animals and in people exposed to large doses of radiation such as the atomic bomb survivors, scientists have made conservative estimates of what might be the largest doses that would be reasonably safe for a person over a lifetime. But these calculations are estimates only, based on mathematical models. Low-level exposures received by the general public have shown no link to cancer induction. Even so, the U.S. Government uses these estimates to set the limits on all potential exposures to radiation for workers in jobs that expose them to ionizing radiation. International experts and various scientific committees have, over the years, examined the massive body of knowledge about radiation effects in developing and refining radiation protection standards.

Should Patients Be Concerned about the Radiation They May Receive from Tests that Their Physicians Have Ordered?

The doses involved in medical procedures that use radiation or radioactive materials have been decreasing over the past two decades as x-ray films and equipment have been improved. Also, the ability to target radiation more precisely to one part of the body has resulted in less exposure to the rest of the body.

It is always wise to avoid unnecessary radiation exposure. Physicians routinely compare the risks of radiation to the benefits derived from a diagnostic use of radiation to ensure that there is more benefit to the patient than risk. In many cases, such diagnostic tests enable doctors to treat the patient without invasive and life-threatening procedures.

Therefore, patients should not be concerned about radiation exposure from medical tests as the benefits of these procedures far outweigh the potential risks from their exposure.

Should People Be Concerned about Ionizing Radiation?

Experts estimate that a person in the United States gets only 20 percent of their radiation exposure, on average, from medical x-rays and other man-made sources. The remaining 80 percent comes from natural—and usually unavoidable—sources, such as radon gas, the human body, outer space, and rocks and soil.

The cancer risk associated with exposure to large doses of ionizing radiation is among the best understood of any relationships involving environmental agents that cause cancer; this relationship continues to be studied and reevaluated. This knowledge is constantly used in evaluating the risks and benefits of the uses of radiation in medicine. In the overwhelming majority of cases where it is used, the benefits of medical radiation far outweigh the risks associated with it, but there is a tradeoff. In this sense, radiation is no different than any other diagnostic or therapeutic agent, except that we have more information than usual.

Properly managed, radiation can be used for great benefit to humanity and with minimal risk, a risk comparable to or lower than those commonly accepted as an ordinary part of daily life such as driving to work.

Section 29.4

Mammogram

Excerpts from "Understanding Breast Changes," National Cancer Institute (NCI), NIH.

Mammography, The Key to Early Breast Cancer Detection

The key to finding breast cancer is early detection, and the key to early detection is screening: looking for cancer in women who have no symptoms of disease. The best available tool is a regular screening mammogram—x-ray of the breast—coupled with a clinical breast exam—by a doctor or nurse.

Mammography. A mammogram is an x-ray of the breast. Cancers that are found on mammograms but that cannot be felt (nonpalpable cancers) usually are smaller than cancers that can be felt, and they are less likely to have spread.

Mammography is not foolproof. Some breast changes, including lumps that can be felt, do not show up on a mammogram. Changes can be especially difficult to spot in the dense, glandular breasts of younger women. This is why women of all ages should have their breasts examined every year by a physician or trained health professional.

A lump should never be ignored just because it is not visible on a mammogram.

Two Kinds of Mammography: Diagnostic and Screening

If a woman visits her doctor because of unusual breast changes such as a lump, pain, nipple thickening or discharge, or changes in breast size or shape, or has a suspicious screening mammogram, the doctor often asks her to have a diagnostic mammogram: an x-ray of the breast to help assess her symptoms. A diagnostic mammogram is a basic medical tool, and it is appropriate for women of any age.

This section discusses screening mammograms: x-rays that are used to look for breast changes in women who have no signs of breast cancer. (Even though the woman has no symptoms of breast disease, a diagnosis of breast cancer can begin with a doctor checking a screening mammogram.

What Are the Benefits of Screening Mammography?

High-quality mammography is the most effective tool now available to detect breast cancer early, before symptoms appear–often before a breast lump can even be felt. Regularly scheduled mammograms can decrease a woman's chance of dying from breast cancer. For some women, early detection may prevent the need to remove the entire breast or receive chemotherapy.

Who Benefits from Screening Mammography?

Studies done over the past 30 years clearly show that regular screening mammography significantly reduces the death rate from breast cancer in women over the age of 50. Recent results from studies show that regular mammography also reduces death rates from breast cancer in women who begin screening in their forties.

The effectiveness of mammography seems to increase as a woman ages, and the time it takes for benefits to emerge appears to take longer in younger women.

Who Is at Average Risk for Breast Cancer?

Simply being a woman and getting older puts you at average risk for developing breast cancer. The older you are, the greater your chance of getting breast cancer. No woman should consider herself too old to need regular screening mammograms.

Who Is at Higher than Average Risk for Breast Cancer?

One or more of the following conditions place a woman at higher than average risk for breast cancer:

- personal history of a prior breast cancer

- evidence of a specific genetic change that increases susceptibility to breast cancer mother, sister, daughter, or two or more close relatives, such as cousins, with a history of breast cancer (especially if diagnosed at a young age)

- a diagnosis of a breast condition that may predispose a woman to breast cancer (i.e., atypical hyperplasia), or a history of two or more breast biopsies for benign breast disease

Also playing a role in a heightened risk for breast cancer is breast density. Women ages 45 or older who have at least 75 percent dense tissue on a mammogram are at elevated risk. And a slight increase in the risk of breast cancer is associated with having a first birth at age 30 or older.

In addition, women who receive chest irradiation for conditions such as Hodgkin's disease at age 30 or younger remain at higher risk for breast cancer throughout their lives. These women require meticulous surveillance for breast cancer.

These factors that increase cancer risk—risk factors—do not by themselves cause cancer. Having one or more does not mean that you are certain or even likely to develop breast cancer. Even among women with no other risk factors except a strong family history—for example, both a mother and a sister or two sisters with early onset breast cancer—three-fourths will not develop the disease.

Clearly, there is much yet to be learned about what causes breast cancer.

On the other hand, not having any of the known risk factors does not mean that you are "safe." Most women who develop breast cancer do not have a strong family history of breast cancer or fall into any special higher risk category.

What Are the Limitations of Screening Mammography?

Early detection by mammography does not guarantee that a woman's life will be saved. It may not help a woman who has a fast-growing cancer that has spread to other parts of her body before being detected. Also, about half of the women whose breast cancers are detected by mammography would not have died from cancer, even if they had waited until the lump could be felt, because their tumors are slow-growing and treatable.

False Negative Mammograms

Breasts of younger women contain many glands and ligaments. Because their breasts appear dense on mammograms, it is difficult to see tumors or to distinguish between normal and abnormal breast conditions. As a woman grows older, the glandular and fibrous tissues of her breasts gradually give way to less dense fatty tissues. Mammograms can then see into the breast tissue more easily to detect abnormal changes. About 25 percent of breast tumors are missed in women in their forties, compared to about 10 percent of women older than age 50. These are called false negatives. A normal mammogram in a woman with symptoms does not rule out breast cancer. Sometimes a clinical breast exam by a doctor or nurse can reveal a breast lump that is missed by a mammogram.

False Positive Mammograms

Between 5 and 10 percent of mammogram results are abnormal and require more testing (more mammograms, fine needle aspiration, ultrasound, or biopsy), and most of the follow up tests confirm that no cancer was present. It is estimated that a woman who has yearly mammograms between ages 40 and 49 would have about a 30 percent chance of having a false positive mammogram at some point in that decade, and about a 7 to 8 percent chance of having a breast biopsy within the 10-year period. The estimate for false positive mammograms is about 25 percent for women ages 50 or older.

Increased Cases of Ductal Carcinoma in Situ (DCIS)

The increased use of screening mammography has increased the detection of small abnormal tissue growths confined to the milk ducts in the breast, called ductal carcinoma in situ (DCIS). Doctors don't know which, if any, cases of DCIS may become life threatening. Usually, the growth is removed surgically, and radiation treatment is often given.

How Mammograms Are Made

Mammography is a simple procedure. It uses a "dedicated" x-ray machine specifically designed for x-raying the breast and used only for that purpose (in contrast to machines used to take x-rays of the bones or other parts of the body). The standard screening exam includes two views of each breast, one from above and one angled from the side. A registered technologist places the breast between two flat plastic plates. The two plates are then pressed together. The idea is to flatten the breast as much as possible; spreading the tissue out makes any abnormal details easier to spot with a minimum of radiation. The technologist takes the x-ray, then repeats the procedure for the next view.

The pressure from the plates may be uncomfortable, or even somewhat painful. It helps to remember that each x-ray takes less than one minute–and it could save your life. It also helps to schedule mammography just after your period, when your breasts are least likely to be tender, or at the same time each year, if you no longer have your period.

Although some women are concerned about radiation exposure, the risk of any harm is extremely small. The doses of radiation used for mammography are very low and considered safe. The exact amount of radiation needed for a specific mammogram will depend on several factors. For instance, breasts that are large or dense will require higher doses to get a clear image. Federal mammography guidelines limit the radiation used for each exposure of the breast to 0.3 rad. (A "rad" is a unit of measurement that stands for radiation absorbed dose.) In practice, most mammograms deliver just a small fraction of this amount.

Specialized mammography facilities have experienced personnel as well as modern equipment that is custom designed for mammograms.

The combination of good technology and expertise makes it possible to obtain good quality x-ray images with very low doses of radiation.

Reading a Mammogram

The mammogram is first checked by the technologist and then read by a diagnostic radiologist, a doctor who specializes in interpreting x-rays. The radiologist looks for unusual shadows, masses, distortions, special patterns of tissue density, and differences between the two breasts. The shape of a mass can be important, too. A growth that is benign (noncancerous) such as a cyst, looks smooth and round and has a clearly defined edge. Breast cancer, in contrast, often has an irregular outline with finger-like extensions.

Many mammograms show nontransparent white specks. These are calcium deposits known as calcifications.

Macrocalcifications are coarse calcium deposits. They are often seen in both breasts. Macrocalcifications are most likely due to aging, old injuries, or inflammations. They usually are not signs of cancer. Macrocalcifications are usually associated with benign breast conditions; many clusters of macrocalcifications in one area may be an early sign of breast cancer.

Microcalcifications are tiny flecks of calcium found in an area of rapidly dividing cells. Clusters of numerous microcalcifications in one area can be a sign of ductal carcino main situ. About half of the cancers found by mammography are detected as clusters of microcalcifications.

Reporting the Results

The radiologist will report the findings from your mammogram directly to you or to your doctor, who will contact you with the results. If you need further tests or exams, your doctor will let you know. If you don't get a report, you should call and ask for the results.

Don't simply assume that the mammogram is normal if you do not receive the results.

Your mammograms are an important part of your health history. Being able to compare earlier mammograms with new ones helps your doctor evaluate areas that look suspicious. If you move, ask your radiologist for your films and hand-carry them to your new physician, so they can be kept with your file. Always make sure that the radiologist who reads your mammogram has the old films to use for comparison.

Mammograms and Breast Implants

A woman who has had breast implants should continue to have mammograms. (A woman who has had an implant following breast cancer surgery should ask her doctor whether a mammogram is still necessary.) However, the woman should inform the technologist and radiologist beforehand and make sure they are experienced in x-raying patients with breast implants.

Because silicone implants are not transparent on x-ray, they can block a clear view of the tissues behind them. This is especially true if the implant has been placed in front of, rather than beneath, the chest muscles.

Experienced technologists and radiologists know how to carefully compress the breasts to avoid rupturing the implant. They can also use special techniques to detect abnormalities, sliding the implant backward against the chest wall, and pulling the breast tissue over and in front of it. Interpreting the mammogram can also be difficult, especially if scar tissue has formed around the implant or if silicone has leaked into nearby breast tissues.

Choose a Mammography Facility

Many places—breast clinics, radiology departments of hospitals, mobile vans, private radiology practices, doctors' offices—offer high-quality mammography. Your doctor can arrange for a mammogram for you, or you can schedule the appointment yourself. You can call NCI's Cancer Information Service (1-800-4-CANCER) to find a mammography facility in your community.

All facilities must be certified by the Food and Drug Administration (FDA). Staff of the facility are required to post the FDA certificate in a prominent place; if you don't see it, you should ask about certification. Without the FDA "seal of approval," it is now illegal for mammographic facilities to operate.

Assuring High-Quality Mammography

To make sure that all women have access to high-quality mammography, a federal law—the Mammography Quality Standards Act—now requires all mammography facilities to be certified by the FDA. Each facility must demonstrate that it meets federal standards for equipment, personnel, and practices.

Equipment must be capable of producing high-quality mammograms with the lowest possible amount of radiation exposure. Furthermore, it must be regularly checked by a radiological physicist and adjusted as necessary to be sure that its measurements and doses are correct.

Doctors and other staff members must be specially trained to perform and interpret breast x-rays. The technologists who take mammograms are certified by the American Registry of Radiological Technologists or licensed by the state; the doctors who read mammograms should be board-certified radiologists who have taken special courses in mammography.

The regulations also specify that mammography facilities must perform mammography regularly and frequently, maintain quality assurance programs, and ensure proper and timely reporting of test results.

Cost of Mammograms

In addition to quality, another important consideration is cost. Most screening mammograms cost between $50 and $150. Most states now have laws requiring health insurance companies to reimburse all or part of the cost of screening mammograms; check with your insurance company. Medicare pays some of the cost for screening mammograms; check with your health care provider or call the Medicare Hotline (1-800-638-6833) for details.

Some health service agencies and some employers provide mammograms free or at low cost. Low cost does not mean low quality, however. A large government survey found that some of the facilities charging the lowest fees (often because they serve large numbers of women) were among the best in terms of complying with high-quality standards.

Your doctor, local health department, clinic, or chapter of the American Cancer Society, as well as NCI's Cancer Information Service at 1-800-4-CANCER (1-800-422-6237), may be able to direct you to low-cost programs in your area.

Schedule a Regular Mammogram

Early detection of breast cancer is crucial for successful treatment, and regular screening mammography is currently the best tool for early detection. A1993 survey by the National Center for Health Statistics found that 60 percent of all women ages 40 to 49 got a mammogram in the preceding 2 years, and 65 percent of women ages 50 to 64 had done so, but only 54 percent of women ages 65 and over had been screened during that time. It is clear that many women still do not get mammograms at regular intervals. Sadly, the women least likely to have regular exams include those at highest risk, women ages 60and older.

The reason women most frequently give for having—or not having—a mammogram is whether or not the doctor suggested it. Although surveys show that more doctors routinely advise women about mammography, some fail to do so—because they forget, or because they assume that another doctor has done so. If your doctor doesn't suggest mammography, it will be up to you to raise the issue.

Other Techniques for Detecting Breast Cancer

Clinical Breast Exam

Most professional medical organizations recommend that a woman have periodic breast exams by a doctor or nurse along with getting regular screening mammograms. You may find it convenient to schedule a breast exam during your routine physical.

The examiner will look at your breasts while you are sitting and while you are lying down. You may be asked to raise your arms over your head or let them hang by your sides, or to press your hands against your hips. The examiner checks your breasts carefully for changes in the skin such as dimpling, scaling, or puckering; any discharge from the nipples; or any difference in appearance between the two breasts, including differences in size or shape. The next step is palpation: Using the pads of the fingers to feel for lumps, the examiner will systematically inspect the entire breast, the underarm, and the collarbone area, first on one side, then on the other.

A lump is generally the size of a pea before a skilled examiner can detect it. Lumps that are soft, round, and smooth tend not to be cancerous. An irregular, hard lump that feels firmly anchored within the breast tissue is more likely to be a cancer. However, these are general observations, not hard and fast rules.

- The only sure way to know if a solid lump is cancer is to have some tissue removed and examined under the microscope.

A breast exam by a doctor or nurse can find some cancers missed by mammography, even very small ones. In addition to the skill and carefulness of the examiner, the success of a physical exam can be influenced by your monthly cycle and by the size of your breast, as well as by the size and location of the lump itself. Lumps are harder to find in a large breast.

Currently, mammography and breast exams by the doctor or nurse are the most common and useful techniques for finding breast cancer early. Other methods such as ultrasound may be helpful in clarifying the diagnosis for women who have suspicious breast changes. However, no other procedure has yet proven to be more effective than mammography for screening women with no symptoms; thus, most alternative methods of breast cancer detection are used primarily in medical research programs.

Section 29.5

Stereotactic Breast Biopsy

Reprinted with permission © 1997 Steven H. Brick, M.D.,GCM Radiology.

Introduction

Breast cancer is the most common malignancy in women. Approximately 200,000 women are diagnosed with breast cancer every year, and this is expected to increase to almost one million new cases each year by the year 2000. Currently, approximately 50,000 women die from breast cancer every year.

It has been proven that the chances of survival from breast cancer are markedly improved by early detection, before the cancer has spread. Mammography is the best test currently available to diagnose early breast cancer, and screening mammograms should be obtained in asymptomatic women beginning at age 35 to 40 (although the age to begin screening mammography is still somewhat controversial). Unfortunately, mammography does not diagnose cancer, it only reveals x-ray abnormalities that might represent cancer. Although many mammographic abnormalities are definitely benign, and others are obviously malignant, there are many lesions in which the diagnosis cannot be made with certainty based on the mammographic appearance alone. In order to ensure early detection of cancer, most of these indeterminate lesions require biopsy, even though they frequently turn out to be benign. This is why, in the United States, 75-80% of all breast biopsies are for lesions that are proven to be benign.

Biopsy of non-palpable mammographic abnormalities (lesions which are found on the mammogram but which cannot be felt by your doctor) has traditionally been performed with surgical excision. The abnormality is usually first located by a wire placed during mammographic guided needle localization. The patient is then taken to the operating room where the surrounding tissue is removed. If the lesion is found to be malignant, the patient usually requires a second surgical procedure (lumpectomy or mastectomy) for definitive treatment. Stereotactic breast biopsy is an increasingly popular alternative to excisional biopsy that permits accurate diagnosis of breast lesions without surgery.

Procedure

Stereotactic breast biopsy requires equipment that has been specifically designed for this procedure and medical personnel (physicians and technologists) who have received special training.

During stereotactic breast biopsy, the patient lies prone with the breast suspended through a hole in the table and compressed by a plate. All images obtained during the procedure are digital x-rays (as opposed to traditional mammograms which use x-ray exposed film), and this considerably decreases the x-ray exposure to the breast and permits the images to be viewed on the computer monitor only seconds after exposure (traditional mammograms require 3 minute development in a processor). The first x-ray locates the abnormality in the breast. Then two *stereo* views are obtained, angled 15 degrees on either side of the initial image. The physician then electronically marks the lesion on each of the stereo images. The computer determines how the position of the lesion has changed on each of the stereo views and can calculate the exact location of the lesion in 3-dimensional space.

The patient's skin is cleaned and a local anesthetic is given. A small skin nick is made. The biopsy device is held in a cradle attached to the machine. The tip of the needle is advanced to the exact coordinates of the lesion as calculated by the computer. The stereo images are repeated and the location of the needle tip in the lesion is confirmed.

Multiple biopsies (usually 5 to 10) are then taken, each obtaining a small core of tissue.

The biopsy needle used is a special needle which consists of an inner needle with an elongated trough and an overlying sheath. This is attached to a spring loaded "gun". When the device is fired, the inner needle shoots forward, the trough fills with tissue, and the outer sheath than shoots forward to cut the tissue and secure it in the trough. This occurs in a split second, and the rapid firing yields excellent cores of tissue with minimal discomfort to the patient. At the conclusion of the procedure, the skin nick is simply covered with a dressing (no sutures are required), and the patient is sent home. She is told to avoid strenuous activity for 24 hours, and can usually resume normal activity the next day.

Results

Stereotactic breast biopsy has been shown to be a very accurate procedure. Correlation between stereotactic and excisional biopsy results have been calculated up to 96% in some studies. The accuracy is known to increase at specific institutions as the operators become more experienced. However, the procedure is not perfect. Occasionally, the lesion might not be adequately sampled, or even missed entirely (although it should be noted that lesions can also be missed during excisional biopsy). There are several safeguards in place to decrease the risk that a cancer might be missed:

- Imaging the specimen: When a nodule is biopsied, an image of the breast after the procedure should show multiple defects in the nodule where tissue was removed. If no defects are seen, the lesion can be re-localized and additional biopsies can be obtained. When microcalcifications are biopsied, the tiny cores of tissue obtained should be x-rayed to ensure that they contain calcifications.

- Correlation with pathology: The final pathology needs to be compared with the diagnosis suspected from the mammogram. If the results are inconsistent, if no definite pathologic diagnosis can be made, or if the pathologic findings reveal atypical cells, the patient should then undergo excisional biopsy.

- Close mammographic follow-up: If the lesion is found to be benign, most patients have a repeat mammogram of that breast in 6 months to ensure the stability of the lesion.

The benefits of stereotactic breast biopsy, compared to surgical excisional biopsy, include:

- Accuracy similar to excisional biopsy.
- Decreased patient discomfort and recovery.
- No cosmetic defect of the breast.
- No distortion of the breast tissue that might make interpretation of future mammogram s difficult.
- Decreased cost.

The limitations of stereotactic breast biopsy include: Not all lesions can be biopsied (see "patient selection" below). The lesion is not completely removed (some patients require complete removal for peace of mind). The pathologic diagnosis is occasionally indeterminate and excisional biopsy would still be required.

Patient Selection

Most mammographic abnormalities (nodules or microcalcifications) can be successfully biopsied using the stereotactic technique. If the mammographic appearance suggests a probably benign lesion, stereotactic biopsy can eliminate the need for surgery. If the mammogram suggests a probably malignant lesion, stereotactic biopsy can replace the initial excisional biopsy, confirm the diagnosis, and allow the patient to undergo definitive surgery as a one-step procedure.

However, two types of abnormalities can be difficult to biopsy with the stereotactic technique:

- Vague asymmetric density without a defined mass or nodule.
- Diffuse, scattered microcalcifications.

In these types of lesions, the abnormalities are so diffuse and poorly defined that accurate localization on the stereo images can be difficult.

The best source of advise as to whether a patient is a candidate for this procedure would be a radiologist with experience in both mammography and stereotactic breast biopsy.

Chapter 30

Ultrasound

Contents

Section 30.1

Ultrasound Safety

Reprinted with permission. © 1998 American Institute of
Ultrasound in Medicine.

Your Doctor Has Requested an Examination of one or more
organs using ultrasound. Although you may have heard about ultrasound, or possibly have been examined with ultrasound in the past,
you may still have questions about you examination. The American
Institute of Ultrasound in Medicine (AIUM), an organization of physicians, sonographers, and scientists, has compiled information for
this section to help answer some commonly asked questions.

What Is Ultrasound?

Ultrasound is like ordinary sound except it has a frequency (or
pitch) higher than humans can hear. When sent into the body from a
transducer (probe) resting on the patient's skin, the sound is reflected

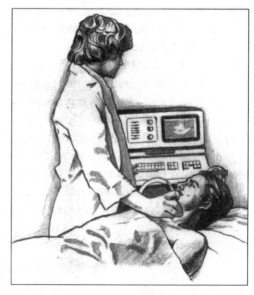

Figure 30.1. *Ultrasound Examination*

off internal structures. The returning echoes are received by the transducer and converted by an electronic instrument into an image on a monitor. These continually changing images can be recorded on videotape or film. Diagnostic ultrasound imaging is commonly called sonography or ultrasonography.

Who Will Perform the Examination?

The examination is usually performed by a specially trained healthcare professional called a sonographer. A series of images will be recorded the sonographer. These images will then be interpreted by a physician. In some cases, you may be examined by a physician to confirm or resolve uncertain findings.

Will It Hurt?

There is no pain involved in an ultrasound examination. You may experience some pressure discomfort when certain areas of the body are scanned. A gel is applied over the area to be examined and the transducer is placed on the skin or, for certain examinations, inserted into the vagina or rectum. The gel may feel cool. It is water-soluble and wipes off easily, but it is a good idea to wear clothing that is easily washable.

When and How Is Ultrasound Used?

There are many medical indications for using diagnostic ultrasound. Pregnancy is probably the most widely recognized reason to have a sonogram. There are, however, many other organs in the body that can be examined with ultrasound. The liver, gallbladder, kidneys, spleen, thyroid, breast, ovaries, uterus, and prostate are a few examples.

Is Ultrasound Safe?

There are no know harmful effects associated with the medical use of sonography. Widespread clinical use of diagnostic ultrasound for many years has not revealed any harmful effects. Studies in humans have revealed no direct link between the use of diagnostic ultrasound and any adverse outcome. Although the possibility exists that biological effects may be identified in the future, current information indicates that the benefits to patients far outweigh the risks, if any.

The AIUM has a Bioeffects Committee that meets regularly to consider safety issues and evaluate reports dealing with bioeffects and the safety of ultrasound.

A United States Food and Drug Administration (FDA) report states that ultrasound has been used for many years with no obvious detrimental effects. Nevertheless, current evidence is considered insufficient to justify an unqualified acceptance of ultrasound safety. The FDA report recommends that ultrasound be used only when a diagnostic benefit is likely, and the exposure should be limited to that required to produce the needed information.

The World Health Organization (WHO) of the United Nations, in its report on ultrasound, recommends prudence in exposure to human subjects but agrees that benefits outweigh any presumed risks. The WHO report states that patients should be examined with ultrasound only for valid clinical reasons.

In conclusion, based on experimental and epidemiological data, there is presently no identified risk associated with diagnostic ultrasound. However, a prudent and conservative approach is recommended in which diagnostic ultrasound is to be used only for medical benefit and with minimal exposure.

Figure 30.2. Ultrasound Image of Fetus.

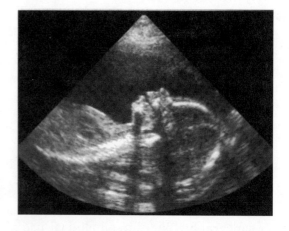

Section 30.2

Abdomen Ultrasound

Why Should I Have an Ultrasound Exam?

In an abdominal examination, ultrasound produces images of the major organs including the liver, gallbladder, pancreas, spleen, kidneys, and large blood vessels.

There are many reasons for examining the abdomen with ultrasound. Among the more common reasons:

- To look for causes of upper abdominal pain which may be related to problem in the liver, gallbladder, pancreas, or kidneys,
- To detect gallstones,
- To determine abnormalities of the liver or spleen,
- To evaluate the kidneys for blockage, or
- To look for enlargements (aneurysms) and other abnormalities of abdominal blood vessels.

Ultrasound will not always be able to provide all the information your doctor requires, in these cases, additional studies may be required.

Are There Any Special Preparations for the Exam?

If the gallbladder is to be examined, you should have nothing to eat or drink except water six hours before the exam. This is because most food and drink cause the gallbladder to contract preventing adequate examination with ultrasound.

Will It Hurt?

There is no pain involved in an ultrasound examination of your abdomen. A gel is applied to your abdomen and the instrument is then placed on the skin surface to provide better contact between the transducer and the skin. This gel may feel cool and, even though it wipes off easily, it is a good idea to wear clothing that is easily washable.

How Long Will It Take?

The length of time for the examination will vary depending on the specific reasons for your examination. For some studies, such as examination of the gallbladder for stones, the study may require only 5–15minute. But, for a complete study of all the abdominal organs, 30 minutes or more may be required.

Who Will Perform the Exam?

In most cases, you will be examined by a sonographer specially trained in ultrasound. A series of images will be recorded by the sonographer. These images will then be interpreted by a physician. In some cases, you also will be examined by a physician to confirm or resolve uncertain findings.

What Are the Limitations of the Exam?

Because bone weakens sound waves, ultrasound cannot be used to examine the bones surrounding your abdomen, such as your ribs. Also, because sound is weakened as it passed through layers of tissue, results from patients who are obese are not of the same quality as those who are thin. In addition, ultrasound cannot image through gas. Thus, bowel gas may limit visualization of some structures of interest.

How Much Does the Exam Cost?

The price of an ultrasound examination varies widely depending on the reason for the exam and the complexity of the equipment used. Generally, insurance companies will help cover the cost of ultrasound examinations.

Section 30.3

Breast Ultrasound

Why Do I Need a Breast Ultrasound Examination?

Information obtained from a breast physical examination alone may be incomplete. Breast ultrasonography, when used in conjunction with a physical exam and/or mammography, can identify cysts, tumors, abscesses, lymph nodes, and very dense breast tissue. In some cases, tissue sample (biopsy) of a suspicious area is required to make a specific diagnosis. If this is needed, ultrasonography can be used to guide the needle biopsy without the need for surgery. Aspiration of breast cysts is commonly performed using ultrasound guidance.

How is Breast Ultrasonography Performed?

You will be asked to remove your top and bra. A paper or cloth gown will be given to you to cover yourself. You will be instructed to lie or sit on an examining table. A gel will be placed on your skin and a transducer (scanner) will be moved over the area to be examined. The

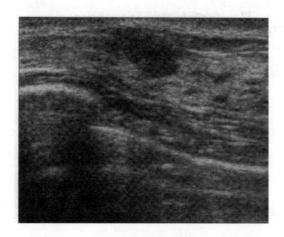

Figure30.3. Ultrasound Image of Breast Tissue.

223

examiner may feel the area for any lumps while performing the examination. No pain is involved in this type of examination. The images obtained are seen on a monitor or stored on film or videotape.

Who Will Do the Examination?

The examination is usually performed by a specially trained healthcare professional called a sonographer or by a doctor trained in ultrasonography. The images obtained from the exam will be interpreted by a physician. A cyst aspiration or biopsy may be recommended, using ultrasound as a guide.

What Are the Limitations of this Examination?

Results of the examination may vary depending on the type of breast tissue you have. In any case, if a suspicious area noted on mammography cannot be seen with ultrasound, it should be evaluated by other means.

Section 30.4

Doppler Ultrasound

Reprinted with permission. © 1992, reviewed 1995, American Institute of Ultrasound in Medicine.

You Have Just Been Sent for an Ultrasound Study of your blood vessels using Doppler ultrasound. Although you may have heard about ultrasound before, or possibly have been examined with ultrasound in the past, you still may have questions about your examination. The American Institute of Ultrasound in Medicine, an organization of physicians, sonographers and scientists, has compiled these questions and answers to explain how ultrasound works.

What Is Doppler?

Doppler ultrasound is a special form of ultrasound. With Doppler ultrasound, it is possible to see the structures inside the body and evaluate blood flow at the same time. In order to do this, the machine uses ultrasound in two ways. One method of evaluation gives us information about the structures within the body and the other method tells us about blood flow. In the first method, the returning echoes are processed by the machine and a picture is made of the area beneath the scanner. The walls of your blood vessels, for example, are seen this way. On the other hand, if sound waves strike moving objects (like the red blood cells), the frequency of the sound is changed. This process is similar to the change in the pitch of an ambulance siren as it passes the listener. The doctor, vascular technologist, or sonographer performing the scan can display this change in frequency in several ways to evaluate blood flow within the body. An audible sound may be used of the flow may be shown as a graph or color display.

Why Should I Have a Doppler Ultrasound Exam?

A doppler ultrasound exam gives your physician a great deal of information about your blood vessels and about the way blood is passing through them. Doppler ultrasound is particularly well suited to evaluating problems within the veins and arteries. Because we have blood vessels throughout the body, Doppler may be used almost anywhere. One of the most common uses of Doppler ultrasound, however, is in the neck to look at carotid arteries. These vessels supply large amounts of blood to the brain and may become blocked. Blockage can lead to stroke.

In the heart, Doppler can tell about the flow of blood and whether it is directed correctly. In the abdomen, Doppler can help evaluate

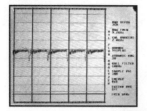

Figure 30.4. Doppler Graph and Image.

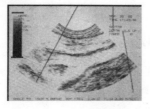

blood flow to the liver and many other abdominal organs. Doppler also is used to evaluate blood flow in the legs and may be helpful in identifying blockages in the arteries and clots in the veins.

Will It Hurt? Are There Any Special Preparations for the Exam?

There is no pain involved in an ultrasound examination and for most Doppler exams, no preparation is necessary. Your doctor may ask you to refrain from eating the morning of the exam if the scan involves the upper abdomen. A gel is applied to your skin and the instrument is then placed on the area to be examined. This gel may feel cool and, even though it wipes off easily, it is a good idea to wear clothing that is easily washable.

What Can I Expect during the Exam?

The pictures made by the returning echoes are displayed on one or more small TV screens which are studied by the specialist performing the scan. In addition, returning sound waves which have been reflected by moving blood can be heard by means of speakers in the instrument. The sounds may be similar to the sound of wind blowing through the trees.

How Long Will It Take?

The average Doppler ultrasound exam takes 30–60 minutes. The length of the exam is dependent upon a number of factors including the portion of the body to be examined and the complexity of the anatomy. With atherosclerosis, or hardening of the arteries, the vessels may be very difficult to evaluate and may require more scanning time.

Who Will Perform the Exam?

Doppler ultrasound may be performed by your physician, a vascular technologist, or a sonographer. The exam will be interpreted by a physician.

Will I Need More Than One Exam?

In many cases, follow-up exams are necessary to evaluate progression of your condition or response to therapy.

How Much Does the Exam Cost?

The price of an ultrasound examination varies widely depending on the reason for the exam and the complexity of the equipment used. Generally, insurance companies will help cover the cost of the examination.

Section 30.5

Echocardiogram and Transesophageal Echocardiogram (TEE)

"Cardiovascular Center Diagnostic Tests," © 1998 Mt. Sinai School of Medicine.

Echocardiogram

An echocardiogram is a sophisticated diagnostic test that employs ultrasound (high-frequency sound waves) to obtain moving and still pictures of your heart.

A transducer wand is a small hand-held device used to produce the sound waves and receive the echoes as they "bounce" off the heart and reflect as images on a screen. The pictures appear on a television screen, but the process doesn't involve exposure to radiation.

An echocardiography examination consists of three elements: M-mode, two-dimensional imaging and Doppler imaging.

M-mode echocardiography is a single beam directed toward the heart. It is most useful in visualizing the left side of the heart. Two-dimensional echocardiograms produce a real-time motion picture of your heart, which is displayed in different cross-sections, depending on the angle of the transducer. Most of the procedure consists of two-dimensional echocardiography. Doppler echocardiography measures the velocity of blood flow and shows the turbulence of blood flowing through the heart.

Why Has My Doctor Ordered an Echocardiogram for Me?

Echocardiography is considered one of the most powerful diagnostic tools in cardiology. Echocardiograms provide both functional and anatomic information about your heart.

227

Echocardiograms can show your physician how well your heart valves are working, how well your heart muscle is moving and how your blood is flowing. They can measure the dimensions of the four chambers of the heart and provide information about your arteries. Echocardiograms can also identify blood clots within the heart chambers.

You might have complained to your physician of shortness of breath, chest pain or other symptoms. Perhaps you had no symptoms, but upon examination, he detected an abnormal or unexpected heart sound called a "murmur," which is often caused by an abnormal pattern of blood flow in the heart. Your doctor could order an echocardiogram to help find the cause of your symptoms.

You might have undergone other diagnostic tests, such as an exercise tolerance test. Based on the results of those tests, your physician has decided that additional information is needed to determine your course of treatment. Echocardiograms can provide that information.

Echocardiograms help doctors distinguish between two or more ailments that have similar symptoms and which may produce similar results on other diagnostic tests.

Finally, an echocardiogram is a safe and painless test. Having this procedure may enable you to avoid more risky, invasive diagnostic procedures.

What Preparations Should I Make before the Echocardiogram?

You will have to undress from the waist up and put on a short hospital gown. If you are a woman, wear a two-piece outfit that fastens in the front.

If you are scheduling an exercise stress test for the same day as the echocardiogram, make sure you have the exercise test after the echocardiogram, or at least two to three hours before. This is to guarantee that the echocardiogram is performed under "at rest" conditions.

Where Are Echocardiograms Performed?

Echocardiograms may be performed in a hospital, test center, or doctor's office.

What Happens during the Echocardiogram?

The operator of the test (usually a trained technician or a physician) will explain the procedure to you and answer your questions.

You will take this test lying down.

The operator will clean three areas on your chest with alcohol on gauze. It may feel a little cool. Then he will place electrodes on these spots, and attach them by leads to an electrocardiogram machine. This machine monitors your heart rhythm throughout the test.

The operator will put conductive gel on your chest. This gel will help the transducer pick up signal. The gel will feel a little cool at first. Then the operator will pick up the transducer. This device looks like a wand or a microphone. The transducer generates and receives the sound signals. The operator will put the transducer on your chest, directly above the structures your doctor wants to visualize. He will press firmly as he moves the transducer in arcs across your chest. This does not hurt.

You may be asked to participate by inhaling, exhaling or holding your breath at various times during the test. For the remainder of the time, you should remain still.

The operator will make moving recordings of various views of your heart, on a video cassette recorder and will also select "freeze" frames for the final report.

How Long Does the Procedure Take?

An echocardiogram may take up to approximately 45 minutes to perform. Allow additional time for check-in.

What Is a Transesophageal Echocardiogram?

Although regular echocardiograms (transthoracic cardiograms), may be performed on everyone, clear pictures may be obtained from only 95 percent of the population. People who have chronic obstructive pulmonary disease (COPD), who have barrel-shaped chests or who are obese, may provide unclear echocardiograms that are of little diagnostic value.

Transesophageal echocardiography (TEE) is a diagnostic ultrasound technique that is very similar to the echocardiogram, but it is one in which images of the heart are acquired from inside the esophagus and stomach rather than from the chest wall.

A small probe will be placed in your esophagus, to enable the operator to visualize your heart and aorta. The esophagus is situated next to the heart and aorta. This proximity allows for the use of a higher frequency transducer. Also, there is no obstruction by air-filled lungs. TEE takes pictures of the heart from behind, which allows excellent resolution of other structures. As a result of these factors, transesophageal provides clearer imaging than a regular echocardiogram.

Some people who have undergone regular echocardiograms also require an esophageal echocardiogram to obtain specific additional information.

Does TEE Involve Any Risks?

Although TEE is considered an invasive procedure, the risk of complications is low. Although the procedure is generally safe, the insertion and manipulation of the TEE probe can result in a number of complications. Some of these are dental injuries or bleeding, injuries to the structures inside your neck and throat, irregular heartbeats (arrhythmias), and respiratory distress. These events are rare.

What Preparations Should I Make for the TEE?

You should fast for at least four hours before the procedure to prevent vomiting during the procedure. You may receive mild sedation during the procedure, and should have someone with you to drive you home afterward.

Discuss your medications with your physician in advance. She may ask you to skip some of them on the day of the procedure.

What Happens during the TEE?

The operator will ask you to remove all oral prostheses and dentures. Then the operator will numb your throat with a local anesthetic spray. In some cases, you may also gargle with an anesthetic for an additional numbing effect.

Once the operator is satisfied that it is OK to proceed, an intravenous line (IV) will be started. Usually, you will be given a mild sedative through the IV line. Your heart rate and blood pressure will also be monitored throughout the procedure.

A small flexible tube (probe) is inserted down your throat. The probe is approximately the diameter of a man's fifth finger.

The operator will then insert a bite block between your teeth to protect the probe.

You will be asked to swallow to facilitate the insertion of the probe. As you swallow, the probe is gently, but firmly, advanced into the esophagus. You may feel uncomfortable during the insertion process.

It is not uncommon to gag because gagging is a normal reflexive re-action to having a foreign object placed in your throat. Because of this, it may take a few tries before the probe is fully inserted, but once it is in place, you should feel only a small sensation of its presence and no pain.

On the end of the probe is a device that transmits and receives the ultrasonic beam, which produces images to create a two-dimensional echocardiogram of your heart. The operator will move the probe to obtain different pictures of your heart.

Once you are stable, the probe will be removed and all monitoring equipment will be disconnected.

What Happens after the Procedure?

You will rest after the procedure, until the sedation has worn off. Your vital signs will be monitored.

You may experience a sore throat and mild difficulty in swallow-ing following the procedure. These reactions are common and rarely last longer than 24 hours.

What Happens Next?

Your doctor will discuss the results of the test with you. He will make recommendations as to further testing (if necessary), and the possible courses of treatment.

Section 30.6

Gynecology Ultrasound

Why Might I Have a Pelvic Ultrasound Exam?

Information obtained from a manual gynecological exam alone may
be incomplete. With pelvic sonograms, anatomy is visualized and may
help explain findings from a manual exam or present additional information.

How Is Pelvic Sonography Performed?

There are two main methods of performing pelvic ultrasound: abdominal (transabdominal) and vaginal (transvaginal, endovaginal).
The same principles of high frequency sound previously described
apply in each technique.

Abdominal or transabdominal ultrasound is performed by a
sonographer or physician who places a transducer on the surface of
the abdomen. A small amount of gel is used on the skin to ensure good

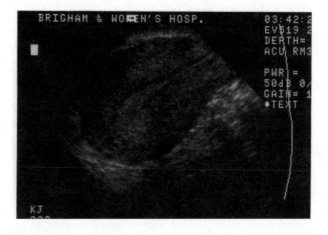

Figure 30.5.
Normal Uterus
by Transvaginal
Scanning.

transducer contact. The transducer slides over the skin, sending and receiving ultrasonic pulses which are then converted into images on a television screen.

Vaginal (transvaginal, endovaginal) sonography involves the insertion of a transducer into the vagina. The tip of the transducer may be circular or oblong but is usually smaller than the standard speculum used when obtaining a routine Pap smear. A protective cover is placed over the transducer, which is then lubricated with a small amount of gel. The transducer is inserted in the vagina either by the physician or sonographer, or you may be asked to insert it as you would a tampon.

How Long Will the Examination Take?

The length of time will vary depending on how easily the necessary information is obtained.

Are There Any Special Preparations?

Abdominal scanning is usually done with the patient lying flat on an examination table. Garments are elevated or pulled down to expose the lower abdomen to the pubic bone. Abdominal scanning may require a full bladder, which provides a "window" through which the pelvic organs may be seen. Therefore you may be asked to drink a large quantity of water and/or refrain from urinating just prior to the examination.

Preparations for vaginal scanning are similar to those for a routine manual pelvic examination. You must disrobe from the waist down. You will need to assume a position similar to the one used for a Pap smear. Either your legs are placed in stirrups or your buttocks elevated by a thick cushion. Your bladder should be nearly or completely empty.

Will I Have an Abdominal or Vaginal Ultrasound Exam (or Both)?

This will depend on the reason the exam has been requested. In some instances, it may only be necessary to perform a pelvic sonogram transabdominally (possibly with a full bladder). In other cases, a vaginal exam alone will be adequate. In still other cases, both transabdominal and transvaginal scans will be necessary.

The decision as to which types of scans are necessary will be made by the examiner. Therefore it makes good sense to arrive for the ultrasound exam with the bladder relatively full.

Is One Exam Preferable to the Other?

Each has its advantages. The transabdominal approach offers a panoramic view of the entire pelvis. This shows where one internal structure is in relation to another. Improved visualization may be achieved using the vaginal approach, since the transducer is brought closer to the area being examined. Thus, it can be very helpful in seeing the fetal heart beat in an early pregnancy, evaluating the uterus, or measuring a cyst in an ovary. The physician or sonographer performing your sonogram will decide whether one or a combination of approaches is best for your particular case.

Is Vaginal Sonography Painful or Harmful?

Although the examination is often performed to look for a cause of pelvic pain, the sonogram itself should not be painful or significantly increase your discomfort. A vaginal sonogram is usually more comfortable than a manual examination.

If you have been experiencing vaginal bleeding, whether pregnant or not, a careful vaginal sonogram will not be harmful and may be helpful in determining the cause of the bleeding.

What Is Doppler Ultrasound?

Doppler ultrasound is a special form of ultrasound. This type of ultrasound is useful in evaluating the blood flow to the pelvic organs. The doctor, vascular technologist, or sonographer performing the scan can display this information in several ways. An audible sound may be used, or the blood flow may be shown as a graphic or color display. It is not painful. The decision to use Doppler will frequently be made at the time of the exam.

Section 30.7

Prostate Ultrasound

Your Doctor Has Requested an Ultrasound Examination of Your Prostate.

The American Institute of Ultrasound in Medicine (AIUM), an organization of physicians, sonographers, and scientists, has compiled information for this chapter to help explain the examination you will receive.

Why Should I Have an Ultrasound of the Prostate?

Many diseases involve the prostate gland, including infection, hypertrophy (enlargement), and cancer. Ultrasound images are used in conjunction with physical examination to localize and identify these disease processes. Specific diagnosis often requires obtaining a tissue sample (biopsy) of a suspicious area. If a biopsy is needed, ultrasound can guide the biopsy needle into the lesion.

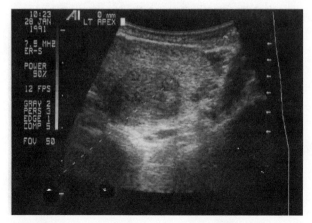

Figure 30.6. Ultrasound image of prostate.

How Is the Examination Sonography Performed?

Because the prostate gland is located immediately in front of the rectum, the transducer is lubricated and placed into the rectum so the sound will only be required to travel a short distance. The image can be obtained from different orientations to get the best view of the prostate gland. Pictures are recorded on film, and occasionally a videotape is taken of the examination as well. If a suspicious lesion is identified by ultrasound or rectal examination, an ultrasound-guided biopsy may be performed. This is accomplished by advancing a needle into the prostate gland while watching with ultrasound. A small amount of tissue is taken for microscopic examination.

Who Should Do the Exam?

The exam may be performed by a physician, usually a radiologist or urologist, or a sonographer. When a sonographer performs the examination, the study will be interpreted by a physician. The findings will be reported to your referring doctor.

Is Specific Preparation Required?

For some patients, an enema is used as a routine preparation for ultrasound of the prostate. If a biopsy is required, you may be given antibiotics by mouth or by injection before and after the procedure. Be sure to inform your doctor of any medications you are currently taking and if you are allergic to any medications.

Will It Hurt?

If no biopsy is required, ultrasound examination of the prostate is similar in discomfort to a rectal examination performed by your doctor. If a biopsy is performed, additional discomfort, due to the needle insertion, is usually minimal because the rectal wall is relatively insensitive in the region of the prostate.

How Long Will It Take?

The amount of time will vary depending on the reason for your examination, the need for biopsy, and how your prostate appears on the ultrasound. The ultrasound scan takes less that 20 minutes to perform, while the procedure may take up 45 minutes if biopsy is required.

How Will I Feel after the Examination?

As after any rectal examination you may experience some mucous discharge or minimal bleeding from your rectum, especially if you have hemorrhoids. In the case of biopsy, many patients will have a small amount of blood in the stool, urine, or semen after the procedure.

—*Contributions from Fred Lee, M.D., FACR, Fred Lee, Jr., M.D., and Deborah J. Rubens, M.D. The second edition is updated with contributions from the members of the Informational Media Committee of the American Institute of Ultrasound in Medicine.*

Chapter 31

CAT Scan/CT Scan

Contents

Section 31.1

History and Description

"CT How It Works," reprinted with permission.
© 1997 Steven H. Brick, M.D

Introduction

In 1972, G.N. Hounsfield, a senior research scientist in Middlesex, England announced the invention of a revolutionary imaging technique that he called computed axial transverse scanning. He presented a cross-sectional image of the head that revealed the internal structures of the brain in a manner previously only seen at surgery or autopsy. Pathologic processes such as blood clots, tumors, and strokes could be easily seen. Structures inside the human body that had never been imaged before could now be visualized.

In the 25 years since Dr. Hounsfield's announcement, his discovery has completely revolutionized the practice of medicine. The name has changed; first to computed axial tomography (CAT), and now to computed tomography (CT). Although the first CT scanners could only image the head, they now have primary roles in diagnosing disorders of the chest, abdomen, and pelvis. The original scanners also took several minutes to acquire a single slice through the brain. The newest scanners can now image the entire body in 1 to 2 minutes.

Equipment

The basic principle behind CT is that the internal structure of an object can be reconstructed from multiple projections of the object. The patient lies on the table within the CT gantry, which is shaped like a giant donut. During each slice acquisition, an x-ray tube circling the patient produces an x-ray beam that passes through the patient and is absorbed by a ring of detectors surrounding the patient. The intensity of the x-ray beam that reaches the detectors is dependent on the absorption characteristics of the tissues it passes through. Since the beam is moving around the patient, each tissue will be exposed from multiple directions. Using a process called Fourier analysis, the computer uses the information obtained from the different amounts of x-ray absorption to reconstruct the density and position of the different structures contained within each slice.

Spiral CT

In standard CT, each revolution of the x-ray tube around the patient produces a single slice that demonstrates the tissue that was traversed by the x-ray beam during that exposure. When imaging the body (i.e. the chest or abdomen), the patient is instructed to hold their breath during the exposure in order to minimize blurring of the image by motion. This exposure usually takes a few seconds. After the exposure, the table moves a small amount so that the next continuous slice of tissue can be exposed. The delay between slices usually takes about 5 to 10 seconds. This process is repeated numerous times until the full extent of the portion of the body being studied is imaged.

The most significant advance in CT technology in the past few years has been the development of spiral (or helical) CT. During spiral CT, the x-ray tube rotates continuously as the patient is smoothly moved through the x-ray scan field. Unlike the separate data sets produces for each individual slice in standard CT, spiral CT produces one continuous volume set of data for the entire region scanned.

Spiral CT has several advantages over standard CT:

- Speed: Since the patient is moving continuously through the scanner, the duration of the exam is markedly shortened. The entire chest or abdomen can be scanned in 30 seconds, usually during a single breath-hold.

- Improved detection of small lesions: In standard CT, the patient holds their breath for a slice acquisition, then breathes, then holds their breath again for the next slice. If they hold their breath slightly differently for each slice, small lesions may fall out of the plane of each contiguous slice and therefore may be missed. Since spiral CT can be performed during a single breath-hold, contiguous slices are truly contiguous. Also, since a volume of data is obtained, the spacing of the acquired slices can be manipulated after the scan is completed. This allows detected lesions to be placed in the middle of the slice, which creates a more accurate image of the lesion.

241

- Improved contrast enhancement: Intravenous contrast is often injected during the CT scan (see below). Since spiral CT can image a region of interest in such a short period of time, the injection of intravenous contrast can be timed to ensure optimal contrast enhancement and improved evaluation of various organs and blood vessels.

- Image reconstruction and manipulation: The volume of data obtained through spiral CT can be manipulated in many fascinating ways by powerful computers connected to the scanner. The transverse images can be reconstructed in any plane. 3-dimensional images can be formed and moved into any position. A surface view of the body can be created, and then skin, muscles, and overlying organs can be stripped away. Contrast enhanced vessels can be isolated and converted into CT angiograms.

Intravenous Contrast

Many patients who undergo CT will receive intravenous contrast. Radiographic intravenous contrast materials all contain iodinated compounds which absorb x-rays. This causes the density of organs or vessels that contain the contrast to increase during the radiographic exam. The contrast used for CT is similar to that used for intravenous pyelography (IVP) and angiography. Intravenous contrast used during CT has two main purposes:

- Vascular enhancement: The enhancement of vessels allow them to be more easily differentiated from adjacent, non-enhancing structures or masses.

- Organ enhancement: Organs such as the liver, pancreas, and kidney will enhance more than tumors in those organs and this makes the tumors easier to identify.

Oral Contrast

Most CT's of the abdomen and pelvis are also performed with oral contrast. This usually consists of a dilute barium solution. Depending on the exam, the patient will drink 1 or 2 bottles of the contrast before the study begins. The oral contrast markedly increases the density of the gastrointestinal tract and allows improved differentiation between bowel and tumors, enlarged lymph nodes, and abscesses.

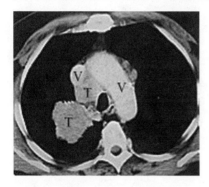

Figure 31.1. Chest CT with Tumor. In this chest CT, the enhancing vessels (V) can be easily separated from the adjacent tumor (T).

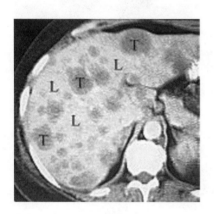

Figure 31.2. Liver CT with Tumor. In the CT of the liver the multiple liver tumors (T) are easily seen because they enhance less than the surrounding normal liver (L).

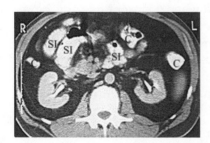

Figure 31.3. CT of the Abdomen. The CT of the abdomen shows oral contrast in the small intestine (SI) and colon (C).

243

Image Orientation

Most CT's are displayed in the axial, or transverse plane. Imagine the patient is lying on their back, and then sliced by a guillotine. The slice is then viewed as if you are standing at their feet, looking up towards the head. Figure 31.4 displays the correct locations on the patient. Anterior refers to the front of the patient, posterior refers to the back.

Figure 31.4. *Tranverse Plane CT*

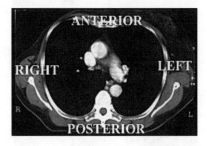

Section 31.2

CT of the Chest

Reprinted with permission. © 1997 Steven H. Brick, M.D.

Introduction

The most frequently performed radiologic exam remains the chest x-ray. It is usually the first test ordered when a patient has any symptoms suggestive of chest disease. However, chest CT has become an essential component in the evaluation of chest disease, both by providing improved characterization of an abnormality seen on chest x-ray, and by permitting visualization of pathologic processes that cannot be detected by chest x-ray. Along with the abdomen, the chest is the most frequent body part imaged by CT in today's medical practice.

Normal Anatomy

CT provides high resolution images of both the lungs and the mediastinum (the central portion of the chest that contains the heart, the large blood vessels going to and from the heart and lungs, the esophagus, the trachea [i.e. windpipe], and lymph nodes). In all CT exams, the image of each slice of tissue is displayed in two sets of "windows". These "windows" present the same data with two different ranges of gray scale, and this allows tissues of markedly different densities to be viewed. With the "mediastinal window" (left), the vascular structures, fat, and lymph nodes in the mediastinum can be differentiated, but the lungs appear mostly black. With the "lung window" (right), the fine details of the lung tissue can be seen, but the mediastinum is mostly white. These images represent a single slice of data, displayed in two different formats.

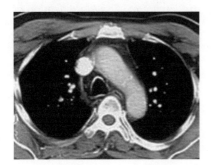 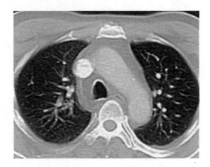

Figure 31.5. Normal CTs of the Chest

Lung Cancer

Lung cancer (also known as bronchogenic carcinoma) remains the most common fatal malignancy in males, and is one of the most common in females. Most lung cancer is easily identified by chest x-ray. However, CT plays a vital role in the management of the lung cancer patient, including:

- Confirmation of a possible abnormality seen on chest x-ray.

- Staging the malignancy (determining how advanced the tumor is) by detection of enlarged lymph nodes (due to spread of the tumor along lymphatic channels), mediastinal or chest wall invasion by the tumor, or additional lesions in the lungs.

- Accurate evaluation of change in size during treatment.

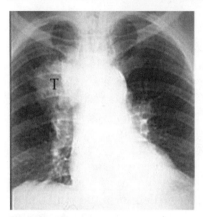

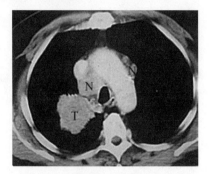

Figure 31.6. Chest X-ray. The chest x-ray reveals an obvious tumor (T) in the right upper lobe.

Figure 31.7. Chest CT. The chest CT better delineates the margins of the tumor (T) and also reveals enlarged lymph nodes (N) from spread of tumor to the mediastinum. The identification of mediastinal metastases helps avoid unnecessary surgery since its presence indicates the patient is not a candidate for surgical resection of the main lung tumor.

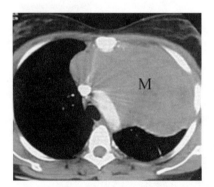

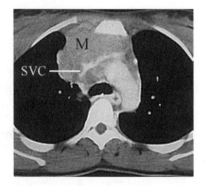

Figure 31.8. Lymphoma Confirmation. The patient on the left has a huge mediastinal mass (M) diagnosed as lymphoma. The patient on the right also has lymphoma, but presented with symptoms of arm and neck swelling due to marked compression of the large veins that return blood from the arms, neck, and head to the heart (one of these vessels is the superior vena cava, or SVC).

Lymphoma

Lymphoma is a type of cancer that arises in the lymph nodes in the body. In the chest, the involved lymph nodes are usually located in the mediastinum, near the trachea and large vessels flowing to and from the heart and lungs. Patients with relatively mild symptoms can frequently present with striking chest x-ray abnormalities. CT is used to confirm the cause of the mediastinal abnormality on CXR, delineate the full extent of tumor, and evaluate complications. CT of the abdomen and pelvis are often performed to stage the tumor and evaluate for involved lymph nodes below the diaphragm.

Pulmonary Metastases

Metastases to the lung (spread of cancer to the lungs from tumors elsewhere in the body) occur in approximately 30% of all cases of cancer, and represent the only site of distant spread in half of those cases. The presence of metastatic disease obviously has a profound effect on the treatment options and life expectancy of cancer patients. Although many lung nodules are detected by chest x-ray, pulmonary metastases are frequently small and can be difficult to identify. CT is considerably more sensitive and it is not uncommon to see multiple lesions on chest CT when the chest x-ray is negative.

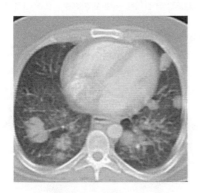

Figure 31.9. Pulmonary Metastases. Typical pulmonary metastases are seen in this patient with colon cancer. Multiple smooth, round nodules of various sizes are seen in both lungs.

Pneumonia

Pneumonia remains a chest x-ray diagnosis and most patients never require CT. However, CT is helpful in some cases when the cause of the chest x-ray findings is not obvious. CT also can provide additional information if there is concern that the pneumonia might be due to a central obstruction (see next section on lobar collapse).

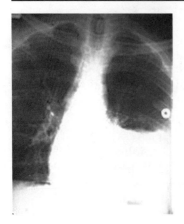
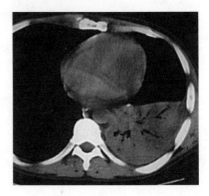

Figure 31.10. X-ray and CT of Pneumonia. This chest x-ray (left) revealed very dense consolidation of the left lung base, and it was uncertain whether this represented pneumonia, pleural effusion (fluid in the space around the lung), tumor, or some combination. The chest CT (right) revealed a very dense pneumonia in the left lower lobe secondary to pneumonia. Note the dark, branching structures called air-bronchograms, which represent air-filled bronchi (branches of the trachea that carry air in and out of the lungs) surrounded by lung tissue completely filled with infected fluid.

Although very rare, a severe complication of pneumonia is the development of a lung abscess. This most frequently occurs as a result of acute staphylococcal pneumonia. CT reveals a large fluid-filled cavity in the lung which develops an air-fluid level when it forms a communication with the bronchial tree. The case below, shown with mediastinal (left) and lung (right) windows, shows the typical appearance of an abscess in the right lower lobe (although the organism in this case was not staphylococcus).

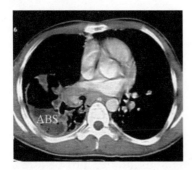
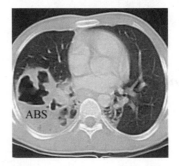

Figure 31.11. Abscess in Right Lower Lobe

Collapsed Lung

Chest x-ray is usually sufficient to diagnose the presence of collapse of a portion of the lung. However, as with pneumonia, chest CT helps to clarify confusing chest x-ray findings and can also demonstrate abnormalities that can cause obstruction of the airways which then leads to collapse (e.g. tumor, enlarged lymph nodes, or, impacted secretions).

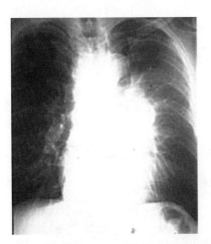
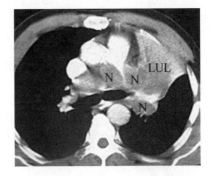

Figure 31.12. X-ray and CT of Collapsed Lung. In this case, chest x-ray shows ill-defined, increased density in the mid left lung field with mediastinal and hilar enlargement (the central, white structures between the darker lungs). CT confirmed that this represented complete collapse of the left upper lobe (LUL) secondary to multiple enlarged lymph nodes (N) in this patient with mediastinal and hilar metastases from lung cancer.

Aortic Dissection

The aorta is the large artery that leaves the heart and carries blood to the entire body. The ascending aorta travels upward in the chest and gives off arteries to the arms, neck, and head. The aorta then turns downward as the descending aorta to supply the rest of the body. If the aorta is diseased, and/or blood pressure is high, a tear can develop in the inner lining of the aorta and blood can dissect and flow between the inner and outer layers of the vessel. This is called an aortic dissection. The patient often presents with severe, "tearing" chest pain which radiates to the back. This is frequently a life-threatening condition which requires rapid diagnosis so that appropriate treatment can be started immediately.

249

Both CT and MRI can be used as a quick, non-invasive diagnostic procedure in the evaluation of this disorder. CT is probably used more frequently since it is often easier to obtain on short notice, is less susceptible to artifacts from patient motion or arrhythmias, and allows easier monitoring of critically ill patients. The main criteria for the CT diagnosis of an aortic dissection is the visualization of contrast enhancement in both the true lumen (the normal path of blood flowing through the artery) and the false lumen (the new path created by the blood flowing between the inner and outer lining of the artery). CT also can determine whether the dissection involves the ascending aorta (Type A—the more dangerous type which usually requires surgical repair), or is limited to the descending aorta (Type B—often doesn't require surgery and is instead treated by control of the patient's high blood pressure).

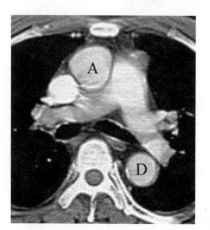 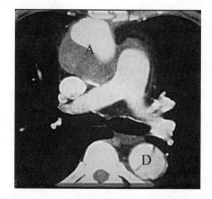

Figure 31.13. Normal and Dissected Aortas. This image on the left shows the normal appearance of the ascending (A) and descending (D) aorta. The patient on the right has a Type A aortic dissection. In the ascending aorta (A), there is normal enhancement of the true lumen and low density, non-enhancing clotted blood in the false lumen. In the descending aorta (D), there is flow in both the true and false lumens, and this outlines the thin flap of tissue that separates the two lumens.

Pulmonary Embolism

Pulmonary embolism is caused by blood clots which form in the deep veins of the legs or pelvis breaking off, flowing completely through the heart, and lodging in the arteries carrying blood from the heart to the lungs. If the clot is big enough, the sudden blockage of blood flow can be fatal. Because the symptoms of chest pain and shortness of breath can be seen in many different disorders, this remains a condition that can be difficult to diagnose clinically. However, rapid diagnosis is important so that treatment with blood thinners can be quickly started.

Most patients with suspected PE are still initially imaged with nuclear medicine lung scan which evaluates the uptake of radioactive materials by the lungs. Unfortunately, this test can be inaccurate. Pulmonary angiography is the most accurate test, but is invasive and carries some risks. The improved vascular enhancement seen with spiral CT has increased its role in the diagnosis of pulmonary emboli, since clots in central pulmonary vessels can frequently be seen. Some centers now feel that the combination of spiral CT to detect clots in the lungs, combined with venous ultrasound of the lower extremities to detect clots in the legs, is the best way to study patients with these disorders and to determine which patients require treatment with blood thinners.

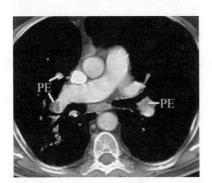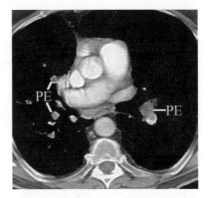

Figure 31.14. *Pulmonary Emboli in Lung Arteries. In this patient with shortness of breath, pulmonary emboli (PE) are seen in multiple pulmonary arteries in both lungs.*

Section 31.3.

CT of the Abdomen

Reprinted with permission. © 1997 Steven H. Brick, M.D.

The development of Computed Tomography (CT) markedly altered the traditional medical approach to the diagnosis of disorders of the abdomen. CT permitted visualization of the abdominal organs with clarity that had been unimaginable in the past and which has not been surpassed since. This non-invasive test now provides such high resolution and accurate images that "exploratory" surgery is now only very rarely performed. CT now plays a critical role in the diagnosis and management of a wide variety of patients throughout the hospital, including the oncology units, the medical and surgical floors, and the emergency room. The ease of CT also allows patients to undergo extensive diagnostic evaluations without requiring hospitalization. CT of the abdomen also permits evaluation of multiple organ systems with a single test, including the liver and biliary tree, spleen, pancreas, adrenal glands, kidneys, vascular and lymphatic structures, and abdominal cavity.

Liver

The liver is the largest organ in the human body. It is responsible for multiple metabolic processes, including synthesis of organic compounds, energy generation and storage, and disposal of toxic substances and waste products. Although relatively insensitive for the detection of diffuse hepatic abnormalities (the term "hepatic" means "relating to the liver") such as hepatitis and cirrhosis, CT is the imaging modality of choice for the detection of tumors and other space-occupying lesions in the liver.

Liver metastases (tumors arising in other organs that have spread to the liver) are found in 25-50% of all cancer patients at autopsy. The most common sites of origin are malignancies of the colon, lung, breast, and pancreas. On an unenhanced CT scan, the density of hepatic metastases can be very similar to the adjacent liver tissue and the lesions can be difficult to detect. Intravenous contrast helps to increase the density differences between the tumor and the normal liver. Although the liver receives 75% of its blood supply from the portal venous system, and 25% form the hepatic artery, most hepatic metastases are supplied by the hepatic arterial circulation. Therefore, following a rapid injection of intravenous contrast, the normal liver will enhance to a greater degree than the metastases and the metastatic lesions will stand out as darker, low density abnormalities. However, some metastases have relatively increased blood flow (renal cell carcinoma, islet cell tumors, melanoma, some breast malignancies) and appear as higher density lesions. One of the advantages of spiral CT is that its speed permits imaging of the liver during both the hepatic arterial and parenchymal phases of contrast enhancement, which improves detection of both types of metastases.

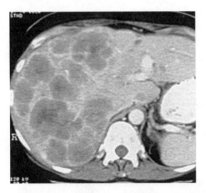

Figure 31.15. *Colon Carcinoma Lesions. Liver metastases can have a wide variety of sizes and appearances. The lesions in the patient with colon carcinoma are fairly large.*

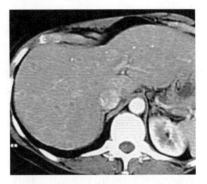

Figure 31.16 *Breast Carcinoma Lesions. The lesions in the patient with breast carcinoma are very small. The rapid injection of intravenous contrast given for the breast exam causes enhancement of the rims of these small lesions and makes them easier to identify.*

Cavernous hemangioma is the most common benign (non-cancerous) liver tumor. The tumor consists primarily of large vascular channels filled with slow-flowing venous blood. Although patients can very rarely present with abdominal pain, a palpable abdominal mass, or intra-abdominal hemorrhage, this usually only occurs with very large lesions. The vast majority of hemangiomata are discovered incidentally when CT or ultrasound of the abdomen is performed in search of other disease processes. The main significance of these lesions is the need to distinguish them from cancerous liver tumors.

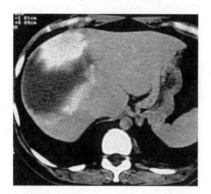 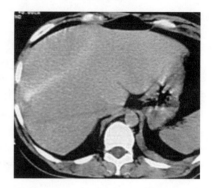

Figure 31.17. Initial and Delayed CT of Benign Liver Tumor. These figures illustrate a case that demonstrates the typical CT appearance of a cavernous hemangioma. The initial study obtained after a rapid injection of intravenous contrast (left) demonstrates a large, low density mass with thick peripheral enhancement in the right lobe of the liver. On the delayed image (right), the slow-flowing vascular channels in the tumor have filled with contrast and the tumor becomes almost identical in density to the surrounding liver.

Liver cysts, which are very common, are frequently discovered during CT or ultrasound of the abdomen. They are benign and are of clinical significance only if they become very large and cause symptoms relating to their size. As with cavernous hemangiomata of the liver, their main significance is the need to distinguish them from liver tumors, especially cystic liver metastases.

Figure 31.18. Hepatic Cyst. This case shows the usual appearance of a simple hepatic cyst. The hepatic cyst is well-defined, with smooth, imperceptible walls and no enhancement. The contents of the cyst are low density, similar to water. Occasionally, differentiation from a cystic tumor can be difficult on CT, and ultrasound or MR can be used for further characterization.

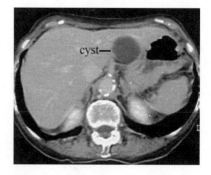

Pancreas

The pancreas was historically considered a "hidden" organ since its location deep in the abdomen made physical detection of abnormalities almost impossible. CT has markedly improved that situation. The pancreas is a complex structure that produces multiple substances required for digestion of food and metabolism and storage of carbohydrates (the best known substance is insulin).

Adenocarcinoma of the pancreas is the most common tumor of the pancreas and has a particularly grim prognosis. Although surgical resection can be successful when the tumor is detected at an early stage, the location of the pancreas is such that symptoms usually do not develop until the tumor is advanced and curative resection is impossible. On CT, most adenocarcinomas of the pancreas demonstrate lower density than the adjacent pancreatic tissue. This differentiation is improved with intravenous contrast because the pancreas will enhance to a greater degree than the tumor (although the more rare pancreatic tumors that arise from the islet cells of the pancreas can be very vascular and tend to enhance more than normal pancreas). CT also is used to stage the malignancy (determine how advanced it is) after it is detected and can identify liver metastases, obstruction of the bile ducts, and direct invasion into adjacent arteries and veins.

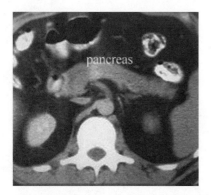 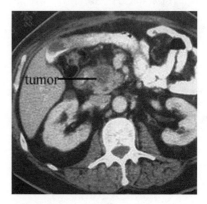

Figure 31.19. Normal Pancreas and Pancreas with Cancer

In the United States, most cases of **pancreatitis** are secondary to either alcohol abuse or biliary tract disease. Other causes include hyperparathyroidism, hypertriglyceridemia, and trauma. The symptoms and complications of pancreatitis are the result of the destructive effects of pancreatic enzymes leaking out of the pancreas into the surrounding tissues. The diagnosis of acute pancreatitis can usually be made based on clinical and laboratory findings alone, and diagnostic imaging is often not required in uncomplicated cases. However, CT is essential to diagnose the possible complications of pancreatitis, including phlegmonous pancreatitis (severe, extensive inflammation) and hemorrhagic pancreatitis, as well as pancreatic abscess and necrosis.

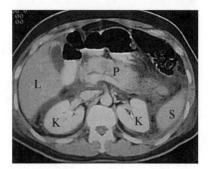

Figure 31.20. Severely Inflamed Pancreas. This Figure demonstrates the typical appearance of phlegmonous pancreatitis. The gray material surrounding the pancreas (P) represents a diffuse inflammatory process from the digestive actions of the pancreatic enzymes leaking out of the pancreas and digesting the surrounding tissues. This process extends to the kidneys (K), liver (L), and spleen (S). As this process progresses, localized fluid collections can form which can become infected and create abscesses. However, sterile and infected fluid collections often have the same appearance on CT and may require CT guided aspiration for diagnosis. If the inflammation is very severe, pancreatic necrosis can occur with irreparable destruction of the pancreatic tissue.

Kidney

CT's main role in imaging the kidney is for the evaluation of **renal cell carcinoma**, which is the most common renal tumor (the term "renal" means "relating to the kidney"). It is not uncommon for CT to detect a renal mass in a patient being evaluated for non-specific symptoms such as weight loss or abdominal. More frequently, the CT is ordered to further investigate an abnormality discovered on an intravenous pyelogram (IVP) or a renal ultrasound. The typical renal cell carcinoma is fairly large by the time it is discovered. CT reveals a large mass either within the renal parenchyma or extending off the kidney. The normal kidney enhances considerably more than the tumor, and the administration of intravenous contrast markedly improves the accuracy of the exam. CT is also very valuable for staging the tumor by detecting tumor extension into the renal vein or inferior vena cava, lymphadenopathy, and direct invasion into adjacent organs (all of which can alter treatment options, surgical approaches, and prognosis).

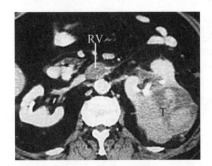 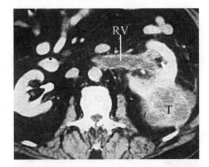

Figure 31.21. Tumor in Left Kidney. *The case above consists of two adjacent images from a patient with a large tumor (T) in the left kidney. There is evidence for tumor invasion into the left renal vein (RV) which is seen as enlargement and diminished enhancement of the vein.*

Trauma

CT has assumed a large role in the management of patients with blunt abdominal trauma. A single test permits evaluation for injuries to the **liver, spleen, kidneys**, and **pancreas,** and also determines whether blood is present in the abdominal cavity. In many cases, it has replaced the need for peritoneal lavage and exploratory laparotomy. However, several important points need to be emphasized:

- This applies to patients with *blunt* abdominal trauma (motor vehicle accidents, falls, assaults, etc.). Patients with *penetrating* abdominal trauma (gunshot, stabbing) usually require surgical exploration.

- Only patients who are hemodynamically stable (stable pulse, blood pressure, respiration) should undergo CT scanning. If they are not stable, they usually belong in the emergency room or operating room.

- The need for surgical repair to an injured abdominal organ should not be based only on the CT findings. Certain injuries can be managed conservatively, without surgery, even if they appear fairly severe on the CT scan, as long as the patient remains stable.

Most injuries to the solid abdominal organs appear as lacerations (breaks in the tissues) or hematomas (blood clots) within the substance of the organs, or as blood clots beneath the capsule of the organ (subcapsular hematoma). Intravenous contrast is required in order to accurately detect these injuries. The case below demonstrates a large hematoma (H) in the spleen, with an associated subcapsular hematoma (S) and free peritoneal hemorrhage (P) around the liver (blood in the abdominal cavity). The case on the right shows a laceration (L) of the left kidney, also with an associated subcapsular hematoma

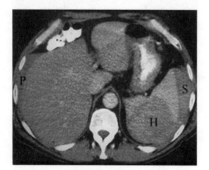 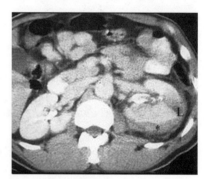

Figure 31.22. *Trauma Injuries: Lacerations and Hematomas*

Section 31.4

CT of the Pelvis

Reprinted with permission. © 1997 Steven H. Brick, M.D.

Introduction

Computed Tomography of the pelvis is usually performed as a continuation of a CT of the abdomen since processes that are diagnosed in the abdomen can often extend inferiorly into the pelvis. Specific pelvic organs are often better evaluated with other imaging modalities. In women, the uterus and ovaries are best seen with ultrasound. In men, the prostate is usually imaged with ultrasound or MRI. However, CT does play a role in the evaluation of some pelvic abnormalities.

Diverticulitis

Diverticula are small outpouchings of mucosa and submucosa of the colon. They are very common in patients over 60 years old, and can frequently be found in younger patients. *Diverticulosis* (which refers simply to the presence of diverticula in the colon) seldom produces symptoms. However, when fecal material becomes trapped in the diverticulum, the lining can rupture and lead to a localized area of inflammation and infection called *diverticulitis*.

CT has replaced the barium enema as the imaging modality of choice for the evaluation of diverticulitis.

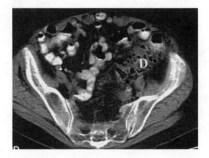

Figure 31.23. Diverticulitis. This patient shows the typical appearance of diverticulitis (D) as a thickened segment of colon with hazy inflammatory changes extending into the surrounding fat.

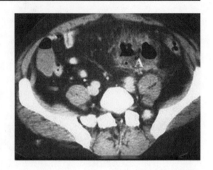

Figure 31.24 Diverticular Abscess. This patient has developed a complication of diverticulitis; the diverticular abscess (A). This appears as a localized collection of gas and fluid outside the colon. These abscesses are frequently drained by placement of a drainage catheter through the skin under CT guidance, which often eliminates the need for surgical drainage.

Tumor

As mentioned in the introduction, most tumors of the male and female pelvis are imaged with other modalities. However, CT plays a role in several situations:

- When a pelvic tumor is very large and ultrasound cannot adequately evaluate its borders and affect on adjacent structures.

- To evaluate tumors in which the CT findings are specific for the type of tumor (e.g. teratoma).

- To identify peritoneal and mesenteric metastases in patients with ovarian carcinoma.

- To identify metastatic lymphadenopathy in patients with carcinoma of the prostate.

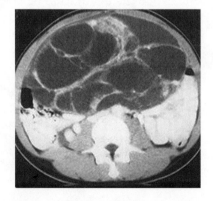

Figure 31.25. Large Pelvic Mass. In this patient, ultrasound revealed a large complex mass in the pelvis. The CT demonstrates a huge, multicystic mass extending out of the pelvis into the abdomen. There was no evidence for spread of tumor outside the large mass. The tumor was a benign cystadenoma at surgery.

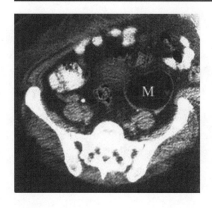

Figure 31.26. Pelvic Teratoma (Benign Ovarian Tumor). In this patient, ultrasound revealed a mass whose characteristics suggested a teratoma (a benign ovarian tumor that often contains fat, teeth, and hair). The CT showed that the mass (M) was composed almost entirely of fat, which confirmed the diagnosis of teratoma. Since this tumor is seldom malignant, and the patient was a poor surgical risk, the CT findings indicated surgery could be safely avoided.

Section 31.5

CT Guided Biopsy

Reprinted with permission. © 1997 Steven H. Brick, M.D.

Introduction

As mentioned in several other CT sections, the development of Computed Tomography permitted visualization of the inner structures of the human body which previously could only be seen at surgery or autopsy. As the resolution of CT improved, and the time required for image acquisition decreased, new diagnostic and therapeutic uses for CT were discovered.

In the past, if a patient had a tumor in the chest, abdomen, or pelvis, surgery was required in order to make a definite diagnosis and determine the specific type of tumor before appropriate therapy could be implemented. This approach is certainly acceptable if the patient would require surgery anyway in order to treat the tumor. However, many patients have types of tumors in which surgery is not indicated (frequently patients with metastatic disease), and other patients are not surgical candidates because of additional medical conditions. CT guided, percutaneous (i.e. through the skin) needle biopsy has developed into the frequently used alternative to open surgical exploration and biopsy.

Indications and Contraindication

Almost any organ or structure in the body can be biopsied percutaneously under CT guidance. This includes the lungs, mediastinum, liver, kidneys, adrenal glands, pancreas, retroperitoneum, and pelvis. The spleen is seldom biopsied because it is a highly vascular organ and the risk of severe post-biopsy hemorrhage is significant. Most biopsies are performed to confirm that a mass is malignant, and to determine the specific type of tumor so that appropriate therapy can be started. Some biopsies are performed to evaluate the type and severity of benign disease (e.g. liver biopsy for hepatitis, renal biopsy for glomerulonephritis).

Relative contraindications to CT guided biopsy include:

- Patients with uncorrectable bleeding disorders. The risk of post biopsy hemorrhage is too high.

- Lesions in which a safe biopsy path cannot be found. This includes deep tumors which the needle could only reach by traversing large blood vessels (in the chest, abdomen, or pelvis), bowel (in the abdomen or pelvis), or other vital organs (e.g. the spleen, heart, aorta).

- Lesions which will be surgically resected regardless of the biopsy result. This applies to many solitary lung and kidney masses.

- Suspected types of lesions in which the risk of life-threatening post-biopsy complications is high. This includes pulmonary arteriovenous malformation, cavernous hemangioma or echinococcal cyst of the liver.

- Patients who cannot cooperate with the exam.

Risks

CT guided biopsy is a relatively safe procedure. The risks are almost always less than surgical biopsy, which would be the most common alternative. The recovery time is considerably less than surgery.

Risks of CT guided biopsy depend somewhat on the site being biopsied. These risks include:

- Bleeding: Most patients have evaluation of their blood clotting status prior to biopsy. Although rare, bleeding can be life-threatening and can require surgery to correct.

- Infection: Infection can develop anytime a needle pierces the skin. However, sterile technique is used during the biopsy and this is a very rare complication.

- Pneumothorax: A reported complication in up to 25% of lung biopsies (although only a few of these patients require a chest tube). Also a risk during biopsies in the upper abdomen (usually liver and adrenal).

- Damage to adjacent organs: Although CT can accurately locate the lesion, the biopsy is not performed under real time imaging. Patient movement and variation in breathing can alter the relationship of the lesion and adjacent organs, including bowel and vascular structures.

Techniques

The technique will vary based on the lesion being biopsied and any limitations of the patient. A generalized sequence is as follows:

- The patient can lie on the CT table on their back, on their stomach, or on either side, depending on the needle path planned. Although systemic anesthesia is usually not required, some patients will receive intravenous sedation and/or pain relief.

- Limited CT scanning is performed, and the lesion is located. The safest and easiest path for the needle is planned.

- The overlying skin is cleaned and draped in a sterile manner. The skin and underlying tissue is anesthetized. Once the depth and angulation of the needle is determined from the CT images, the needle is placed through the skin into the body.

- Additional CT images are obtained to confirm that the tip of the needle lies in the lesion. Adjustments to the needle position are made as necessary.

- When the tip of the needle is shown to lie in the proper position, the biopsy is obtained. Different types of needles are available. Some are for aspiration (obtains scattered cells from the lesion), and others are cutting needles which obtain a small core of tissue.

- A preliminary evaluation of the specimen is frequently performed by the pathologist. If there is sufficient tissue for diagnosis, the procedure is terminated. If not, additional biopsies will be obtained.

- The patient is observed either in the department or in a short-stay nursing unit for 2 to 4 hours, and then sent home. If there are no complications, admission to the hospital is seldom required.

Sample Cases

Adrenal biopsy: The case below is a patient with lung cancer and a mass in the adrenal gland which could represent a benign adenoma or a metastasis. Figure 31.27 shows a small mass in the left adrenal gland (M). Figure 31.28 shows the patient was placed on her stomach for the biopsy. The needle can be seen extending into the mass (M). Note how the needle path just barely avoids the lower aspect of the left lung (L). The biopsy of the adrenal revealed metastatic lung cancer.

Figure 31.27. Adrenal Gland Mass

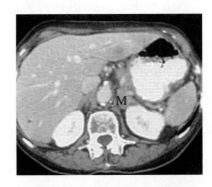

Figure 31.28. Needle Biopsy of Adrenal Gland

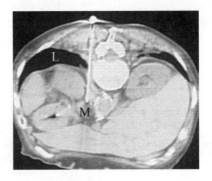

Chapter 32

Viewing the Blood Vessels, Angiography

Contents

Section 32.1

Introduction and Procedure Description

"Diagnostic Angiography," reprinted with permission.
© 1997 James Spies, M.D.

Introduction

Angiography is a diagnostic procedure that allows direct visualization of blood vessels in the body. It is performed by the injection of radiographic contrast material (dye) into the blood vessels via a catheter that is placed directly into the artery or vein. The catheter, which is a very thin flexible tube, is passed into the vessel through a needle puncture site in the vessel. An angiogram is an "invasive" procedure, in that a catheter is passed inside the bodies' blood vessels. It is generally performed to detect abnormalities of the blood vessels themselves, or to evaluate the vascular supply to various organs in the body. While it is not as frequently performed as other radiographic studies, such as chest X-rays or CT scans, angiograms are very important in diagnosing and treating a wide variety of medical problems.

Angiography is a generic term that refers to diagnostic studies of both arteries and veins. **Arteriography** is the more specific term for the study that visualizes the arteries. It is common, however, that these terms will be used interchangeably by physicians when discussing diagnostic studies of the arteries. **Venography**, or a study of the veins using radiographic contrast, is another type of angiogram.

Procedure Description

Most arteriograms are performed as an outpatient procedure, although the patient usually needs to be monitored in a short stay unit for several hours after the procedure. With the time required to register in the morning, the time for the procedure itself, and the post procedure monitoring, you may anticipate being at the hospital most of the day. The post-procedure period, usually between four and six hours, is necessary to be sure that there is no bleeding from the puncture site. After this period, it is usually safe to go home.

The procedure itself will take from one to two hours. It is performed in angiography suite, which is a special type of radiology room. You will be lying on a movable table. An intravenous line will be used to give sedatives and other medications as needed. The artery that is usually used to access the vascular system is in the groin region, at the top of the leg. If you feel carefully, you may be able to feel this artery's pulse in that region. For a number of reasons, this is the safest route to enter the arterial system. If the arteries in the groins are not open, alternative routes include the arteries under the arm or at the elbow.

Sedatives are used to relax you during the procedure. The most common drug used is Versed, which is a drug like Valium but with a shorter duration of action. You will not be asleep during the procedure because your cooperation is needed during the procedure. The intent of the sedation is to relieve any anxiety that you may have at the beginning and during the procedure. In order to ensure the safety of the sedatives, your heart rate and rhythm, breathing, and oxygen level will be monitored during the procedure.

After the sedation is started, the groin area will be washed with a sterile solution. A small amount of hair may have to be clipped. After the cleansing, a sterile drape will be applied to the area. The radiologist will then use a local anesthetic, usually Xylocaine, to anesthetize ("numb") the skin and deeper tissues in the groin, A tiny nick will be made in the numbed area with a scalpel. Then, using the palpable pulse as a guide, the radiologist will puncture the artery. Once the tip of the needle is within the vessel, a wire will passed into the vessel. The needle is then removed with the wire remaining in place This will provide an access for a catheter to be passed over the wire and into the vessel. Once the catheter is in place, fluoroscopy (live X-ray imaging) can be used to guide the catheter to the proper position. When the catheter is in place for injection, contrast can be injected and X-ray images taken. These are taken very rapidly (usually one or two pictures per second). The contrast is injected into the blood stream and the normal flow of the blood causes it to be carried to the entire distribution that the blood vessels supplies. The contrast fills the vessels and allows them to be seen on the X-rays. There is no pain associated with the injection; usually there is only a mild warm sensation.

Once all the pictures are completed, the catheter is removed and pressure is applied by hand over the puncture site. If this were not done, the artery would bleed freely because there is considerable pressure within the blood vessel. After ten to fifteen minutes of pressure,

a clot will have formed in the hole in the artery and will have sufficient strength to allow the pressure to be removed. However, it will
take several hours for the clot that is sealing the puncture site to
mature and to have sufficient strength to allow you to walk or bend
at the hip without the bleeding restarting. While you will be awake
after the procedure, you must stay in bed and will have to use a uri-
nal or bedpan during that period. You will be able to resume your
normal diet immediately after the procedure. Usually four to six hours
of bed rest in the hospital is required before it is safe to go home. Even
after that, a patient's activity must be limited for the first twenty-
four hours after the procedure, and vigorous activity should be avoided
for 48 to 72 hours post procedure.

Usually, the radiologist will be able to review the study immediately and give you an initial impression of his or her findings. A final
written report will be sent to the doctor that requested the procedure.

Section 32.2

Patient Preparation

Reprinted with permission. © 1997 James Spies, M.D.

Patients are encouraged to make an appointment to go to the hospital on a day prior to the procedure to meet the radiologist and to
discuss the procedure. During this visit the radiologist may perform
a limited history and physical examination. This allows the radiologist to understand the symptoms that have led to the request of the
study and to confirm that an arteriogram is the best test to better
define your problem. During this visit, you will be asked for a list of
your current medications. If you don't know the doses, you may bring
the bottles themselves and the information will be recorded.

You will be given specific instructions during your pre-procedure visit.
If you are unable to go in ahead of time, here are the usual instructions:

- You will be told the time your procedure is scheduled by the
  staff in your doctor's office or by the radiology department staff.
  You need to arrive at the hospital an hour and a half ahead of

time at admissions. This allows time for you to be admitted and for the nursing staff to get you ready for the procedure. Often laboratory tests are needed prior to the procedure and these will be obtained at that time.

- On the morning of the procedure, do not eat any solid food. You may take any oral fluids except milk, juices, or alcohol.

- If you are diabetic and take insulin, you need to talk to your doctor or radiology department to get special instructions on diet and insulin dose.

- Take all your normal medications, particularly any blood pressure medications. However, if you take Coumadin (generic name Warfarin), you should not take it ahead of time and it may need to be stopped 2 to 3 days in advance. Please talk to your doctor or radiology department ahead of time for special instructions.

- You will need to stay in the hospital for at least four to five hours after the procedure. Please schedule to have the entire day free for the procedure and the post-procedure care. In addition, you will need to restrict your activity severely for the night of the procedure and to a lesser extent the next day. You may need to take the day after the procedure off from work and you should plan not to drive the day after the procedure.

- You need to arrange for someone to drive you home after the procedure. Ideally, a responsible adult should stay with you for the night of the procedure. On rare occasions, a patient may not be able to arrange transportation and will have to take a cab home. This is a less than ideal circumstance, but most insurers will not pay for hospitalization after an arteriogram and there may be little choice. You should make a concerted effort to have a family member, friend, or neighbor help transport you home after the procedure.

- The radiologist will discuss the preliminary results of the study with you when it is finished. He or she will also call your doctor with a verbal report. A final written report will be sent to you doctor shortly after the procedure.

- If you have questions regarding these instructions or any other special problems you may have, we encourage you to call your doctor or the hospital where your procedure is scheduled in order to discuss your questions or to arrange a visit ahead of time.

Section 32.3

Risks of Angiography

Reprinted with permission. © 1997 James Spies, M.D.

Complications from an arteriogram are very rare, but because this is an invasive procedure there is some risk. Most problems that occur can be detected at the time of the procedure or in the immediate post-procedure period. Most minor complications can be managed with observation overnight. Rarely, they may result in the need for surgery, transfusion or prolonged hospitalization. The range of potential complications is summarized below.

The artery may be injured where it is punctured or along the artery where the catheter is passed. It also could be injured where the contrast is injected for the images. The injury could result in the artery closing down, decreasing blood flow to the area supplied by it. A clot or piece of plaque from the artery wall could float down the leg or into an internal organ, resulting in blockage. These complications may resolve on their own, or with medicine. However, they often require surgery to repair the injury. The chance of this type of complication is less than one percent.

The artery may also bleed at the puncture site during the procedure or afterwards. This is the primary reason that bed rest is required for several hours after the procedure. Usually the bleeding can be controlled with direct pressure at the puncture site. In unusual circumstances, such as in patients with severe high blood pressure, bleeding may be difficult to control. Transfusion or surgery may be needed to control the bleeding. This again is quite rare, occurring in less than one percent of cases.

The contrast agent (dye) used to make the arteries visible on X-rays can also cause problems. Patients can be allergic to the contrast. The most common allergic reaction is hives, which usually goes away by itself or after a dose of Benadryl. Very rarely, about one in ten thousand people, an anaphylactic reaction can occur. This type of reaction can usually be treated, but there is a chance of death from such severe reactions. The dye can also cause an injury to the kidneys, most commonly in patients that already have limited kidney function. For this reason, in most cases your kidney function will be checked with a blood test prior to the procedure. If you know that you have kidney disease be sure to mention it to the radiologist. We usually will be able to proceed with the procedure, but may need to take special precautions before and during the procedure.

Just like contrast, patients may be allergic to the sedatives or local anesthetic used during the procedure. The chance of an allergy and the types of reactions are similar to those seen with contrast. In addition, patients have a variable response to sedatives. In patients who are very sensitive to the medications, it is possible that the blood pressure could drop or the breathing slow or even stop from just a small dose. For this reason, you will monitored closely during the procedure. In almost all cases these problems can be safely managed with reversal medications and supplemental oxygen. Rarely, severe cardiac or respiratory problems can result in cardiac arrest and death.

There are also complications that can occur with certain types of arteriograms that are not usually seen with others. The most important example of this is carotid arteriography, which is a study of the arteries in the neck that supply the brain. Similar to other arteriograms, debris from the walls of the vessels or a tiny clot from the catheter can detach. However, because the catheter is in the carotid artery, it is possible that this debris can lodge in an artery in the brain. This can result in a stroke or a temporary stroke. We take special precautions to try to prevent this severe complication and fortunately they are very rare. The chance of a stroke is about one in five hundred patients. A temporary stroke occurs in one in one hundred and usually resolves in a few hours.

Many complications are easily treated and do not result in serious or permanent injury. Unfortunately, with any complication there is always a chance that it not be easily treated and may result in permanent injury, limb loss or even death. These outcomes are very rare and often occur in patients with multiple pre-existing medical problems.

It is important that you understand the spectrum of risks associated with a procedure. This understanding can help you in making an informed decision as to whether the benefits of the procedure are worth the risk, however remote, of a complication. Usually an arteriogram is ordered when a surgical or interventional procedure is being considered or when a diagnostic problem exists that cannot be resolved with other non-invasive tests. Most commonly, an arteriogram is necessary and not having the study will prevent the planned treatment. When weighing the pros and cons, you should talk to your

271

doctor who can help put these issues in perspective. We are, of course, always available to answer any questions you have in this regard.

Section 32.4

Carotid Arteriography

Narrowing of the carotid arteries is one of the most common reasons that people have strokes. This can happen because if the artery is narrowed by an atherosclerotic plaque (hardening of the arteries), the blood supply is diminished to the brain. This can lead the artery to clot off, or allow small bits of blood clots or other debris to float from the plaque to the brain. Any of these events can lead to a stroke or to a temporary stroke, called a transient ischemic attack (TIA). A TIA might cause a patient to have slurred speech temporarily, have difficulty feeling or moving an arm or leg, or any number of other symptoms. This is clearly a warning sign that the patient is at risk for a stroke. Stroke symptoms may be identical to a TIA, but persist for weeks or months and may be permanent. Narrowing of the arteries of the neck can also result in an abnormal sound, called a bruit

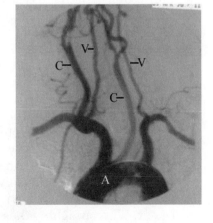

Figure 32.1. *Blood Supply to the Brain. The carotid arteries (C) are the main blood supply to the brain. There are two of them, one on the right and one on the left side of the neck. They arise from the thoracic aorta (A), which is the large artery that receives the blood from the heart and delivers it to the head, arms, abdomen and legs. There are two other arteries that supply the brain, called the vertebral arteries (V). These are in the back of the neck and are much smaller than the carotid arteries.*

(rhymes with phooey). If a doctor hears such a sound, he or she may decide to investigate it further.

When a patient's symptoms or examination raises the possibility of narrowing the carotid arteries, the first test usually done is a duplex scan, which is a type of non-invasive test that uses ultrasound. This will allow the physician to determine if the artery is significantly narrowed. If a significant narrowing is detected, confirmation with an arteriogram is usually the next step. Confirmation is needed because there is a ten percent error rate with duplex scans and we need to be certain that a narrowing is present prior to surgery or any other treatment.

The goal of all these tests is to prevent strokes. A patient's chance of stroke is increased when a severe narrowing is detected. When a severe narrowing is present, surgery is usually recommended to clean out the plaque in the artery and therefore reduce the chance of stroke.

Carotid arteriography is the most definitive test to confirm the presence of a narrowing in the arteries. This usually is only performed if surgery is planned. It gives an accurate picture of the severity of the narrowing as well as its exact location and length. Because the thoracic aorta and limited views of the vessels in the brain are also obtained, narrowing of the vessels at sites not visible to the ultrasound may also be detected.

The figures on the next page are examples of carotid arteriograms.

Occasionally a severely narrowed artery clots off and this may cause a TIA or a stroke. On other occasions, an occlusion occurs without any symptoms. If an occluded artery is discovered during arteriography, no further therapy is usually needed. Reopening the vessel will not usually improve function or reduce the risk of stroke.

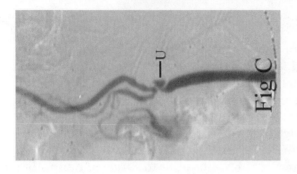

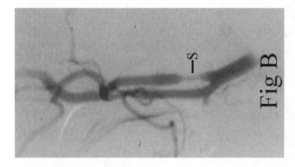

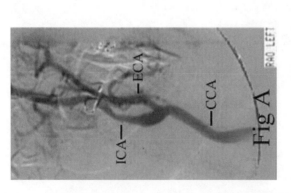

Figure 32.2. Carotid Arteriograms. Figure A shows a normal arteriogram of the carotid artery in the neck. There are two main branches of the main or common carotid artery (CCA), the external carotid artery (ECA) and the internal carotid artery (ICA). Narrowing most commonly occurs at the branch point. Notice that the artery at the level of the base of the brain is also seen. This level cannot be seen with the ultrasound and is one reason that arteriograms provide additional information. Figure B shows a severely narrowed internal carotid artery. The narrowing is called an area of stenosis (S). This is the type of narrowing that usually would be operated upon. Figure C shows a similar narrowing with an ulcer (U) or crater within it. The ulcer allows debris that collects within the plaque to float to the brain. Ulcerated plaques are more likely to cause strokes than smooth plaques like that in Figure B.

Section 32.5

Angiogram of the Legs, Peripheral Arteriography

Reprinted with permission. © 1997 James Spies, M.D.

By far the most common reason to obtain a peripheral arteriogram (angiogram of the legs) is to evaluate for atherosclerosis or hardening of the arteries. Blockage of the arteries of the legs can cause a number of symptoms. The most common and mildest symptom is claudication or pain in the legs after walking. It may feel like a cramp, a tired feeling or a heaviness in the leg. It might be only in the calf, or the thigh or even in the buttocks, depending on the level of the arterial blockage. It occurs because the arteries are narrowed or blocked to the degree that they cannot supply enough blood to the muscles of the leg when the increase demand of exercising or walking occur. Typically the symptoms slowly go away once a patient stops walking or sits down. When the walking starts again, the pain will usually occur after walking a similar distance.

As the blockage progresses, the distance that can be walked without pain decreases. It may progress to the point that just a few steps causes the symptoms or pain may start occurring at rest. Rest pain in the legs that is caused by arterial blockage is a sign of severe disease that must be evaluated by a physician. If not treated, it can lead to limb loss. Claudication is a less severe symptom that should be evaluated by a physician but is not the imminent threat to the leg that rest pain represents.

Another sign of severe arterial blockage is the development of sores or areas of skin breakdown on the feet and ankles that do not heal. This is particularly common in diabetics, who are at increased risk for peripheral vascular disease and limb loss from gangrene. If you have a non-healing sore or painful area on the foot or ankle, it must be evaluated by a physician.

If the physical examination or non-invasive testing of the legs confirms the presence of blocked arteries in the legs, arteriography is usually the next step. It is the best test for evaluating the extent and

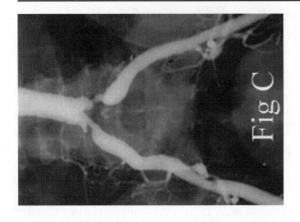

Fig C

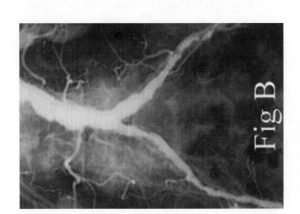

Fig B

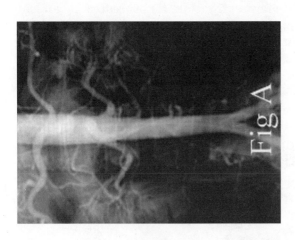

Fig A

Figure 32.3. *Abdominal Aorta Angiograms. In these figures, Figure A shows a normal arteriogram of the abdominal aorta. Notice that it is smooth and gently tapered without a strictures or narrowings. Figure B shows a study of the abdominal aorta of a patient with severe artery blockage and severe pain in the legs after just walking across the room. Notice the multiple areas of irregularity and narrowing of the abdominal aorta and its main branches. Figure C shows a mostly normal vessel with severe narrowings in the two main branches of the aorta, the common iliac arteries. These are the type of lesions that might cause claudication after two or three blocks of walking.*

location of the blockage. It provides a "road map" of the vessels and thus allows a decision to be made on the best types of treatment. The treatment options may include exercise therapy in mild cases, with balloon angioplasty or surgery in more advanced cases.

Section 32.6

Renal Arteriography, Angiogram of the Kidneys

Reprinted with permission. © 1997 Steven H. Brick, M.D.

There are two common reasons that an arteriogram of the kidneys may be required; to evaluate for a potential cause for high blood pressure and to evaluate tumors or possible tumors of the kidney.

While the majority of people with high blood pressure do not have a specific cause that can be identified, some people have a narrowing of one or both of the arteries that results in high blood pressure. The reason for this involves some pretty complex physiology, but it may be simplified as follows:

- The kidney has sensors that help the body regulate blood pressure. When the kidney detects that blood pressure is low, it secretes chemicals that cause the body to retain fluid and raise the volume of the blood and thus increase the pressure within the blood vessels. When one or both of the arteries to the kidneys are narrowed, the pressure within the arteries of the kidney (beyond the narrowing) is decreased and this makes that kidney think that the entire body has low blood pressure. It secretes chemicals to raise the blood volume to more than normal. This results in high blood pressure.

Since a narrowing of the renal artery is a treatable cause of high blood pressure, it is important to identify people that have such a narrowing. There are several signs that suggest narrowed arteries of the kidney. If the high blood pressure occurs in a young person, or has rapidly developed or suddenly become worse, or if the high blood pressure is hard to control, then it is more likely that a narrowing of the renal artery may be the cause. There are several non-invasive tests that can also suggest a narrowed artery. The most commonly used are a nuclear renal scan or a duplex ultrasound test. While not 100% accurate, these tests are often done as a screen for patients that may have a narrowed artery. If one of these tests is positive, or the patient's pattern of high blood pressure matches the criteria described above, an arteriogram is usually done.

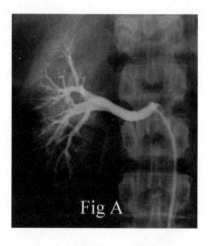

Figure 32.4. Renal Arteriograms: Normal and with Atherosclerosis. Figure A reveals a renal arteriogram in a normal patient. Notice that the vessel is smooth without any areas of constriction. Contrast that appearance with Figure B, where there is a severe narrowing from atherosclerosis or hardening of the arteries. This narrowing is very likely a primary cause of this patient's severe high blood pressure.

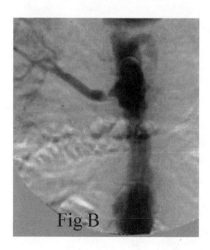

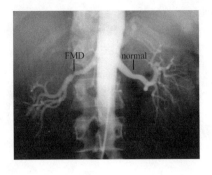

Figure 32.5. Fibromuscular Dysplasia (FMD). This figure shows another type of renal artery narrowing that causes high blood pressure, most commonly in women between the ages of 20 and 50. It is called fibromuscular dysplasia, or FMD. The cause for this type of narrowing is not known, but this is readily treatable with balloon angioplasty. A successful procedure often results in cure of the hypertension and it is rare to recur. The narrowing involves a lengthy segment of the vessel with a series of web-like narrowings interspersed with dilated areas, often called a "string-of-beads" appearance as seen in the right renal artery in this patient. The left renal artery is normal.

The other major reason to perform a renal arteriogram is to either diagnose a renal tumor or to better define the vascular supply of a tumor that is already known to be present.

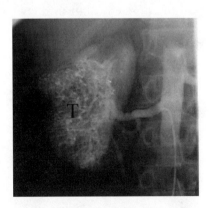

Figure 32.6. Renal Cell Carcinoma. This figure shows a large tumor (T) in the kidney with abnormally increased blood vessels. This is an example of renal cell carcinoma, the most common cancer of the kidney.

Section 32.7

MR Angiography

Reprinted with permission. © 1997 James Spies, M.D.

MR angiography (MRA) permits imaging of the blood vessels in several parts of the body with diagnostic accuracy similar to contrast angiography (the injection of x-ray dye directly into blood vessels, usually with a catheter inserted into the artery in the upper thigh), but at a fraction of the time and cost, and with none of the risk. The most frequent vessels studied include the brain and the neck.

The physics of MRA is extremely complex, but a simplified explanation will be attempted. The basic principle is that special pulse sequences are used by the MR scanner which causes flowing blood to appear very bright and all stationary tissue to appear very dark. If arterial structures are being studied, additional pulses are applied to erase the signal in veins. Multiple very thin slices are obtained at adjacent levels through the region of interest. An extremely powerful computer then stacks these images on top of each other and creates a 3D image similar in appearance to a contrast angiogram. *No radiographic contrast is used.* The constructed images can be rotated 360 degrees so that the vessels can be studied in all projections.

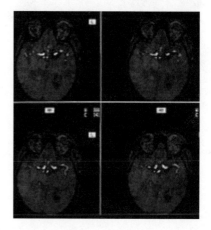

Figure 32.7. MR Scanner Images. This is an example of the raw images created by the scanner. Note that the vessels are bright and all of the surrounding tissues are dark.

The images below demonstrate the appearance of the MRA after computer processing. The same data is used to create sagittal (top), transverse (middle), and coronal images (bottom). Remember, no contrast is injected.

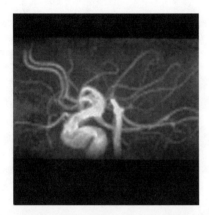

Figure 32.8. MRA Sagittal Images

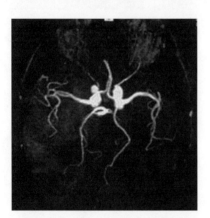

Figure 32.9. MRA Transverse Image

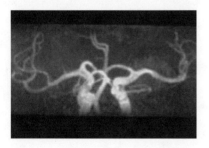

Figure 32.10. MRA Coronal Image

The following case demonstrates the accuracy and sensitivity of MRA. A tiny aneurysm (a localized weakening and enlargement of a blood vessel) enlargement is seen arising from an artery deep in the brain. Cerebral aneurysms can rupture without warning, which can cause severe neurologic damage or death, and often are surgically repaired shortly after they are discovered.

Figure 32.11. *Cerebral Aneurysm*

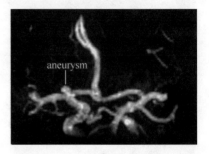

Chapter 33

Nuclear Imaging

Contents

Section 33.1

Nuclear, SPECT, and PET Scans

Excerpts from "A Primer on Medical Imaging—Part Two," *FDA Consumer* (May 1989) by Egon Weck, reviewed for currency 1999.

Nuclear medicine emerged after World War II when radionuclides (radioactive isotopes, which emit ionizing radiation) became available. At first, radiation from radionuclides was used to destroy cancerous tissue inside the body. In 1963, however, a body scanner using radionuclides was developed. Unlike an X-ray machine, which beams radiation at the body from outside, a nuclear scan places the source of radiation inside the patient.

To prepare for nuclear scans (also known as scintigrams), a very small and virtually harmless amount of a radionuclide is administered by mouth, injection, or inhalation. A variety of radionuclides, such as technecium and thallium, are available; each has a special affinity for a different organ or part of the body.

A "camera" or scanning device then picks up the radiation being emitted from the body and transforms it into an image. Nuclear scans lack the clear definition of structure visible on an X-ray. But they can reveal areas of an organ, such as the liver, that are not functioning normally.

Some radionuclides that concentrate in diseased areas, such as tumors, show them as hot spots on a scintigram. Others concentrate in healthy, functioning tissues to reveal areas of disease as cold spots.

SPECT (Single Photon Emission Computed Tomography) and Stroke

The single photon emission computed tomography (SPECT) scan is a refinement of nuclear scanning. SPECT employs some of the same radionuclides, but it uses a more sophisticated camera to pick up the radiation. SPECT resembles the CT (computed tomography) scan inasmuch as the signals picked up by the "camera" are fed to a computer, which performs countless computations and transmits the results to a TV screen to produce either a slice-like cross-section or a 3-D image.

While some of the radionuclides used in nuclear scans are employed in SPECT, newer ones have been developed especially for SPECT. One injectable imaging agent, called SPECTamine, is specifically designed to pass intact through the blood-brain barrier (which keeps many chemicals out of the brain). When used by skilled specialists, this agent can help make quick, accurate assessments of the effects of a stroke, showing which blood vessels have been affected and the nature and extent of brain damage.

PET (Photon Emission Tomography) for Early Signs

In diseases like cancer, by the time the structural damage shows up on X-rays, it may be too late to effect a cure. So medical investigators are constantly looking for ways to detect early signs of disease.

Another drawback with X-rays is that mental and nervous system disorders seldom produce visible anatomical changes. What is needed is a form of medical imaging capable of visualizing metabolic processes. Enter PET: positron emission tomography.

PET scans employ radionuclides with positrons attached to them. Positrons are subatomic particles that resemble electrons but carry a positive instead of a negative charge. When a positron collides with an electron, the particles are annihilated and transformed into two photons (photons are a form of radiant energy). Because they travel in opposite directions, the source of each pair of photons can be identified with great precision.

As in other forms of tomography, a computer processes the information picked up by a PET scanner and produces an image on a TV screen. The resulting image can be color-coded to differentiate distinct areas of the target.

To prepare for a PET scan, a positron-labeled compound is administered, often by inhalation. The positron tagging is carried out in a machine called a cyclotron, which generates charged atomic particles. The tagged compounds emit their positrons in a matter of minutes, so it takes highly skilled teams working with nearby cyclotrons to perform a PET scan.

"PET's great promise rests with the capability of imaging metabolic rather than anatomical detail," notes Dr. Ronald G. Evens, professor and head of radiology at Washington University's School of Medicine in St. Louis. "Processes such as oxygen uptake, blood flow, glucose metabolism, and drug interaction could give us early warning to diseases that produce no anatomical changes.

"For example, we know that cancers start in small metabolic patterns. It would be extremely useful to get a handle on these early signs," Dr. Evens explains.

PET scans are being applied to the study of brain function and disorders such as schizophrenia and Parkinson's disease. In other areas, the scans are giving medical scientists a closer look at the mechanism that causes strokes and heart attacks, and the clogging process that gradually narrows arteries.

Section 33.2

Bone Imaging

Reprinted with permission © The Society of Nuclear Medicine.

Bone scans are used to detect arthritis, osteoporosis, fractures, sports injuries, tumors and even cases of child abuse. Bone scans may also be used to evaluate unexplained bone pain, malignancies in the breast, prostate or thyroid and certain types of heart or brain damage.

Test Preparation

For most bone studies, you will be asked to drink as many fluids as possible, both before and after the procedure.

Exam Procedure

During the first part of the test, the tracer is injected. It generally takes about two hours for the tracer to be absorbed by the bones. The technologist will let you know if it is okay to eat during this waiting period. During the waiting period, you should try to urinate as often as possible because it will help eliminate the tracer from your body that is not going to the bones.

Depending on the study, the technologist may take pictures of your bones as the tracer is moving through your bloodstream before it reaches your bones. It takes about 30 minutes to complete the images.

In most bone studies, however, the imaging portion takes much longer, from two to four hours. For most bone scans, you will lie on the imaging table with the camera positioned above or below you. Several images may be taken or the camera may move slowly, imaging the entire length of your body. Although the imaging session takes a long time, it is extremely important that you remain as still as possible so that the scan results are accurate.

For children, the procedure is the same as for adults, except that after the tracer injection, the child may be given a sedative. If the child is given a sedative, he or she will have to remain in the nuclear medicine department until they are fully awake. After the test, the child should be able to resume daily activities, and there are no restrictions to eating, drinking or contact with others. If the child has been sedated, you may wish to let him or her rest for a day before resuming normal play activity.

Section 33.3

Brain Imaging

Reprinted with permission © The Society of Nuclear Imaging

A brain scan may be necessary to investigate problems within the brain itself or in blood circulation to and from the brain (perfusion imaging).

Test Preparation

Generally, no special preparation is needed. If special preparation is required, your doctor will let you know.

Exam Procedure

Perfusion Imaging: After relaxing in a dimly lit room, the tracer is injected in the arm. Thirty to 60 minutes after the injection, you will lie on your back under the camera and pictures of your brain will be taken for 30 to 60 minutes. You will be asked not to move, touch your head or cough while the pictures are being taken.

Stress/Rest Test: Most brain scans are taken while the patient is resting, but some medical conditions require evaluation of different activity levels of the brain during active and rest periods. This test is performed using a special drug or while doing certain tasks that activate brain function. The test is performed in two parts: first, a rest image is obtained, and the next day, the necessary stress test is performed.

Cisternography: This test determines if there is abnormal flow of cerebral spinal fluid around or in the brain. The tracer is injected into the lower back region by a doctor. After the injection, you will lie still for a few hours. It usually takes two to three days to complete the images.

Section 33.4

Breast Imaging

Reprinted with permission © The Society of Nuclear Medicine

Nuclear medicine breast imaging is a diagnostic tool used in conjunction with mammograms to more accurately identify and locate cancerous tissue in the breasts. The test is particularly useful when the mammogram results are difficult to interpret because of previous biopsy or breast cancer surgery or dense breast tissue.

Test Preparation

No special preparation is required. However, you may want to avoid eating a large meal before the procedure because you will have to lie on your stomach 15-20 minutes, or longer, if a different type of camera is used.

Exam Procedure

Breast imaging is performed in two parts. First, a medical history is taken. You will then be given two hospital gowns to put on and you will be asked to remove all jewelry and clothing from the waist up, and if you are wearing pantyhose, you may be asked to remove them. The tracer is then injected in either an arm or foot vein. Five or ten minutes after the tracer injection, the images are obtained. For this portion of the imaging session, you will lie face down on a special table that allows the camera to be as close as possible to the breasts. You will be positioned so that your breasts will hang through an opening in the table. Images are obtained of each breast. For the second part of the exam, you will sit on a chair or stool, and the camera will be placed against your chest with your face turned to the side. Pictures are taken of your chest while your arms are raised and wrapped around the camera.

Section 33.5

Cardiac Stress Rest Test

Reprinted with permission © The Society of Nuclear Medicine

This diagnostic procedure measures the distribution of blood flow to your heart in two stages: during some type of stress (such as exercise) and while you are resting.

Test Preparation

Preparation for the test will depend on several factors, including age, fitness level and pre-existing medical problems. You may be asked to:

- Not eat anything three to four hours before the test is performed because images of your heart will be easier to interpret if your stomach is empty. Also, some people may get an upset stomach if they exercise too soon after eating.

- Discontinue taking previous medications, particularly heart medicine, because they may interfere with the accuracy of the test results. You must check with your doctor to find out whether you should stop taking your medications.

- Wear shorts or slacks for the exercise portion of the test, although the technologist will provide you with a hospital gown for the imaging session. Be sure to wear comfortable shoes, such as sneakers or running shoes, because you may have to do your exercising on a treadmill or stationary bicycle.

Exam Procedure

For the exercise test, small pads called electrodes are placed on your chest so that an electrocardiogram (EKG) can monitor your heart rhythm while you exercise. An intravenous tube is placed in your arm for tracer administration, which occurs about one minute before the end of the exercise session. The exercise may consist of walking on a treadmill or riding the stationary bicycle. As the exercise continues, it becomes more difficult (similar to walking up a hill). As the exercise progresses, the heart rate and blood pressure rise. You will be asked to exercise as long as you can.

If a previous medical problem prevents you from exercising, your doctor may request that using a special medication instead of exercise induce the stress symptoms.

About 30 minutes after the tracer injection, pictures of your heart will be taken.

For the resting portion, you may or may not receive a second injection of tracer, depending on the type of tracer used. As with the imaging portion for the exercise images, pictures will be taken of your heart. This imaging session may take 15 to 30 minutes to complete.

Section 33.6

Liver and Hepatobiliary Imaging

Reprinted with permission © The Society of Nuclear Medicine

Liver scans help diagnose disorders such as cirrhosis, hepatitis, tumors and other problems in the digestive tract. Gallbladder scans are used to evaluate upper abdominal pain, determine causes of jaundice and identify obstruction in the gallbladder.

Test Preparation

For the liver scan, no special preparation is required. If you are having a liver/spleen test, however, you should not have any gastrointestinal tests with barium at least 24 hours before the liver test.

For the gallbladder scan, you may be asked to:

- Not eat or drink for two to four hours before the test because contents in the stomach will alter the test results.

- Stop taking current medications because certain drugs affect how the tracer flows through the biliary tract.

- Remove metal accessories as they may interfere with the study.

Exam Procedure

Liver Scan: After an injection of tracer into your arm, you will wait 10 to 15 minutes for the tracer to be absorbed by the liver. You will then lie on your back on the table, and pictures will be taken of your abdomen from several positions.

Liver/Spleen Scan: Tracer is injected in your arm. Ten to 15 minutes after the injection, you will lie on your back and images from different positions will be taken of your liver and spleen.

Gallbladder Scan: After tracer injection (in the arm), you will lie on your back on the imaging table and multiple images of the abdominal area will be taken. For this test, the images are taken immediately after the tracer injection. Imaging takes one to two hours (or longer) because it is not possible to determine how long it will take your liver to excrete the tracer or when your gallbladder will be visible to the camera.

Gallbladder Scan in Children: The procedure is the same as for adults, except that children under age 3 may require sedation. Also, the imaging time for children is not as long, lasting 45 minutes to 1 hour.

Section 33.7

Ovarian Cancer/Colorectal/ Prostate Cancer Imaging

Reprinted with permission © The Society of Nuclear Medicine

These imaging tests use monoclonal antibodies, which are special disease-fighting substances. When combined with a radioactive tracer, they are quite useful for detecting various tumors, especially those in the ovaries, colon or prostate. You may need a monoclonal antibody scan if you have a history of ovarian, colorectal or prostate cancer, or if your doctor wants to check for recurrences.

Test Preparation

Generally, no special preparation is required. You should, however, tell the technologist if you:

- have had a nuclear medicine test recently

- have been given other murine monoclonal antibody products (ask your doctor, if you are not sure)

- have had previous surgery

- have had a colostomy (if so, you may need to bring an extra bag with you so that you can change it before the imaging session begins

- are allergic or sensitive to any substances or drugs.

If special preparation is required, your doctor will let you know.

Exam Procedure

Monoclonal antibody scans take about three days to perform. You should plan on being at the hospital two to four hours for each session, although it may not take that long.

On the first day of the test, you will get an injection of tracer in your arm. During the injection, and for a short time after it, the technologist will monitor you. You will then be told when to return for the imaging portion of the test (generally two but sometimes up to five days after the injection). You may be asked to take a laxative (or be given an enema) before the imaging session to remove any bowel material so that the pictures are as clear as possible.

Imaging Session: Before the images are taken, you will be asked to empty your bladder (void). For some patients, it may be necessary to insert a catheter. You will also need to remove any gold or metal objects from the neck to the hips (e.g., gold necklace, coins or keys in pocket, belt with metal buckle). You will lie on your back under the camera, and several images will be taken of different areas of your body. After the first set of images are taken, additional imaging sessions may be scheduled the next day.

Section 33.8

Frequently Asked Questions

Reprinted with permission © The Society of Nuclear Medicine

Why May Several Different Tests Be Needed?

Sometimes a variety of diagnostic tests are performed to determine the nature of a medical problem and the most appropriate treatment. Although a diagnosis is usually made with one nuclear medicine test, it may be necessary to confirm the test results with another test or studies.

Are Nuclear Medicine Procedures Safe?

Nuclear medicine procedures are very safe. A patient only receives an extremely small amount of tracer, just enough to provide accurate diagnostic information. The amount of radiation in a nuclear medicine test is no more than that received during an x-ray.

Who Performs Nuclear Medicine Tests?

A nuclear medicine technologist, a health care professional trained and experienced in the theory and practice of nuclear medicine procedures, performs the test by administering the tracer, positioning the patient under the camera and operating the equipment used in the test.

A nuclear medicine physician, who is specially trained in physics and chemistry and is licensed to use tracers, interprets the images.

How Should I Prepare for the Test?

Generally, no special preparation is required, but if preparation is needed, you will be notified before the test. Certain tests may require some slight preparation. For example, if you are having a cardiac stress-rest test, you may be asked not to eat three to four hours before the test because the pictures of your heart will be easier to interpret if the stomach is empty. Or, if you are having a prostate, ovarian or colorectal cancer scan, it is important to let the technologist know if you have had a nuclear medicine test recently, have had previous surgery or are allergic or sensitive to any substances or drugs.

You need not worry about stopping your regular, daily activities or stop taking previously prescribed medications. Although you should check with your doctor, most medications generally do not affect the accuracy of the test results.

The key to having a successful nuclear medicine test is to remain as still as possible. Any movement may distort the image results, making them difficult to interpret and increasing the possibility of redoing the test. Be sure to dress comfortably so that you are relaxed during the test. You should also dress warmly since some imaging rooms may be cold. Also, if lying on your back for long periods of time causes discomfort, you may take a pain reliever before the test is performed.

What Should I Tell My Doctor before the Test Is Scheduled?

You should tell your doctor if you are pregnant or think that you are pregnant. You should also tell your doctor if you are breastfeeding.

Why Do Nuclear Medicine Tests Take a Long Time to Perform?

The amount of time needed for a procedure depends on the type of test. Nuclear medicine tests are performed in three parts: tracer administration, taking the pictures and analyzing the images. For many tests, a certain amount of time is needed (from a few hours to a few days) for the tracer to accumulate in the part of the body being studied before the pictures can be taken. During the imaging session, the time needed to obtain the pictures (from minutes to hours) will vary depending on the test.

Does the Tracer Cause Side Effects?

Adverse reactions, or side effects, are rare, but do let the technologist know if you experience any symptoms during or after the tracer injection.

What Happens after the Test?

When the exam is completed, the nuclear medicine physician reviews your images, prepares a report and discusses the results with your doctor. Your doctor will explain the test results to you and discuss what further procedures, if any are needed.

After the test, should I avoid physical contact with others? No. If you have had radioiodine treatment, however, there are guidelines that your doctor may recommend that you follow to reduce the chance of radiation exposure to others. In general, the tracer you are given will remain in your body for a short period of time and is cleared from the body through natural bodily functions. Drinking fluids will help eliminate the tracer more quickly.

Can I Resume My Daily Activities after the Test?

You should be able to resume your daily activities after a nuclear medicine test. If you were temporarily asked to stop taking any medication prior to the test or if your doctor changed your usual dosage because of the test, be sure to ask when and if you should resume taking your medication(s).

Are Nuclear Medicine Tests Performed on Children?

Yes, scans are performed on children. The tests are usually done to evaluate bone pain, injuries, infection or kidney or bladder functions. The amount of tracer is carefully adjusted based on the child's size. Sedation is sometimes required, depending on the child and type of test being given.

What You Should Know

- Remember to remain still while the pictures are being taken. Movement may distort the images and make the test results difficult to interpret.

- Do not worry about the amount of radiation you will receive during the test. It is no more than what you would receive from similar x-ray procedures.

- Be sure to tell your doctor if you are pregnant, think you are pregnant, or are a nursing mother.

- Let the technologist know if you experience any symptoms during or after the tracer is administered.

- The radioactive tracer remains in your body for a short time and it is cleared from the body through natural bodily functions. Drinking plenty of fluids will help the tracer clear through your body more quickly.

- Ask the technologist to explain any part of the procedure that you do not understand.

Nuclear Medicine Procedures

Scans may be used to diagnose a host of medical problems. Some of the more frequently performed tests include:

- Bone scans to examine orthopedic injuries, fractures, tumors or unexplained bone pain.

- Heart scans to identify normal or abnormal blood flow to the heart muscle, measure heart function or determine the existence or extent of damage to the heart muscle after a heart attack.

- Breast scans which are used in conjunction with mammograms to more accurately detect and locate cancerous tissue in the breasts.

- Liver and gallbladder scans to evaluate liver and gallbladder function.

- Ovarian and colorectal cancer imaging to detect tumors and determine the severity (staging) of various types of cancer.

- Prostate cancer imaging to detect tumors and to determine the extent and spread of various types of cancers.

- Brain imaging to investigate problems within the brain itself or in blood circulation to the brain.

- Renal imaging in children to examine kidney function.

Other commonly performed procedures include thyroid uptake scans to analyze the overall function of the thyroid and show the structure of the gland; lung scans to evaluate the flow of blood and movement of air into and out of the lung as well as determine the presence of blood clots; gallium scans to evaluate infection and certain types of tumors; and gastrointestinal bleeding scans.

Nuclear medicine can also be used for treatment (therapy). Radio-iodine treatment for the thyroid is a common therapeutic procedure.

The material presented here is for informational purposes only and is not intended as a substitute for discussion between you and your physician. Be sure to consult with your physician or the nuclear medicine department where the test will be performed if you require more information about specific nuclear medicine procedures.

Chapter 34

Magnetic Resonance Imaging (MRI Scan)

Contents

Section 34.1

How MRI Works

Reprinted with permission. © 1997 Steven H. Brick, M.D.

Equipment

Magnetic resonance imaging (MRI) scan requires the use of a very strong magnetic field. Unlike other devices used in radiology, MR imaging uses no radiation. The magnet is contained in the housing of the scanner and this creates a magnetic field oriented down the center of the magnet. The patient is placed within the magnetic field by lying on a table which is placed through the center of the opening of the magnet, similar to lying on a road running through a tunnel. The strength of the magnetic field is measured in units called *gauss or Tesla*: 10,000 gauss equals 1 Tesla. The earth's magnetic field is approximately 0.6 gauss. The strongest magnetic field permitted in MRI scanning of humans is 1.5 Tesla (1.5T).

Three types of magnets are available for use in MRI. The strongest is a *superconducting* magnet. This is a type of electromagnet in which current flowing in a circular direction in a coil of wire creates a magnetic field oriented down the core of the coil. In superconducting magnets, the wire conducts the current without significant resistance because it is cooled to a temperature close to absolute zero by being bathed in a jacket of liquid helium and/or liquid nitrogen. Most MR scanners in use today are superconductng magnets. *Resistive* magnets are electromagnets, similar to superconducting magnets, but

Figure 34.1. *Magnetic Resonance Scanner*

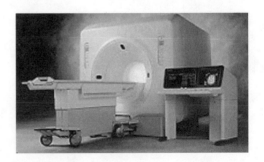

they are air cooled therefore have greater resistance to current and create weaker magnetic fields. *Permanent* magnets are made of solid magnetic material, similar to bar magnets, and create the weakest magnetic fields. However, they can be arranged in a configuration that doesn't require the patient to be surrounded by the magnet and are used in Open MR scanners.

Creating an Image

The physics of MRI are extremely complex, but an extremely simplified explanation will be attempted. When a patient is placed within an MR scanner, the protons in the patient's tissues (primarily protons contained in water molecules) align themselves along the direction of the magnetic field. A radiofrequency electromagnetic pulse is then applied, which deflects the protons off their axis along the magnetic field. As the protons realign themselves with the magnetic field, a signal is produced. This signal is detected by an antenna, and with the help of computer analysis, is converted into an image.

Figure 34.2. Longitudinal Relaxation

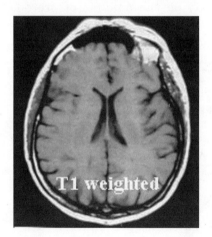

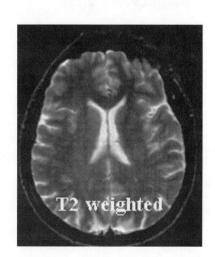

Figure 34.3. Transverse Relaxation

The process by which the protons realign themselves with the magnetic field is referred to as *relaxation*. The protons undergo 2 types of relaxation: T1 (or longitudinal) relaxation and T2 (or transverse relaxation) relaxation. Different tissues undergo different rates of relaxation, and these differences create the contrast between different structures, and the contrast between normal and abnormal tissue, seen on MR scans. *T1 weighted images* emphasize the difference in T1 relaxation times between different tissues. In these images, water containing structures are dark. Since most pathologic processes (such as tumors, injuries, and Cardio-Vascular Aneurysms CVA), involve edema (or water), T1 weighted images do not show good contrast between normal and abnormal tissues. However, they do demonstrate excellent anatomic detail. *T2 weighted images* emphasize the difference in T2 relaxation times between different tissues. Since water is bright on these images, T2 weighted images provide excellent contrast between normal and abnormal tissues, although the anatomic detail is less then that of T1 weighted images. *Proton density images* emphasize neither T1 nor T2 relaxation times, and therefore produce contrast based primarily on the amount of protons present in the tissue.

Intravenous contrast is often used to improve the sensitivity of MR imaging, especially in the brain and spine. MR contrast agents contain gadolinium, which increases T1 relaxation and causes certain abnormalities to "light up" on T1 weighted images. These agents contain no iodine, and allergic reactions are extremely rare.

Image Orientation

MRI images can be obtained in any imaging plane without moving the patient. However, three standard views are usually used:

- **Transverse (axial):** *Imagine the patient is lying on their back and is sliced across from right to left. You are viewing from the patient's feet.*

- **Coronal:** *Imagine the patient is standing in front of you and is sliced across from right to left. You are viewing from the front of the patient.*

- **Sagittal:** *Imagine the patient is standing sideways and is sliced across from front to back. You are viewing from the side of the patient.*

302

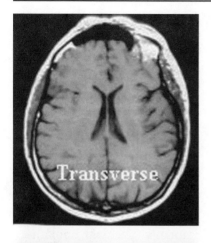

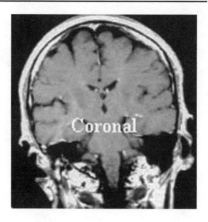

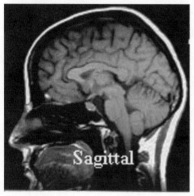

Figure 34.4. MRI Imaging Orientations

Safety

Although multiple studies have been performed, no significant biological hazards have been demonstrated as a result of exposure to patients from the magnetic fields or radio frequency electromagnetic pulses used in magnetic resonance imaging. However, there can be adverse effects on various medical devices implanted into patients and therefore all patients must be carefully screened to determine if MR scanning can be safely performed. All patients will be asked to complete a questionnaire prior to undergoing an MR scan. This may be provided either at your doctor's office or at the site of the MR scanner. It is critical that all questions be answered completely and honestly. If you have any questions, be sure to ask the staff at the MR scanner. Potential risks fall into the following categories:

- Cardiac pacemakers: Absolute contraindication. These patients cannot be scanned.

- Cerebral aneurysm clip: Most patients who have had surgical repair of a cerebral (brain) aneurysm are not permitted to have an MR scan (the clip used to repair the aneurysm might move and bleeding could occur).

- Implanted electromagnetic devices: Medication or insulin pumps, biostimulators, and neurostimulators can be damaged by the magnetic field and those patients should not be scanned.

- Prosthetic heart valves: Most are safe, but check with the MR staff.

- Magnetically activated or supported implants (Cochlear implants, some dental and ocular implants): Should not be scanned.

- Orthopedic devices (Joint replacements, plates, screws, etc.): All are safe.

- Metal fragments in body (bullet, BB, shrapnel, etc.): Safe, unless in contact with vital organ, such as heart, spinal cord, eye.

- Surgical clips: Safe.

- Intravascular coils, filters, or stents: Safe if in place more than 1 week.

Section 34.2

MRI of the Brain

Reprinted with permission. © 1997 Steven H. Brick, M.D.

Introduction

The brain is the most complex organ in the human body. The development of Computed Tomography (CT) in the 1970's revolutionized imaging of the brain. However, MRI has taken those advances several levels higher and has replaced CT as the imaging modality of choice for most disorders of the nervous system.

Normal Anatomy

MRI demonstrates normal anatomy of the brain in a manner far superior to CT. In addition to providing improved anatomic detail and improved contrast between normal and abnormal tissue, MR permits imaging in multiple planes without re-positioning the patient (CT is usually limited to the transverse plane).

A wide variety of intracranial abnormalities can be accurately diagnosed with MRI, and many are demonstrated below, including primary brain tumor, metastatic disease (spread of tumor to the brain from cancer elsewhere in the body), cerebral infarct (stroke), multiple sclerosis, and cranial nerve tumors. Other pathologic processes include hemorrhage, vascular abnormalities, and pituitary and sellar masses.

It should be noted that CT still has a primary role in imaging the patient with an acute neurologic event. Since MR is relatively insensitive to the detection of hyperacute hemorrhage (bleeding less than

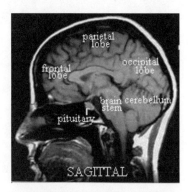 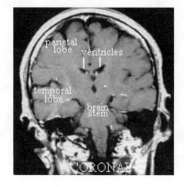

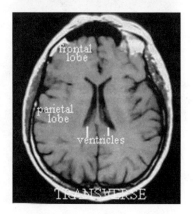

Figure 34.5. Normal Brain Anatomy

24 hours old), patients in whom very acute or post-traumatic hemorrhage is suspected should still be imaged initially with CT.

Brain Tumor

Glioblastomas comprise more than 50% of all brain tumors and occur most frequently in middle age. The tumor itself is of varying intensity on different MR images, but frequently shows enhancement from contrast. Surrounding edema (swelling of the brain) is often present and is best seen on T2-weighted images, although it can be difficult to separate the edema from the tumor prior to contrast administration. Mass effect (pressure from the tumor) and hydrocephalus ("water on the brain") are well demonstrated by MR's multiplanar capabilities.

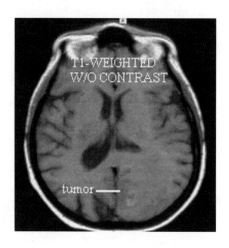

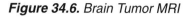

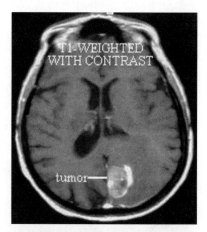

Figure 34.6. Brain Tumor MRI

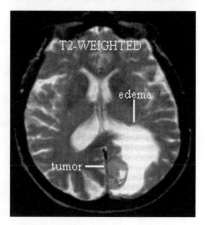

Cerebral Metastases

Cerebral metastases (spread of tumor to the brain from cancer elsewhere in the body) are a significant cause of morbidity and mortality (illness and death) in cancer patients. Early detection has a considerable effect on treatment and prognosis. MRI with contrast is considerably more sensitive than CT for the detection of cerebral metastases. The lesions often are invisible without contrast and therefore it is imperative that all cancer patients have MR of the brain performed with intravenous contrast.

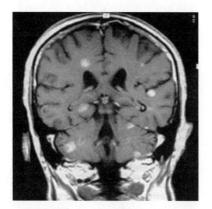
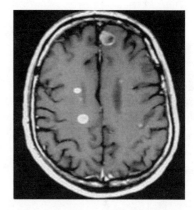

Figure 34.7. Metastasized Cancer in the Brain. These T1-weighted images with contrast in the coronal (left) and transverse (right) planes show the typical appearance of cerebral metastases as multiple small, round enhancing nodules. They are frequently located at the gray matter-white matter interface (the outer layer of the brain) and may be associated with edema (swelling) and/or hemorrhage (bleeding).

Stroke

Cerebral infarction (stroke) is a major cause of morbidity, mortality, and disability in the elderly population. As newer treatment options are being developed, the early and accurate diagnosis of stroke becomes more critical. MRI is the imaging modality of choice for the detection of cerebral infarction, and also provides vital information concerning the size and location of the infarct. MR also can demonstrate complications of infarction, such as hemorrhage, mass effect, and herniation (movement of the brain from increased pressure in one area).

Figure 34.8. Infarct (Stroke) Images. These transverse proton-density (left) and T2-weighted (right) images demonstrate an acute left temporal lobe infarct as swelling and edema of the cortical gray matter (the outermost layer of the brain) along the distribution of a branch of the left middle cerebral artery. Although not used in this case, intravenous contrast is usually administered in the evaluation of infarction since it can both aid in the detection of an early infarct and can help determine the age of the infarct. Although hyperacute hemorrhage (less than 24 hours ago) can be difficult to detect, MR is very sensitive for the detection of even small amounts of hemorrhage after the first day.

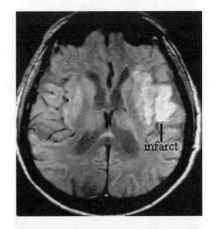

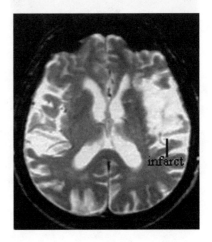

Multiple Sclerosis

Multiple sclerosis (MS) is a common disorder caused by plaques of inflammation and "demyelination" of the myelin sheaths of neurons (lining of nerve cells) in the central nervous system white matter. It predominately affects young and middle aged patients of Northern European extraction. The diagnosis is usually made on clinical findings, with intermittent symptoms implicating specific sites of central nervous system (CNS) involvement separated by time and place. The initial relapsing and remitting course frequently shifts into a chronic progressive course in later years. MRI is the first imaging modality that permits direct visualization of the MS plaques in the CNS.

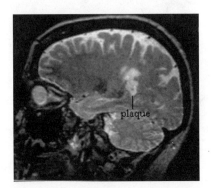 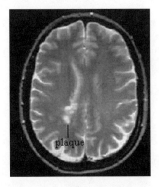

Figure 34.9. MS Plaques in the Central Nervous System. These T2-weighted sagittal (left) and transverse (right) images show a single large plague adjacent to the right lateral ventricle. Several additional lesions were seen on other slices. The classic MR appearance of MS plagues shows multiple focal periventricular lesions (the ventricles are inter-connecting spaces of spinal fluid within the brain) that are increased signal on proton-density and T2-weighted images, creating a "lumpy-bumpy" configuration. The lesions are usually small and homogeneous. Active lesions can enhance with contrast.

Acoustic Schwannoma

Acoustic schwannomas (previously called acoustic neuromas) are benign tumors that arise from the sheath of the eighth cranial nerve, usually within the internal auditory canal (IAC). These structures are found in the bones at the base of the brain. Patients can present with unilateral (one-sided) hearing loss and/or tinnitus (ringing in the ear). MRI is far superior to CT in evaluating these lesions since CT is severely limited by artifact from the dense bones at the skull base and restriction to the transverse plane.

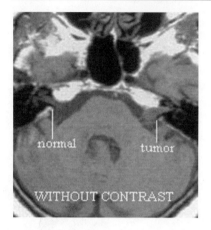

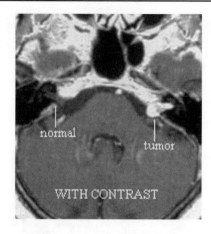

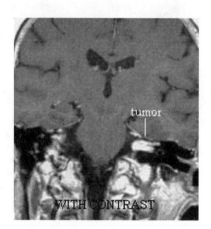

Figure 34.10. Benign Tumor in the Auditory Canal. The above pre-contrast T1-weighted axial (upper left) and post-contrast T1-weighted axial (above right) and coronal (immediate left) images demonstrate the classic appearance of an acoustic schwannoma in the left internal auditory canal. The normal right IAC is seen on the axial images. The tumors are usually round or oval shaped, can be small or large, can be limited to the internal auditory canal or extend into the space next to the canal, and demonstrate diffuse enhancement with contrast.

Section 34.3

MRI of the Spine

Reprinted with permission. © 1997 Steven H. Brick, M.D.

Introduction

MRI has become the main diagnostic test for imaging the spine and has eliminated the need for CT and myelography in many clinical settings. Detailed studies of the cervical (neck), thoracic (upper back), or lumbar spine (lower spine) can be easily obtained. Surveys of the entire spine can also be obtained in a single exam. The superior contrast and spatial resolution of MRI, along with the capability of presenting images from many different views, allows exquisite display of normal spinal anatomy. The most frequent pathologic conditions seen are secondary to degenerative disc disease, including herniated disc (sometimes referred to as "ruptured disc") and spinal stenosis. Other disorders that can be studied include metastatic disease (spread of cancer in a different part of the body to the spine), infection, and trauma.

Normal Anatomy

The spine consists of 29 bones called vertebrae stacked one on top of the other extending from the base of the skull down to the coccyx (tail-bone). Most of these vertebrae have 2 components: the vertebral body and the posterior elements. The vertebral bodies are square shaped bones filled with bone marrow. The fat in the marrow is bright on T1-weighted MR images. The vertebral bodies are separated by discs, which serve as cushions for the spine. The discs can be thought of as jelly donuts, with a gelatinous center (the nucleus propulsus) surrounded by a fibrous capsule (the annulus fibrosis). The posterior elements have a ring-like configuration with the spinal cord running down the center of the stacked rings. The spinal cord is surrounded by a thin walled tube filled with cerebrospinal fluid (CSF) called the thecal sac. The nerve roots leave the spinal cord through openings called foraminae in between adjacent vertebrae and then spread out to muscles and organs throughout the body. Each vertebrae is assigned a number (e.g. C5 is the fifth cervical vertebrae from the top). The discs are labeled according to their adjacent vertebrae (e.g. L3-4 is the disc between the third and fourth lumbar vertebrae).

The cervical cord can be followed from its origin from the brain stem to its junction with the thoracic cord.

The thoracic spine consists of 12 vertebrae; T1 through T12 (no images of the thoracic spine are included here).

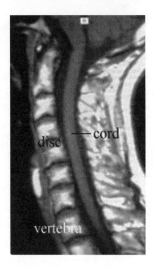 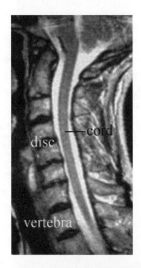

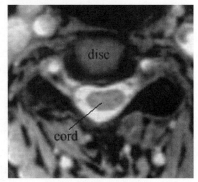

Figure 34.11. Normal Anatomy of the Cervical Spine. The cervical spine consists of 7 vertebrae; C1 through C7. The above images include T1-weighted sagittal (upper left), T2-weighted sagittal (upper right), and T2-weighted transverse images (right).

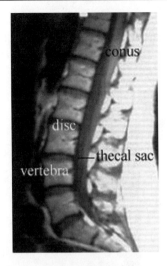 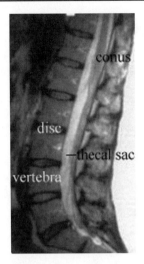

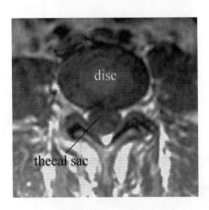

Figure 34.12. Normal Anatomy of the Lumbar Spine. The lumbar spine consists of 5 vertebrae; L1 through L5. These images include T1-weighted sagittal (upper left), T2-weighted sagittal (upper right), and T2-weighted transverse images (left). The spinal cord usually ends at the L1-L2 level in a structure called the conus medullaris. Below this level, the nerve roots extend inferiorly in the cauda equina, surrounded by the CSF filled thecal sac until they exit the spine through their respective neural foramen.

Herniated Disc

In the intervertebral disc, the annulus fibrosis (the donut in the jelly donut model) serves as the retaining capsule of the nucleus propulsus (the jelly). The medical term for a "ruptured" disc is a herniated nucleus propulsus (HNP), or simply a herniated disc. This occurs when the "jelly" in the center of the disc squirts through a tear in the "donut". As this material pushes into the spinal canal, it can compress the nerve roots either as they descend in the thecal sac, or as they leave the sac. In the neck, these nerves innervate the shoulders and arms. In the back, these nerves innervate the legs and compression can cause the typical pain of sciatica which radiates down one leg. Your doctor can frequently tell which nerve is being affected because compression of a specific nerve will cause pain or numbness in a specific part of the arm or leg.

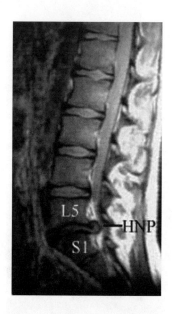

Figure 34.13. Left Sided Herniated Disc. These sagittal (upper right) and transverse (lower right) images of the lumbar spine demonstrate a left sided herniated disc (HNP) at L5-S1. The sagittal images are best to delineate the herniation of the nucleus propulsus through the annulus fibrosis. The transverse images best define the compression of the thecal sac and the left S1 nerve root.

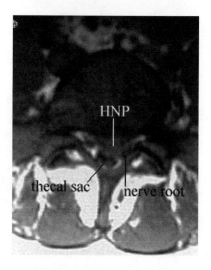

Spinal Stenosis

Spinal stenosis is due to narrowing of the spinal canal, usually secondary to degenerative disc disease. The canal is usually narrowed in the front by a bulging or herniated disc. This is frequently accompanied by narrowing of the sides and back of the canal from enlargement of the supporting bones and ligaments that form the protective ring around the spinal canal. Patients frequently have pain in both arms or legs, often exacerbated by standing.

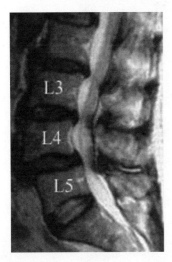 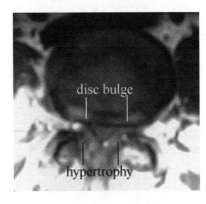

Figure 34.14. Spinal Stenosis (Narrowing of the Spinal Cord). This case demonstrates spinal stenosis at L3-4 and L4-5. The sagittal image (left) shows the stenosis at L4-5 is at least partly due to anterior displacement of L4 on L5 (this slip is called "spondylolisthesis"). The transverse image (right) shows the typical triangular configuration of the narrowed thecal sac.

Metastases to the Spine

The most common tumors that tend to spread to the spine arise in the prostate, breast, and lung. Metastatic tumors demonstrate decreased signal on T1-weighted images and are well seen when contrasted against the high signal fatty marrow in the vertebrae. Since the presence of metastases has such a great impact on the prognosis for a cancer patient, MRI is frequently used to further evaluate suspected lesions seen on x-ray or bone scan. MRI also serves a vital role in evaluating the cancer patient with suspected cord compression (tumor that pushes against the spine and which can lead to permanent paralysis). MRI can survey the entire spine in less than one hour with minimal discomfort to the patient. The location of metastases can be accurately identified and, more importantly, the sites of compression of the spinal canal or spinal cord can be delineated prior to surgery or radiation therapy.

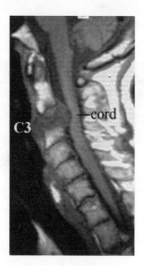 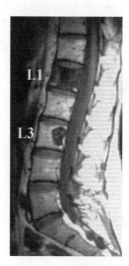

Figure 34.15. Metastatic Tumors in the Spine. Metastases to the spine are seen in these two different patients. The low signal of the tumors involving the cervical spine at C3 (left) and the lumbar spine at L1 and L3 (right) can be easily separated from the high signal of the normal marrow. The lesion at C3 is causing significant compression of the spinal cord in this patient who presented with rapidly worsening weakness of the arms and legs.

Spinal Infection

Spinal infection (infective spondylitis) can be extremely difficult to diagnose clinically because its symptoms are very similar to other, more common causes of back pain. Infection frequently begins in the vertebral body, but can also originate in the disc, epidural space (the space between the thecal sac and the vertebra), or paraspinal soft tissues. Mechanisms of infection include blood borne organisms, spread from an adjacent site, or direct implantation (trauma, post-operative).

In addition to diagnosing the presence of infection, MRI can evaluate for the extent of bone and disc destruction. It can also detect any extension of infection into the epidural space (epidural abscess) with secondary thecal sac or spinal cord compression that might require surgical decompression.

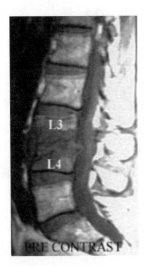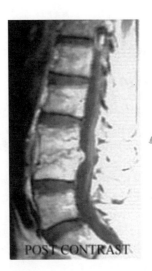

Figure 34.16. Spinal Infection. This case presents the typical MRI findings of spinal infection. The non-contrast T1-weighted sagittal image (left) shows destruction of the L3-4 disc and the adjacent vertebral body endplates with replacement of the normal marrow signal. After contrast is administered (right), there is diffuse enhancement of the entire mass of infected material. A small epidural abscess can also be seen extending posteriorly from the disc into the spinal canal.

Section 34.4

MRI of the Knee

Introduction

The availability of MR scanning has allowed imaging of disorders of the knee with detail that could only previously be seen at surgery. Normal anatomy can be demonstrated with exquisite detail. Injuries such as tears in the meniscus (also known as torn cartilage) or the anterior cruciate ligament are demonstrated below. Other disorders that can be diagnosed include collateral ligament tears, occult fractures (very subtle fractures that aren't seen on x-rays), avascular necrosis (death of a small portion of bone near the joint), chondromalacia (softening of the cartilage of the patella), and tumors.

Normal Anatomy

The human knee permits flexion and extension of the leg. The proper functioning of its many components are required for motion, stabilization, and cushioning. These components include:

- Bony structures and their overlying cartilage: femur (thigh bone), tibia (thick bone in lower leg), fibula (thin bone in lower leg), patella (kneecap)

- Motion-producing muscles and tendons: flexor - bend the knee (biceps femoris, semimembranous, semitendinous, sartorius, gracilis) and extensor - straighten the knee (quadriceps, patellar)

- Stabilizing components: medial and lateral collateral ligaments (MCL and LCL), anterior and posterior cruciate ligaments (ACL and PCL), medial and lateral menisci, patellofemoral mechanism, joint capsule.

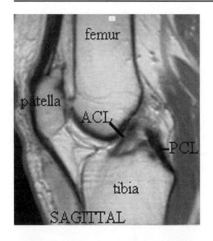

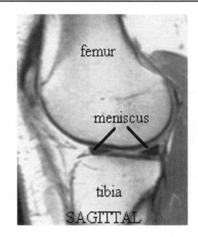

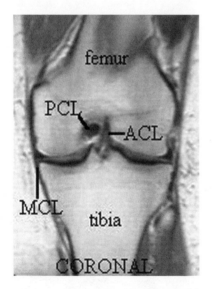

Figure 34.17. Normal Anatomy of the Knee

Torn Meniscus

The medial and lateral menisci are C-shaped structures composed of fibrocartilage that fill in the space at the articulation between the end of the femur at the top of the tibia. They serve to stabilize the joint, absorb shock, and guide the movements of the joint. Meniscal tears can develop as the result of an acute injury. However, many tears are degenerative in origin and are the result of years of chronic stress

319

on the joint during normal use. The normal meniscus has a dark, triangular appearance. MRI has been proven to be highly sensitive (up to 95% sensitivity) and accurate for the diagnosis of meniscal tears.

On MR scans, a torn meniscus appears as linear increased signal within the meniscus that extends to an articular surface (Grade III signal) and this corresponds to a tear that can be detected at arthroscopy in over 90% of cases. Areas of increased signal in the meniscus that do not extend to the surface are labeled Grade I (round or globular signal) or Grade II (linear signal) and are not felt to be significant since they usually cannot be identified at arthroscopy.

Figure 34.18. Torn Meniscus

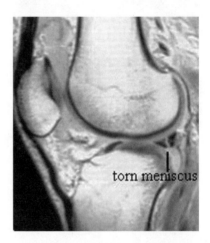

Figure 34.19. Torn Anterior Cruciate Ligament

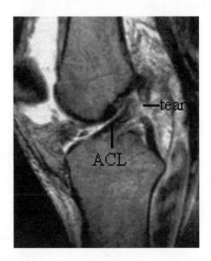

Torn Anterior Cruciate Ligament

The anterior cruciate ligament (ACL) extends from the inner aspect of the lateral femoral condyle posteriorly, to its attachment on the tibial plateau just anterior and lateral to the anterior tibial spine. It serves to control anterior motion of the tibia in relation to the femur, especially during extension (straightening of the leg).

On MR images, a torn ACL can appear as discontinuity or complete absence of the ligament, which is frequently replaced by an amorphous collection of edematous tissue. Associated findings often include lateral bone bruises (tiny microfractures in the femur or tibia), anterior displacement of the tibia in relation to the femur, and buckling of the posterior cruciate ligament.

Section 34.5

MRI of the Shoulder

Reprinted with permission. © 1997 Steven H. Brick, M.D.

Introduction

The shoulder is the most mobile joint in the body. MRI permits non-invasive imaging the many interconnected structures of the shoulder with resolution and tissue contrast unattainable with CT. Highly detailed images of the normal shoulder anatomy can be obtained. The most common application for MRI of the shoulder is to detect rotator cuff tear. Prior to MRI, the rotator cuff could only be imaged by arthrography, which involves inserting a needle into the joint and injecting radiographic contrast ("X-ray dye"). MRI allows evaluation of the cuff in a completely non-invasive manner. Another common use is to evaluate for cartilage tears in patients with recurrent dislocations of the shoulder.

Normal Anatomy

The rotator cuff consists of a group of tendons that arise from four different muscles (the supraspinatus, infraspinatus, subscapularies and teres minor muscles). It covers the top of the shoulder joint and serves mainly to raise the arm away from the body and to turn the arm outward. It also serves as a stabilizer of the shoulder joint. The glenoid labrum is a fibrous ring attached to the glenoid process of the scapula (the shoulder blade) and along with the joint capsule and various ligaments, serves to stabilize the humeral head in the shoulder joint (keep the arm in its socket). Important bony structures include the humeral head, scapula, and acromioclavicular joint.

Figure 34.20. *Normal Rotator Cuff*

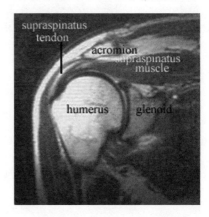

Figure 34.21. *Rotator Cuff Tear*

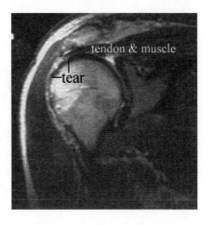

Rotator Cuff Tear

The general public often thinks of rotator cuff tears as season or career ending injuries suffered by major league pitchers. However, this condition is considerably more common in the older population. Causes of disorders of the rotator cuff include pressure from degenerative changes from adjacent structures (impingement from the acromioclavicular joint), occupational or athletic overuse, or primary degeneration of the tendon (probably related to poor blood supply). Rotator cuff pathology progresses through several stages, from edema and hemorrhage (Stage I), to fibrosis (scarring) and thickening (Stage II), to partial or complete tear (Stage III). Rotator cuff tears almost always begin in the supraspinatus tendon, although extension into the other tendons of the cuff can also be seen.

On MRI, rotator cuff tears appear as areas of increased signal in the tendon. Tears can be full thickness or partial. In full thickness tears, the muscle can pull away from the joint because the tendon no longer anchors it to the humerus. MRI also reveals the extent of impingement on the rotator cuff from the acromioclavicular joint, findings that are important to note when surgical repair is being considered.

Section 34.6

MRI of the Hip

Reprinted with permission. © 1997 Steven H. Brick, M.D.

Introduction

The most frequent parts of the musculoskeletal system that are imaged with MRI are the knee and shoulder. However, MRI has also been used to study almost every joint in the body, including the hip. The most common clinical indications for MRI of the hip are to determine the presence of avascular necrosis and occult hip fracture.

Avascular Necrosis

Avascular necrosis (AVN) is due to poor blood supply and eventual death of the cellular elements in the bone marrow of the femoral head (the top part of the thigh bone that forms the ball in the "ball-in-socket" hip joint). The main clinical symptom is pain. Predisposing conditions include steroid use, trauma, alcohol abuse, pancreatitis, and sickle cell anemia. By the time changes of AVN are seen on x-rays, bone destruction has usually already occurred. MRI permits diagnosis at much earlier stages, with early treatment hopefully preventing joint destruction and the need for hip replacement.

Early changes of AVN on MRI consist of alterations in the homogeneous marrow signal seen in the normal femoral head. In more advanced cases (such as this patient's left hip) flattening and irregularity of the femoral head can be seen due to subtle microfractures and collapse of the joint surface.

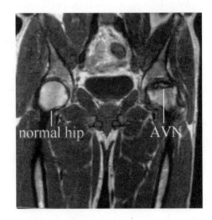

Figure 34.22. MRI of Hip

Occult Hip Fracture

The great majority of hip fractures are obviously diagnosed with plain x-rays. However, some patients have hip fractures which cannot be seen (these are called "occult" hip fractures). The evaluation of these patients includes a variety of options. Nuclear medicine bone scan is frequently used, but can be negative for up to four days after the injury. Plain tomography and CT can be helpful, but they mainly image cortical bone and subtle fractures can be difficult to diagnose with certainty.

MRI requires no time delay and has proven to be an extremely accurate method to diagnose occult hip fractures. As shown in the following T1-weighted coronal (right) and transverse (left) images, the fracture line can be easily seen extending through the marrow space of the left femoral neck. Even if no hip fracture is present, MR can frequently diagnose the cause of the patient's pain by seeing other findings including bone bruise, joint effusion, soft tissue hematoma, and pelvic fractures.

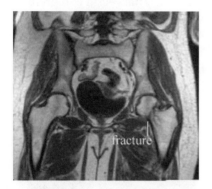 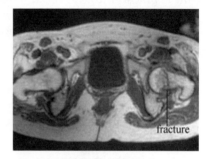

Figure 34.23. *MRI of Hip Fractures*

Section 34.7

MRI of the Prostate

Reprinted with permission. © 1997 Steven H. Brick, M.D.

Adenocarcinoma of the Prostate

Adenocarcinoma of the prostate is the most common non-skin malignancy in U.S. men and is the second leading cause of death by cancer. Prostatic carcinoma is being detected more frequently than in the past as the result of increased use of annual rectal exams, serum prostate-specific antigen (PSA) levels, and ultrasound studies of the prostate. The choice of appropriate treatment is mainly determined by the life expectancy of the patient and by whether the tumor is confined to the gland and its capsule (the fibrous covering of the gland). If the tumor is confined to the gland, surgery (radical prostatectomy) is often the treatment of choice. However, if the tumor extends through the capsule, surgery is not recommended and radiation therapy is usually advised. Hormonal therapy is preferred when the cancer spread to other parts of the body.

Tumor spread outside the prostatic capsule has traditionally been detected by the examiner's finger during rectal exam. MRI has attempted to improve the accuracy of those findings. In order to best evaluate the prostate, MRI is performed with a special surface coil that is placed into the rectum during the exam. This rectal coil greatly improves the sensitivity of the study when compared to traditional imaging with the body coil. However, at the conclusion of the study, images of the abdomen and pelvis with the body coil are performed in order to detect any enlarged lymph nodes that might represent distant spread of tumor.

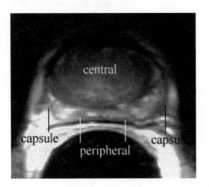 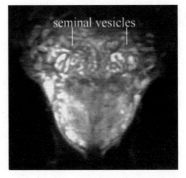

Figure 34.24. MRI of Normal Prostate. The above transverse (left) and coronal (right) of the normal prostate show the rounded, lower signal peripheral zone which is the frequent site of benign prostatic hypertrophy (BPH). Prostatic carcinoma is usually found in the peripheral zone, which has a more homogeneous, higher signal appearance. The prostatic capsule is seen as a thin, low signal line surrounding the gland. The coronal images are best for evaluation of the seminal vesicles and direct invasion of these structures would be a contraindication for surgery.

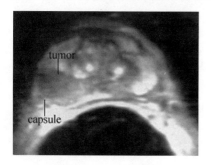

Figure 34.25. *Prostate Carcinoma. This transverse image shows the prostatic carcinoma in the right peripheral zone as a low signal lesion. The tumor extends to the prostatic capsule, but not through it. This patient would be a candidate for surgical treatment.*

Section 34.8

Open MRI

Reprinted with permission. © 1997 Steven H. Brick, M.D.

As discussed in the "MRI: How It Works" section of this chapter, most MR scanners in use today are superconducting magnets in which the magnet field is generated down the bore of an electromagnetic coil. By design, these scanners are shaped like a tunnel and are enclosed on all sides (although they are open at the top and bottom). Some patients, especially those with claustrophobia, are uncomfortable with the enclosed feeling created by the MR scanner. Many can undergo the exam without difficulty by taking an oral sedative (e.g. Valium, Ativan) prescribed by their doctor prior to the exam. Most facilities also are equipped to safely administer intravenous sedation when needed. Almost all claustrophobic patients are able to undergo the MR scan successfully with one of the sedative approaches.

However, there is an alternative to the traditional enclosed MR scanner. **Open MRI** scanners use permanent magnets above and below the patient, usually supported by widely spaced columns. This permits the sides of the scanner to almost completely open and markedly decreases the enclosed feeling. The magnet used in open MRI in considerably weaker than a superconducting magnet. This lowers the resolution of the images created, although diagnostic studies can usually be produced. Therefore, open MRI is recommended only when the patient cannot undergo a traditional scan and these types of patients usually include:

- Claustrophobic patients *who either do not want to receive sedation or in whom sedation is inadequate or unsafe.*

- Obese patients *who are either too large to fit in an enclosed magnet or whose weight exceeds the limit of the table on the enclosed magnet.*

Part Five

Electrical Tests

Chapter 35

Electrocardiogram (ECG) and Signal-Averaged ECG

Electrocardiogram

An electrocardiogram (ECG) is a graphic recording of your heart's electrical activity. Normally, electrical impulses move unimpeded throughout the heart and play an important role in causing the heart to beat. An electrocardiogram can give your doctor considerable information about the health and functioning of your heart. Your doctor can learn about your heart rhythm, the chambers of your heart, the functioning of your heart muscle and whether you had a heart attack in the past.

Why Does My Doctor Want to Perform an ECG?

The reasons for ordering an ECG vary. If this is a new doctor, or if you have never had this test, an ECG may be performed as part of a complete history and physical examination. The ECG reading will give the doctor a baseline picture of your heart's activity. Future ECGs will be compared to ascertain if changes have taken place, or if you have had an intervening heart attack.

You may have complained to your physician of symptoms such as chest pain, palpitations, fainting or irregular heartbeats. You doctor will have this test performed to rule out certain cardiac diseases or determine if additional testing is necessary.

"Cardiovascular Center Diagnostic Tests," © 1998 Mt. Sinai School of Medicine.

Signal-Averaged Electrocardiogram

This type of ECG, a signal-averaged electrocardiogram, can tell your doctor if you are at risk for developing potentially lethal heart rhythms. It is a technique that amplifies low amplitude ECG signals, and reduces random noises surrounding these signals. These signals are called "late potentials." The ECG is filtered and parts of it are averaged, allowing identification of late potentials.

Late potentials represent delayed conduction through diseased heart muscle. Late potentials may be present in a variety of situations, a few of which are arrhythmias (irregular heart rhythms), heart chamber abnormalities, syncope (loss of consciousness), and scar tissue from prior heart attacks.

Why Has My Doctor Ordered a Signal-Averaged ECG?

If you recently had a heart attack or have undergone open heart surgery, your doctor may want to evaluate your heart rhythms to rule out life-threatening arrhythmias.

You may have symptoms such as syncope of unknown origin and/ or palpitations. The signal-averaged electrocardiogram will help your doctor determine whether further testing (e.g. electrophysiology study), is required.

Are There Any Risks Associated with an Electrocardiogram or Signal-Averaged Electrocardiogram?

Both of these tests are safe and painless. There are no known risks associated with the ECG or the signal-averaged ECG, and you will not have to sign a consent form.

What Preparations Should I Make before the Test?

At the commencement of the test, you will be asked to undress from the waist up. Women should wear a two-piece outfit that buttons or zips in the front.

What Happens during the Test?

After you have removed your garments, a nurse or technician will clean areas of your chest, back and limbs where the electrodes will be placed.

Then the nurse or technician will place the electrodes on your body and attach the leads to the ECG machine. The electrodes are usually thin, gel-backed, self-sticking rectangles, about an inch long. The gel may feel a little cool at first.

Then you will lie down for a few minutes, while the technician enters information into the ECG computer.

Next the technician will press a button, and you will be asked to lie still for less than a minute while your heart's electrical activity is recorded. You will not feel anything. The whole tests lasts from 30 to 60 minutes.

What Happens after the Test?

Sometimes your doctor will examine you immediately after the test. Sometimes you will get dressed and your doctor will discuss the results of the test at another time.

What Will My Physician Do with this Information?

Based on the ECG, your history and physical examination, your doctor will determine if additional testing is necessary. She may prescribe medication for you or decide that no further action is required.

Chapter 36

Electroencephalograph (EEG)

What Is the EEG?

The EEG (electroencephalogram) displays the electrical activity of the brain. Nerve cells in the brain are constantly creating very small electrical signals, whether a patient is waking or sleeping. The EEG machine contains amplifiers which make these signals, or brainwaves, big enough so we can see them. The electrical signals are picked up by electrodes glued to the scalp, and travel to the amplifiers of the EEG machine and then are either written out on paper or saved on the hard drive of a computer and displayed on the computer's monitor. There are two electrodes plugged into each amplifier on the EEG machine. The amplifier looks at the two electrode signals coming into it and cancels out signals that are the same. So, the signal that you see on the paper or on the computer screen is actually the difference between the electrical activity picked up by two electrodes. The placement of the electrodes is important because the closer the electrodes are to each other the less differences in their brainwaves. Therefore, if the electrodes are too close, the EEG will look like a straight line

---

This chapter combines text from "EEG Questions and Answers" by Seline Haines, R.EEG.T., Head EEG Technician at the Epilepsy Center at Barnes Hospital and a member of the professional advisory board of the Epilepsy Foundation of the St. Louis Region (EFS), reprinted with permission; and "Electroencephalography (Brain Monitoring)," used with permission from *Everything You Need to Know about Medical Tests*, © 1996 Springhouse Corporation.

instead of showing the brainwaves. This is why the technician measures the head of each patient. Measuring the electrode placements allows the technician to have equal distances between all the electrodes to get clear and symmetrical brainwaves. The technician also has to constantly watch the EEG to make sure the electrodes are working properly and to eliminate any artifact or electrical interference that might occur.

Why Is This Test Done?

An electroencephalograph may be performed for the following reasons:

- To determine the presence and type of seizures

- To help diagnose brain abscesses and tumors

- To evaluate the brain's electrical activity in head injury, meningitis, encephalitis, mental retardation, and psychological disorders

- To confirm brain death.

What Should You Know before the Test?

- Don't drink caffeine-containing coffee, tea, colas, or other beverages beforehand. Otherwise, you can follow your usual diet.

- Thoroughly wash and dry your hair to remove hair sprays, creams, or oils.

- Tell the doctor or nurse if you take any medications—especially drugs for seizures, anxiety, insomnia, or depression. You may have to stop taking any of these medications for a day or two before the test.

- If you're going to have a "sleep electroencephalograph," you'll need to stay awake the night before the test. Just before the test, a nurse will give you a sedative to help you sleep during the test.

- You'll be asked to sign a form that gives your permission to do the test. Read the form carefully and ask questions if any portion of it isn't clear.

What Happens during the Test?

- During the test, you relax in a reclining chair or lie on a bed, and electrodes are attached to your scalp with a special paste. The electrodes don't cause any electric shocks.

- Before the recording procedure begins, close your eyes, relax, and remain still. Don't talk.

- The recording may be stopped now and then to let you rest or reposition yourself.

- After the initial recording, you may be tested under various stress-producing conditions to elicit patterns not observable while you're resting. For example, you may be asked to breathe deeply and rapidly for 3 minutes, which may elicit brain wave patterns typical of seizures or other problems. Or a bright light may be shone at you.

What Happens after the Test?

- The nurse will remove the electrode paste from your hair.

- If you received a sedative before the test, you'll feel drowsy afterward.

- The nurse will tell you when you can take any medications that were suspended for the test.

Does the Test Have Risks?

An electroencephalograph can cause seizures in a person with a seizure disorder. If a seizure occurs, the doctor will treat it right away.

What Are the Normal Results?

An electroencephalograph records a portion of the brain's electrical activity as waves. Some of the waves are irregular, while others demonstrate frequent patterns. Among the basic waveforms are the alpha, beta, theta, and delta rhythms. Alpha waves occur at a frequency of 8 to 12 cycles per second in a regular rhythm. They're present only when you're awake and alert but your eyes are closed. Usually, they disappear with visual activity or mental concentration. Beta waves occur at a frequency of 13 to 30 cycles per second. They're generally associated with anxiety, depression, or the use of sedatives. Theta waves occur at a frequency of 4 to 7 cycles per second. They're most common in children and young adults. Delta waves occur at a frequency of 0.5 to 3.5 cycles per second. Normally, they occur only in young children and during sleep.

What Do Abnormal Results Mean?

Usually, about 100 pages of recording paper are evaluated, with particular attention paid to basic waveforms, symmetry of brain activity, brief bursts of energy, and responses to stimulation. In seizure disorders, the electroencephalograph pattern may identify the specific type of seizure. In absence seizures, the electroencephalograph shows spikes and waves at a frequency of 3 cycles per second. In generalized tonic-clonic or grand mal seizures, it usually shows multiple, high-voltage, spiked waves in both hemispheres of the brain. In complex partial seizures, the electroencephalograph usually shows spiked waves in the affected region. And in focal seizures, it usually shows localized, spiked discharges. In brain tumors or abscesses, the electroencephalograph may show slow waves (usually delta waves, but possibly beta waves). Generally, any condition that causes a diminishing level of consciousness alters the electroencephalograph pattern in proportion to the degree of consciousness lost. For example, if a person has meningitis or encephalitis, the electroencephalograph shows generalized, diffuse, and slow brain waves.

How Can the EEG Help in the Treatment of Seizures?

The EEG is still the leading test used to help diagnose seizures. Many people do not have a detectable brain lesion causing their seizures, and tests like the MRI and CT scan show normal brain structure. The EEG, however, can show abnormal electrical function of the brain even when these other tests are normal.

The EEG of persons with epilepsy can be divided into two categories, the interictal and ictal EEG. The interictal (routine) EEG is the EEG recording taken when the patient is not having seizures. Most patients with seizures will have at least one routine EEG. This test is done to look for interictal epileptiform abnormalities, that is, abnormal activity that can occur in a patient with epilepsy in the absence of an actual seizure. Sometimes the patient is asked to attempt to go to sleep, or to hyperventilate, or a strobe light is flashed in his or her eyes to try to bring out these abnormalities. Finding these abnormalities confirms that the patient has seizures, and helps the doctor determine what type they are.

The ictal EEG is the EEG recording taken during an aura and/or a seizure. This is done when a patient's seizures fail to respond to treatment, and the doctor wants to confirm the diagnosis, or possibly determine if brain surgery can be used to treat the seizures. Usually, ictal EEG recordings need to be made during closed-circuit television monitoring in an Epilepsy Center. For these tests, the person is usually admitted to the hospital and has their EEG and their video recorded continuously to capture actual seizure events. In our center [Epilepsy Center at Barnes Hospital], it typically takes about 1 or 2 days to confirm a patient's seizure diagnosis, while it takes an average of 5 days in the hospital to evaluate a patient for epilepsy surgery.

What Does the EEG Tell the Doctor?

The most common interictal EEG abnormality in persons with epilepsy is a spike, which is a burst of electrical activity which stands out from the normal EEG patterns. These spikes can be confined to one area of the brain (focal), or can occur in several areas of the brain independently of each other (multifocal), or come simultaneously from wide areas of the brain (generalized). The pattern of interictal abnormalities can determine if the person has focal or generalized epilepsy. These types of epilepsy have different causes, and may respond to different drugs.

The ictal EEG abnormalities are a little more complicated. These abnormalities can show rhythmic activity but can also show other EEG patterns depending on whether the recording was done from scalp electrodes or from electrodes implanted on the brain itself. The ictal EEG of the person with generalized epilepsy will usually show widespread brain involvement from the onset of the seizure. The ictal EEG of the person with focal epilepsy will usually show the seizure starting from a specific brain area but it can then spread to involve other areas, or even the whole brain. These patterns can tell the doctor which part of the brain is causing the seizure and how much of the brain becomes involved during it.

Chapter 37

Exercise Stress Test

Cardiologists employ a number of stress tests with the common goal of measuring how your heart and blood vessels respond to physical exertion and, in some cases, how strong your heart is after heart attack or surgery.

During these diagnostic tests, you will wear electrodes, which are connected by leads to a monitor. By observing this monitor, the physician can record your heartbeat during the test.

The most common of these tests is known as an exercise stress test, an exercise tolerance test or a stress electrocardiogram. Other stress tests are nuclear stress tests and stress echocardiograms. In some cases, as when people can't exercise because of other medical problems such as arthritis, a variety of drugs can be used to simulate the effect of exercise on the heart.

Why Does My Doctor Want Me to Undergo this Test?

You may have symptoms of heart disease, such as chest or arm pain, shortness of breath, dizziness, fatigue, or swelling of your feet and ankles. Based upon your symptoms, your doctor may want to determine whether you have heart disease, such as coronary artery disease.

Coronary artery disease, or atherosclerosis, occurs when a buildup of fat, cholesterol and other substances on the inner walls of the

---

"Cardiovascular Center Diagnostic Tests," © 1998 Mt. Sinai School of Medicine.

coronary arteries blocks the flow of oxygen-rich blood. If blood flow is completely blocked, the heart doesn't get the oxygen it requires, and the heart muscle may become permanently damaged.

If you have known coronary artery disease, the stress test can also provide some information to your physician as to the severity of the disease.

An exercise stress test can be used to measure your exercise capacity, if you have disease of your heart valves, or if you have heart failure.

Your doctor may order a stress test after you have undergone corrective surgery, such as coronary bypass surgery or balloon angioplasty, to help her design a safe rehabilitation program for you.

Is It a Risky or Dangerous Test?

An exercise stress test is extremely safe. There are some risks associated with the test. They include dizziness, falling down, chest pain and shortness of breath. These events are rare. Death is very rare. The doctor will explain the risks and benefits of the procedure and obtain your informed consent before the test.

You should not undergo exercise stress testing if you have any of the following conditions: severe congestive heart failure, life-threatening abnormal heart rhythms, heart infection, severe valve disease, severe hypertension or any medical condition that precludes you from walking safely on a treadmill.

What Preparations Should I Make before the Test?

Don't eat, drink, smoke or have any caffeine for four hours before the test. Caffeine is found in coffee, tea, chocolate and cola drinks, and in some over-the-counter pain relievers. If you have diabetes, ask your physician what you may eat.

Discuss with your doctor any medications you are currently taking. You may take approved medications with small sips of water.

Wear comfortable clothing. If you are a female, wear a two-piece outfit. You may have to undress from the waist up to put on a short hospital gown.

Wear rubber-soled shoes or sneakers.

How Long Will the Test Take?

The entire test, including preparation, takes about 45 minutes. Allow extra time for check in.

What Will Happen during the Test?

The areas where the electrodes will be placed are first cleaned with alcohol and then with a slightly abrasive material. This may hurt a little bit. The number and type of electrodes vary among practitioners. Most doctors use at least three electrodes.

Before the treadmill test begins, the electrodes will be placed on your chest and back. The electrodes are wired to an electrocardiograph, which records your heart's electrical activity.

A blood pressure cuff will be placed around your arm so that your blood pressure can be measured throughout the test.

Before the test, a resting ECG, blood pressure reading and pulse levels are taken. ECG leads are kept in place during the exercise and for 10 minutes or more after, as some changes may take longer to appear.

Then the physician will show you how to use the treadmill. During the test, he will increase the speed and incline of the treadmill every two to three minutes. If you're at high risk for coronary artery disease or in poor physical condition, the grade and speed may be increased in smaller increments. Most stress tests last six to 10 minutes.

While you exercise, your doctor or a technician will look for changes in ECG patterns and blood pressure levels that may indicate your heart is not getting enough oxygen. Other signs of coronary artery disease include chest pain and unusual shortness of breath.

Feelings of fatigue, shortness of breath and sweating are normal during testing. Your doctor will terminate the test early if he believes it's unsafe for you to continue.

At the end of the test your doctor may provide a cool-down phase of approximately three minutes. Alternatively, he may ask you to lie down. It's also possible that he will want you to sit upright for a few minutes instead.

Do I Have Any Additional Responsibilities during the Test?

You should tell the doctor if you feel any of the following symptoms during the test: chest, arm or jaw discomfort; severe shortness of breath; fatigue; dizziness; or leg cramps or soreness.

What Happens after the Test?

When the test is over, you may eat, drink and return to your normal routine. Ask your doctor about resuming your medications. Active

343

exercise should be postponed until your doctor has reviewed the test results with you.

The test results will help your doctor plan your treatment and determine whether additional testing is necessary. Additional testing may include cardiac catheterization. During cardiac catheterization, a dye is injected—via long catheters that are inserted in the groin—directly into the arteries that feed the heart muscle. X-ray movies are obtained, which enable the doctor to visualize your arteries and any blockage of blood flow.

Your doctor may order another exercise stress test called "nuclear" stress testing.

What Is "Nuclear" Stress Testing?

A nuclear stress test allows your doctor to see pictures of your heart when you are at rest and immediately after you have exercised. The test can give information about the size of the heart's chambers, the pumping action of the heart, and the blood supply to the heart muscle.

This test is very similar to the exercise stress test, but differs in a few ways. You will receive an intravenous injection of a small amount of a radioactive substance (thallium or Sestamibi) shortly before the end of the test.

As in the exercise stress test, you will have electrodes placed on your chest and back and you will walk on a treadmill.

After the exercise portion of the test, you will leave the treadmill and go into another room, where you will lie flat on a narrow bed. The physician will use a gamma-ray camera to take pictures of your heart.

The nuclear substance is taken up by your heart muscle, so that images are picked up by the camera and visualized on the monitor. The gamma-ray camera is round. It passes over your body as it takes pictures.

This part of the test takes about 15 to 20 minutes.

Then you will leave the testing area for three or four hours. You can walk around, but don't exercise. You may eat a light meal, but refrain from drinking caffeinated beverages. When you return, you will receive another injection of radioactive material, and the scan will be repeated to show pictures of your heart while you are at rest.

Your doctor will discuss the results of the nuclear stress test with you in a day or two. If the test shows that blood flow is normal during rest but abnormal during exercise, then the heart isn't receiving enough blood when you work harder than usual. If the test is abnormal during both exercise and rest segments, there probably is limited blood flow to a part of the heart at all times. If no radioactive substance is seen in a part of the heart muscle, it is indicative of a prior heart attack.

What If I Am Unable to Exercise?

If you are too sick to perform an exercise tolerance test, your doctor can use a drug that increases blood flow to the heart and thus "mimics" the test. Then the nuclear portion of the test can be performed as usual.

You should not eat, drink, smoke or have any caffeine for four hours before test. Some over-the-counter pain relievers may contain caffeine. If you have diabetes, consult your physician about eating.

What Is a Stress Echocardiogram?

An echocardiogram is a diagnostic test that employs ultrasound (high frequency sound waves) to obtain moving and still pictures of your heart. It is a safe and painless procedure.

A transducer wand is moved across your chest, to produce the sound waves and receive the echoes as they "bounce" off the heart and reflect as images on a television-like screen. The pictures are similar to X-ray images, but the process doesn't involve exposure to radiation. The pictures are recorded on videotape and paper.

Some of the information that stress echocardiography can provide includes size measurements of the heart's four chambers, pictures of the appearance and motion of the heart valves, and indications as to how forcefully the heart contracts and forces blood throughout the body.

What Happens during the Stress Echocardiogram?

The treadmill portion of the test resembles that of the exercise tolerance test. In this case, after your heart rate reaches a certain limit, you will be asked to lie down for the echocardiography portion of the test.

The echocardiograph operator will place three electrodes on your chest, and attach them by leads to an ECG machine so that your heart rhythm can be monitored throughout the test.

The operator will put a harmless, odorless gel on your chest. The gel will feel a little cool and moist at first. The gel helps the transducer pick up the sound waves from your heart. This device looks like a wand or a microphone. The transducer both generates and receives the sound signals.

The operator will put the transducer on your chest, directly above the structures your doctor wants to visualize. He will press firmly as he moves the transducer in arcs across your chest. This does not hurt.

You may be asked to participate by inhaling, exhaling or holding your breath at various times during the test. For the remainder of the time, you should remain still.

A stress echocardiogram takes approximately 60 minutes to perform.

What Is a Dobutamine Stress Echocardiogram?

If you are unable to exercise, you may be given a drug such as Dobutamine, which mimics the effect of stress on the body. The echocardiogram procedure is the same as above, except that slowly you will be given Dobutamine intravenously.

As in the drug-induced stress test, you should refrain from eating, drinking or ingesting caffeine for four hours before the test. Again, if you have diabetes, consult your physician about eating.

Chapter 38

Electrophysiology Study

An Electrophysiology Study (EPS) is a procedure used to evaluate and record the electrical activity of your heart. It is not a surgical procedure. It is a diagnostic test that provides a considerable amount of information about your heart rhythm (the speed and pattern of your heartbeat).

During the EPS, special thin, long, flexible insulated wires (electrode catheters), are inserted in the veins in your groin or neck. Sometimes the physician will insert the wire in a vein on the side of your neck or in a vein in the area just below your collarbone. The catheters' movements are monitored by X-ray pictures on a video screen. These catheters are used to locate the site of the abnormal rhythm. Then the doctor will place a special catheter at the insertion site, and electrical signals will be sent through the catheter to stimulate your heart. The electrophysiologist will try to reproduce the rhythm disturbances you might have had before the study.

What Is an Abnormal Heart Rhythm?

Your heart's electrical system creates signals that tell the chambers of the heart to contract. Sometimes problems with the heart's electrical signals lead to abnormal heart rhythms, rate, or both. These are referred to as "arrhythmias." Some of these conditions are life-threatening without treatment.

"Cardiovascular Center Diagnostic Tests," © 1998 Mt. Sinai School of Medicine.

Arrhythmia can produce the following symptoms: fainting, dizziness, weakness, shortness of breath, palpitations, anxiety, chest pain or chest discomfort.

You may have an arrhythmia called "ventricular tachycardia" (VT or V-tach). This consists of very fast but regular heartbeats originating from the lower chambers of your heart. Your heart will not pump as efficiently as it does during a normal rhythm. You may feel it pound. You may feel faint or dizzy.

You may have an arrhythmia called "atrial fibrillation." This occurs when the atria (upper chambers of the heart) rapidly quivers. This may last for a few seconds to hours or may be continuous all the time.

Another type of arrhythmia is called "ventricular fibrillation" (VF). VF is an unstable heart rhythm during which your heart doesn't beat, but quivers. Your heart will stop pumping blood and you will suffer a temporary loss of oxygen. You will usually pass out within a few seconds.

There is another type of arrhythmia that is called "Paroxysmal supraventricular tachycardia." This consists of rapid heartbeat of sudden onset and termination.

Sometimes the heart beats too slowly. This is called "bradycardia." If you have bradycardia, your blood may not move through the heart and to the body the way it should.

One form of bradycardia, called "heart block," occurs when electrical signals fail to travel from the upper chambers of the heart to the lower chambers.

You may have Wolff-Parkinson-White Syndrome, wherein an extra pathway exists between the upper and lower chambers of the heart. Electrical signals may pass back and forth via this abnormal connection between the upper and lower chambers. This can cause the heart to speed up.

You may have an arrhythmia that is not presented here. Your doctor can discuss your condition with you and address your questions and concerns.

Why Did My Doctor Order this Test for Me?

Your doctor ordered this test because other tests may not have provided sufficient information about your heart rhythm problem. The other diagnostic tests you might have had include Holter monitoring, an electrocardiogram, an echocardiogram or a signal averaged electrocardiogram (amplified electrocardiogram).

An Electrophysiology Study can often determine exactly what your rhythm problem is and what should be done to control it.

There are many reasons for performing an EPS. These include:

1. To learn the origin of your heart rhythm disturbance.

2. To learn the nature of your heart rhythm disturbance.

3. To find a possible cause of your dizzy spells or blackouts.

4. To evaluate how well your medication or medications are controlling your arrhythmia.

5. To find out the best treatment for your arrhythmia.

Does this Procedure Involve Any Risks?

The risks for this procedure are low. They include bleeding, blood clots, perforation of the heart muscle or a blood vessel, stroke, heart attack and death. These events are rare. After explaining the risks to you, the electrophysiologist will ask you to sign a consent form.

What Preparations Should I Make before the EPS?

- Consult your physician about your current medications well in advance. He may tell you to stop taking certain medications two to three days before the procedure.

- Don't eat or drink anything after midnight before the procedure. You may take approved medications with a small sip of water.

- Bring someone with you to drive you home after the procedure.

- You should leave all valuables and money at home or with a relative. Do not wear any jewelry to the hospital. You may wear dentures or dental bridges.

- Empty your bladder prior to the test.

- You will probably have blood tests, an electrocardiogram and a chest X-ray taken prior to the procedure.

- You may receive a mild sedative to help you relax. You will stay awake throughout the study.

What Happens during the Electrophysiology Study?

Electrodes will be placed on your back, shoulders and chest area to monitor your heart rhythm at all times. A blood pressure cuff will be placed around your arm so that your blood pressure may be monitored, as well. You will have an intravenous line to give you fluids and medication, if necessary.

The catheter site, in your groin or neck, will be shaved and cleansed. You will be covered with sterile sheets. The electrophysiologist will give you medication to numb the catheter insertion area(s). The numbing medicine will cause you to feel stinging for a short while, but you won't feel any pain. When the electrophysiologist uses a special needle to find the vein, you will feel some pressure. Let her know if you feel pain at that point. If you do, you will receive more medication.

Part of the X-ray machine that guides the electrophysiologist will be placed directly over your body.

After the catheters are in place, the electrophysiologist will evaluate your heart rhythm by giving your heart small electrical impulses to make it beat at different speeds. It's very important to let her know how you feel throughout the procedure.

You may feel your heartbeat changing or your heart racing from time to time. Some people faint when their hearts beat fast. If this occurs, the electrophysiologist may give you some medication, or she may deliver an electrical impulse called a countershock to change your heart rhythm back to normal.

When the procedure is complete, the electrophysiologist will remove the catheters and apply pressure to the area for five to 10 minutes to prevent bleeding. Then a dressing will be applied to the area.

How Long Does the Procedure Take?

An EPS usually takes two to four hours.

What Happens after the Procedure?

After the procedure, your blood pressure, heart rate, and maybe your catheter insertion sites, will be checked at regular intervals.

You will rest for about four hours. You must keep your legs straight; do not bend your knees. You are allowed to roll back and forth on the bed. You may move your feet and wiggle your toes to relieve stiffness.

You will leave with a dressing on the catheter insertion site(s).

Your doctor will review your test results and discuss them with you. She will explain your treatment options.

Usually, you will be able to go home on the day of the procedure.

What Should I Do at Home?

When you are at home, contact your doctor if you notice any bleeding at the insertion site, shortness of breath, coldness or numbness of your arm or leg, increase in bruising or swelling, a fever over 100 degrees F, or if you feel chest pain.

Avoid heavy lifting for a few days.

You will probably be able to resume your normal activities in a day or two.

Chapter 39

Holter Monitor Test

A Holter monitor test is a daylong continuous recording of your heart's electrical activity, made by a small strap-on recorder that operates while you go about your daily routine.

How Does It Work?

You will be asked to wear a portable recording instrument, the "Holter" monitor. This instrument may be worn by a strap over your shoulder or attached around your waist. It looks like a slightly over-sized Walkman in a canvas case. When the nurse or technician opens the Holter monitor, you will see that it takes a standard-sized audiotape. It is powered by a nine-volt battery.

The monitor has five or seven lead wires that will be attached to electrodes, which you will wear on your chest.

You will wear the monitor for 24 hours.

Why Does My Doctor Want Me to Undergo this Test?

The reasons for ordering a Holter monitor test vary. You may have complained of certain symptoms such as chest pain, palpitations, fainting or irregular heartbeats. If you are using a pacemaker, your physician may want to assess its functioning over a 24-hour period of time.

If you are unsure as to your physician's reason for ordering this test, discuss it with him or her.

"Cardiovascular Center Diagnostic Tests," © 1998 Mt. Sinai School of Medicine.

What Are the Risks or Dangers of this Test?

This is a noninvasive procedure. There are no risks or dangers.

What Preparations Should I Make before the Test?

It's a good idea to shower or bathe beforehand, because you will have to refrain from these for the 24 hours of the test.

What Should I Wear to the Test?

You will be asked to remove your clothing above the waist, so wear items that are easy to remove.

How Long Will the Test Take?

You will have to report to your doctor to be fitted with the monitor. The test is usually performed for a period of 24 hours, but occasionally a physician may order it for 48 hours. You will report back to your doctor after the test to return the equipment and the tape recording.

Must I Sign a Consent Form?

You will not have to sign a consent form for this test.

Will I Be Given Local or General Anesthesia?

You will not need or be given any anesthesia for this test.

What Will Happen on the Day of the Test?

After you have removed the garments above your waist, a nurse or technician will clean the areas of your chest where the electrodes will be placed. If you are a male, the first step will be to shave those areas with a disposable safety razor. Some men find this to be unpleasant. The nurse or technician will shave as little hair as possible.

Next, the nurse or technician will clean the areas with alcohol. If you have a scratch, it will sting a little. Then he or she will use gauze to dry the areas.

Then the nurse or technician will place five or seven electrodes on your chest. These will usually be round disks with a gel on one side and a snap on the other. The gel is sticky and will feel cold for a second. The snap is attached to a lead wire, which is attached to the portable monitor. One of the wires is a ground wire.

Sometimes, the nurse or technician will loop the wires near the electrodes and tape the electrodes to your chest. This will prevent the wires from shaking and adversely affect the recording. The monitor may feel a little heavy, but it is perfectly safe and comfortable.

Who Will Be in the Room with Me during the Test?

Usually a nurse or technician will perform the test.

Will I Have Any Responsibilities during the Test?

The nurse or technician will provide you with a diary or log to complete. You will make an entry every time you have any of the following symptoms: pain, headache, dizziness, shortness of breath. You will also record any strong emotion (crying, anger, laughing, etc.) or other physical symptoms. For each entry you will be asked to record the time it occurred and what your activity was at the time.

You should also record the following activities: eating, sleeping, exercising, moving bowels, engaging in sexual activity, drinking (especially alcohol or caffeinated beverages), and taking medications.

Is There Anything I Shouldn't Do during this Test?

- During the 24 hours of Holter monitoring, you should not shower, bathe or swim, as any moisture will loosen the electrodes. You may sponge bathe.

- Do not use any body powder or talcum.

- Avoid using electric blankets, as they may interfere with the recording.

- Do not remove the monitor. Keep the strap around your waist or shoulder while moving about.

- Do not remove any tape that has been placed over the lead wires.

- Do not shake the wires.

- If a lead wire comes unsnapped from an electrode, just snap it back on and record this in your diary.

- Do not open the monitor. This may cause it to fail to record.

- Do not drop the monitor.

The nurse or technician may provide you with some tape in case the tape comes off a wire. This could happen in the summer when the moisture from perspiration may loosen the tape.

Otherwise, you may engage in normal activities.

What Will I Feel during this Test?

You will not feel anything during the Holter monitoring.

What Happens after the Test?

After 24 hours, the battery will give out and the tape will be full. Return to your doctor's office, where a nurse or technician will remove the electrodes. This part of the test may hurt briefly, particularly if you have hair on your chest and there is tape on the electrodes. It feels like a bandage being pulled off.

What Should I Do after the Test Is Finished?

After the recording is completed and the electrodes have been removed, you may have temporary red marks where the electrodes were placed. Don't scrub them, because the skin may chafe. Gently wash these spots a little bit each day. If you have sensitive skin, it may break out. You may wish to use a skin care product to soothe any skin irritation.

What Happens Next?

A technician will analyze the information on the tape recording. A report will be provided to your physician.

What Kinds of Information Will the Test Give My Doctor?

The test will let your doctor know if your have any arrhythmias (irregular heart beats) or myocardial ischemia (decreased oxygen to the heart).

What Will My Doctor Do Next?

Your doctor will explain the results of the test to you. If necessary, he or she may order additional tests, prescribe medications or recommend another form of treatment.

Chapter 40

Sleep Studies

What Is Insomnia?

Insomnia is the perception or complaint of inadequate or poor-quality sleep because of one or more of the following:

- difficulty falling asleep

- waking up frequently during the night with difficulty returning to sleep

- waking up too early in the morning

- unrefreshing sleep

Insomnia is not defined by the number of hours of sleep a person gets or how long it takes to fall asleep. Individuals vary normally in their need for, and their satisfaction with, sleep. Insomnia may cause problems during the day, such as tiredness, a lack of energy, difficulty concentrating, and irritability.

Insomnia can be classified as transient (short term), intermittent (on and off), and chronic (constant). Insomnia lasting from a single night to a few weeks is referred to as transient. If episodes of transient

This chapter contains text from the following National Heart, Lung, and Blood Institute publications; "Facts About Insomnia," NIH Publication No. 95-3801, "Sleep Apnea: Is Your Patient at Risk?," NIH Publication No. 95-3803, and "Facts About Sleep Apnea," NIH Publication No. 95-3798.

insomnia occur from time to time, the insomnia is said to be inter-mittent. Insomnia is considered to be chronic if it occurs on most nights and lasts a month or more.

How Is Insomnia Diagnosed?

Patients with insomnia are evaluated with the help of a medical history and a sleep history. The sleep history may be obtained from a sleep diary filled out by the patient or by an interview with the patient's bed partner concerning the quantity and quality of the patient's sleep. Specialized sleep studies may be recommended, but only if there is suspicion that the patient may have a primary sleep disorder such as sleep apnea or narcolepsy.

What Is Sleep Apnea?

Sleep apnea is a serious, potentially life-threatening condition. It is a breathing disorder characterized by repeated collapse of the up-per airway during sleep, with consequent cessation of breathing. Vir-tually all sleep apnea patients have a history of loud snoring. They may also unknowingly experience frequent arousals during the night, resulting in chronic daytime sleepiness or fatigue.

If a patient complains of sleepiness but does not have other signs and symptoms suggestive of sleep apnea, a review of sleep habits may be helpful (e.g., how many hours of sleep the patient averages per night, recent changes in schedule, recent lifestyle changes). The patient may simply need to consider ways in which to increase the daily amount of sleep. If the patient is getting sufficient sleep, then other conditions such as narcolepsy or depression should be consid-ered.

Sleep apnea is also seen in children. Tonsillar hypertrophy is the most common cause. Children with sleep apnea may exhibit differ-ent signs and symptoms than adults. During sleep, children exhibit snoring and labored breathing. Features compatible with sleep ap-nea include weight loss or failure to gain weight, poor school perfor-mance, secondary enuresis, and behavioral problems.

Early recognition and treatment of sleep apnea is important be-cause it may be associated with irregular heartbeat, high blood pres-sure, heart attack, and stroke. If there is a high suspicion of sleep apnea after evaluating a patient, a sleep study is indicated to estab-lish a diagnosis.

How Is Sleep Apnea Diagnosed?

Polysomnography

In addition to the primary care physician, pulmonologists, neurologists, or other physicians with specialty training in sleep disorders may be involved in making a definitive diagnosis and initiating treatment. Diagnosis of sleep apnea is not simple because there can be many different reasons for disturbed sleep. Several tests are available for evaluating a person for sleep apnea. Currently polysomnography, which requires an overnight stay in a sleep laboratory, is the optimum test for diagnosing sleep apnea.

Polysomnography is a test that records a variety of body functions during sleep, such as the electrical activity of the brain, eye movement, muscle activity, heart rate, respiratory effort, air flow, and blood oxygen levels. These tests are used both to diagnose sleep apnea and to determine its severity.

Multiple Sleep Latency Test (MSLT)

The Multiple Sleep Latency Test (MSLT) measures the speed of falling asleep. In this test, patients are given several opportunities to fall asleep during the course of a day when they would normally be awake. For each opportunity, time to fall asleep is measured. People without sleep problems usually take an average of 10 to 20 minutes to fall asleep. Individuals who fall asleep in less than 5 minutes are likely to require some treatment for sleep disorders. The MSLT may be useful to measure the degree of excessive daytime sleepiness and to rule out other types of sleep disorders. Diagnostic tests usually are performed in a sleep center, but new technology may allow some sleep studies to be conducted in the patient's home.

Where Will a Sleep Study Be Done?

Diagnostic tests usually are performed in a sleep center, but new technology may allow some sleep studies to be conducted in the patient's home. A variety of home monitors are currently available or being developed that can record both cardiopulmonary parameters (for example, airflow, ventilatory effort, heart rate, and oxygen saturation) and sleep parameters and may be useful in diagnosing sleep apnea.

It is imperative that a sleep study be interpreted by someone with expertise in sleep disorders since an accurate diagnosis is crucial to avoid undertreatment or overtreatment of patients.

The severity of symptoms will determine how quickly a sleep study should be obtained and therapy initiated. Patients who report falling asleep while driving or those with heart failure angina are high priority for a sleep study and rapid intervention. Symptom severity along with availability of resources will determine the type of study and referral options.

For More Information

National Center on Sleep Disorders Research
Two Rockledge Centre Suite 7120
6701 Rockledge Drive MSC 7920
Bethesda, MD 20892-7920
(301) 435-0199
(301) 480-3451 (fax)

NHLBI Information Center
P.O. Box 30105
Bethesda, MD 20824-0105
(301) 592-8573
(301) 592-8563 (fax)
E-mail: nhlbiinfo@rover.nhlbi.nih.gov
Website: http://www.nhlbi.nih.gov

Part Six

Tests of Blood and Other Body Fluids and Tissues

Chapter 41

Blood Tests

Contents

Section 41.1

What Is a Blood Test?

A blood test is a laboratory test that is done on the blood that your doctor draws from your arm. Although blood might appear to be a uniform red liquid, more than half of it is made up of a straw-colored, watery fluid called "plasma." The remainder is made up of different types of cells that are suspended in the plasma. Hemoglobin in the cellular portion of the plasma makes the blood appear red. Blood travels throughout your body in blood vessels called veins and arteries. Since blood travels throughout the body, your doctor gains a lot of information from blood tests. Blood tests are an important part of your physical examination.

What Is a "Normal Range" for a Blood Test?

Results from blood tests done on active, healthy people fall within a specific range. This range of values is considered to be the "normal" range. When someone has a disease or health problem, some of their blood test results may be higher or lower than normal. When your doctor sees that a blood test is out of the normal range, he or she may order additional tests to determine the cause of the abnormality.

What Blood Tests Are Most Common?

There are hundreds of blood tests, but your doctor can gain much of the information needed by ordering 10 to 20 tests. The most commonly ordered blood tests include:

- complete blood cell (CBC) count
- cholesterol and triglyceride
- electrolytes (sodium, potassium, chloride, carbon dioxide)
- blood glucose (or blood sugar)
- hepatitis
- kidney function tests (blood urea nitrogen [BUN], creatinine)

- liver function tests (ALT, AST, gamma GT, bilirubin)
- prostate specific antigen (PSA)
- thyroid function tests (TSH, T3, T4)

—by Jan Hodnett

This content has been medically reviewed by Brian S. Bull, MD Chairman, Department of Pathology and Laboratory Medicine, and Karen Hay, MS, MT(ASCP), Technical Specialist Hematology Research Loma Linda University Loma Linda, Calif.

Section 41.2

Complete Blood Cell Count

The complete blood count, which is called a CBC, is one of the most common blood tests and is usually done as part of a routine checkup. In the CBC test, the different types of cells in the blood are counted and examined by a machine. The six tests that make up a CBC are:

- Red blood cell (RBC) count
- Hematocrit
- Hemoglobin
- White blood cell (WBC) count
- Differential blood count (Diff)
- Platelet count

Red Blood Cell Tests

Red Blood Cell (RBC) Count

Red blood cells are the most common type of cell in the blood. Your body contains millions upon millions of these disc-shaped cells. Your doctor orders a RBC to determine if the number of red blood cells in your body is low (called anemia) or high (called polycythemia). Your doctor may also learn about the size and shape of your red blood cells from an RBC. Women are more likely than men to have anemia because of the loss of blood each month through menstruation.

Common causes of an abnormal RBC:

- Anemia

  1. Iron deficiency anemia
     - In adults, most often due to chronic blood loss (eg, menstruation, small amounts of bleeding due to colon cancer); occasionally due to a diet lacking iron.
     - In small children, most often due to a diet lacking iron.
  2. Acute blood loss (eg, acute bleeding ulcer, trauma)
  3. Hereditary disorders (eg, sickle cell anemia, thalassemia)

- Polycythemia (relatively uncommon)

Hematocrit

A hematocrit is another way to determine whether your red blood cell count is high, low, or normal. The hematocrit measures how much of your blood is made of red cells. A hematocrit can be done by pricking your finger with a needle and drawing a drop of blood up into a glass tube, which looks like a small straw. The red cells in this tiny sample of blood are packed down and measured by spinning the glass tube in a centrifuge. This is easier and faster than drawing a tube of blood from your arm and is often done on children so a blood sample can be taken from a finger prick.

Common causes of an abnormal hematocrit:

- Anemia

  1. Iron deficiency anemia
     - In adults, most often due to chronic blood loss (eg, menstruation, small amounts of bleeding due to colon cancer); occasionally due to a diet lacking iron
     - In small children, most often due to a diet lacking iron
  2. Acute blood loss (eg, acute bleeding ulcer, trauma)
  3. Hereditary disorders (eg, sickle cell anemia, thalassemia)

- Polycythemia (relatively uncommon)

Hemoglobin

Hemoglobin—found in the red blood cell—gives blood its red color. It is the chemical compound that combines with oxygen from your lungs and carries the oxygen to cells throughout the body. The oxygen is used by the cells to produce energy. The blood also brings carbon dioxide—the waste product of this energy production process—back to your lungs, where it is exhaled.

People with a low hemoglobin level have anemia. When a person has a low hemoglobin level, he or she usually also has a low red blood cell count and a low hematocrit.

Common causes of an abnormally low hemoglobin:

* anemia

* iron deficiency anemia, which may be caused by an diet poor in iron-containing foods

* loss of blood through internal bleeding, such as an ulcer, or external bleeding, such as trauma

White Blood Cell Tests

White Blood Cell (WBC) Count

Another type of cell in the blood is known as a white blood cell. These cells lack hemoglobin. When using a special stain and looked at under a microscope, white blood cells appear light beige or blue, with a dark blue-stained nucleus. There are far fewer white cells than red cells in the blood. White blood cells are your body's protectors. When you have an infection, increased numbers of white blood cells are sent from the bone marrow to attack the bacteria or virus that is causing the infection. A low white blood cell count makes it harder for your body to fight off an infection. People with a low WBC are more likely to catch colds or other infectious diseases and are said to be immunocompromised.

Low WBC counts may be seen in:

* overwhelming infections
* AIDS
* cancer

High WBC counts may be seen in:

- infections
- leukemia

Differential Blood Count (Diff)

White blood cells come in several shapes and sizes. The different types of white blood cells can be identified by examining a blood sample under a microscope or using a laboratory instrument known as a hematology analyzer.

There are five different kinds of white blood cells:

- neutrophils
- lymphocytes
- monocytes
- eosinophils
- basophils

Your doctor orders a differential blood count in order to help him or her make a diagnosis.

- A high eosinophil count often indicates allergies, skin diseases, or parasitic infections.

- A low lymphocyte count may be seen in AIDS.

- A high monocyte count usually indicates an infection, often one caused by bacteria.

- A high neutrophil count is seen in infections, some cancers, arthritis, and sometimes when the body is under stress (for example, after surgery, trauma, or a heart attack).

- Immature (or young) white cells of all types may be seen in bacterial infections and leukemia.

Platelet Count

Platelets are the smallest type of cell found in the blood. Platelets help stop bleeding after an injury by gathering around the injury site, plugging the hole in the bleeding vessel and helping the blood to clot more quickly.

Platelet counts are often done if you are prone to bruising or if you are about to have surgery. A low platelet count is called thrombocytopenia.

Common causes of a low platelet count: patients undergoing cancer treatment:

- some leukemias
- certain types of cancer
- immune system disorders, when the body will sometimes destroy its own platelets.

This content has been medically reviewed by Brian S. Bull, MD Chairman, Department of Pathology and Laboratory Medicine, and Karen Hay, MS, MT(ASCP), Technical Specialist Hematology Research Loma Linda University Loma Linda, Calif.

Section 41.3

Blood Cholesterol

Excerpts from "Facts about Blood Cholesterol," National Heart, Lung, and Blood Institute (NHLBI), NIH Publication No. 94-2696, revised 1994, reprinted 1996.

Why Blood Cholesterol Matters

Blood cholesterol plays an important part in deciding a person's chance or risk of getting coronary heart disease (CHD). The higher your blood cholesterol level, the greater your risk. That's why high blood cholesterol is called a risk factor for heart disease. Did you know that heart disease is the number one killer of men and of women in the United States? About a half million people die each year from heart attacks caused by CHD. Altogether 1.25 million heart attacks occur each year in the United States.

Even if your blood cholesterol level is close to the desirable range, you can lower it and reduce your risk of getting heart disease. Eating in a heart-healthy way, being physically active, and losing weight if you are overweight are things everyone can do to help lower their levels. This fact sheet will show you how. But first, a few things you ought to know.

The Blood Cholesterol—Heart Disease Connection

When you have too much cholesterol in your blood, the excess builds up on the walls of the arteries that carry blood to the heart. This buildup is called "atherosclerosis" or "hardening of the arteries." It narrows the arteries and can slow down or block blood flow to the heart. With less blood, the heart gets less oxygen. With not enough oxygen to the heart, there may be chest pain ("angina" or "angina pectoris"), heart attack ("myocardial infarction"), or even death. Cholesterol buildup is the most common cause of heart disease, and it happens so slowly that you are not even aware of it. The higher your blood cholesterol, the greater your chance of this buildup.

Other Risk Factors for Heart Disease

A high blood cholesterol level is not the only thing that increases your chance of getting heart disease. Here is a list of known risk factors:

Factors You Can Do Something About

- Cigarette smoking
- High blood cholesterol (high total and LDL-cholesterol)
- Low HDL-cholesterol
- High blood pressure
- Diabetes
- Obesity/overweight
- Physical inactivity

Factors You Cannot Control

- Age:
  - 45 years or older for men
  - 55 years or older for women
- Family history of early heart disease (heart attack or sudden death):
  - father or brother stricken before the age of 55
  - mother or sister stricken before the age of 65

The more risk factors you have, the greater your chance of heart disease. Fortunately, most of these risk factors are things you can do something about.

Who Can Benefit From Lowering Blood Cholesterol?

Almost everyone can benefit from lowering his or her blood cholesterol. Lowering cholesterol slows the fatty buildup in the arteries, and in some cases can help reduce the buildup already there. And, if you have two or more other risk factors for heart disease or already have heart disease, you have a great deal to gain from lowering your high blood cholesterol. In this case, lowering your level may greatly reduce your risk of any more heart problems.

Many Americans have had success in lowering their blood cholesterol levels. From 1978 to 1990, the average blood cholesterol level in the U.S. dropped from 213 mg/dL to 205 mg/dL.

Cholesterol—In Your Blood, In Your Diet

Cholesterol is a waxy substance found in all parts of your body. It helps make cell membranes, some hormones, and vitamin D. Cholesterol comes from two sources: your body and the foods you eat. Blood cholesterol is made in your liver. Your liver makes all the cholesterol your body needs. Dietary cholesterol comes from animal foods like meats, whole milk dairy foods, egg yolks, poultry, and fish. Eating too much dietary cholesterol can make your blood cholesterol go up. Foods from plants, like vegetables, fruits, grains, and cereals, do not have any dietary cholesterol.

LDL-and HDL-Cholesterol: The Bad and The Good

Just like oil and water, cholesterol and blood do not mix. So, for cholesterol to travel through your blood, it is coated with a layer of protein to make a "lipoprotein." Two lipoproteins you may have heard about are low density lipoprotein (LDL) and high density lipoprotein (HDL). LDL-cholesterol carries most of the cholesterol in the blood. Remember, when too much LDL-cholesterol is in the blood, it can lead to cholesterol buildup in the arteries. That is why LDL-cholesterol is called the "bad" cholesterol. HDL-cholesterol helps remove cholesterol from the blood and helps prevent the fatty buildup. So HDL-cholesterol is called the "good" cholesterol.

Things That Affect Blood Cholesterol

Your blood cholesterol level is influenced by many factors. These include:

- **What you eat**—High intake of saturated fat, dietary cholesterol, and excess calories leading to overweight can increase blood cholesterol levels. Americans eat an average of 12 percent of their calories from saturated fat, and 34 percent of their calories from total fat. These intakes are higher than what is recommended for the health of your heart. The average daily intake of dietary cholesterol is 220-260 mg for women and 360 mg for men.

- **Overweight**—Being overweight can make your LDL-cholesterol level go up and your HDL-cholesterol level go down.

- **Physical activity**—Increased physical activity lowers LDL-cholesterol and raises HDL-cholesterol levels.

- **Heredity**—Your genes partly influence how your body makes and handles cholesterol.

- **Age and Sex**—Blood cholesterol levels in both men and women begin to go up around age 20. Women before menopause have levels that are lower than men of the same age. After menopause, a woman's LDL-cholesterol level goes up—and so her risk for heart disease increases.

Have Your Blood Cholesterol Checked

All adults age 20 and over should have their blood cholesterol (also called "total" blood cholesterol) checked at least once every 5 years. If an accurate HDL-cholesterol measurement is available, HDL should be checked at the same time. If you do not know your total and HDL levels, ask your doctor to measure them at your next visit.

Total and HDL-cholesterol measurements require a blood sample that is taken from your arm or finger. You do not have to fast for this test. If you have had your total and HDL-cholesterol checked, check the chart to see how they measure up.

Blood cholesterol levels of under 200 mg/dL are called "desirable" and put you at lower risk for heart disease. Any cholesterol level of 200 mg/dL or more increases your risk; over half the adults in the United States have levels of 200 mg/dL or greater. Levels between 200 and 239 mg/dL are "borderline-high." A level of 240 mg/dL or greater is "high" blood cholesterol. A person with this level has more than twice the risk of heart disease compared to someone whose cholesterol is 200 mg/dL. About one out of every five American adults has a high blood cholesterol level of 240 mg/dL or greater.

Unlike total cholesterol, the lower your HDL, the higher your risk for heart disease. An HDL level less than 35 mg/dL increases your risk for heart disease. The higher your HDL level, the better.

In certain cases, it may be necessary to have your LDL-cholesterol checked, too, because it is a better predictor of heart disease risk than your total blood cholesterol. You will need to fast. That means you can have nothing to eat or drink but water, coffee, or tea, with no cream or sugar, for 9 to 12 hours before the test.

If your doctor has checked your LDL level, use the chart below to see how it measures up.

Table 41.1. LDL-Cholesterol Categories

LDL Level	Risk Level
Less than 130 mg/dL	Desirable
130 to 159 mg/dL	Borderline–High Risk
160mg/dL and above	High Risk

Note: These categories apply to adults age 20 and above.

If your LDL-cholesterol level is high or borderline-high and you have other risk factors for heart disease, your doctor will likely plan a treatment program for you. Following an eating plan low in saturated fat and cholesterol and increasing your physical activity is usually the first and main step of treatment. Some people will also need to take medicine. *(If you have high blood cholesterol and would like more details on what it means and what you should do about it, contact the NHLBI Information Center.)*

What about Cholesterol Levels in Children?

Most children do not need to have their blood cholesterol checked. But, all children should be encouraged to eat in a heart-healthy way, along with the rest of the family. Children who should be tested at age 2 or older include those who have any of these conditions:

• at least one parent who has been found to have high blood cholesterol (240 mg/dL or greater), or

• a family history of early heart disease (before age 55 in a parent or grandparent).

Also, if the parent's medical history is not known, the doctor may want to check the child's blood cholesterol level, especially in children with other risk factors like obesity.

How High Is a Child's "High" Blood Cholesterol?

If your child does need to have a cholesterol test, it can be part of a regular doctor's visit. Your doctor will likely measure your child's total cholesterol level first. However, if your family has a history of early heart disease, the doctor may measure the LDL–cholesterol level right from the start. Otherwise, your child's LDL–cholesterol level should be measured if his or her total cholesterol level was checked and found to be 170 mg/dL or greater. The blood cholesterol categories for children from families with high blood cholesterol or early heart disease are shown in the table below.

Table 41.2. Total and LDL-Cholesterol Levels in Children and Teenagers from Families with High Blood Cholesterol or Early Heart Disease.

Risk Level	Total Cholesterol	LDL–Cholesterol
Acceptable	Less than 170mg/dL	Less than 110 mg/dL
Borderline	170 to 199 mg/dL	110–129 mg/dL
High	200 mg/dL or greater	130 mg/dL or greater

Note: These blood cholesterol levels apply to children 2 to 19 years old.

Should You Know Your Cholesterol Ratio?

When you have your cholesterol checked, some laboratories may give you a number called a cholesterol ratio. This number is your total cholesterol or LDL level divided by your HDL level. The idea is that combining the levels into one number gives you an overall view of your risk for heart disease. But the ratio is too general: It is more important to know the value for each level separately because LDL- and HDL-cholesterol both predict your risk of heart disease.

What Are Triglycerides?

Triglycerides are the form in which fat is carried through your blood to the tissues. The bulk of your body's fat tissue is in the form of triglycerides. Your triglycerides are measured whenever your LDL-cholesterol is checked. Triglyceride levels less than 200 mg/dL are considered normal.

It is not clear whether high triglycerides alone increase your risk of heart disease. But many people with high triglycerides also have high LDL or low HDL levels, which do increase the risk of heart disease.

Will Lowering My Blood Cholesterol Help Me Live Longer?

Many studies show that lowering cholesterol levels reduces the risk of illness or death from heart disease, which kills more men and women each year than any other illness. If you have heart disease, lowering your cholesterol level will probably help you to live longer. If you don't have heart disease, the studies so far do not show that you will live longer, but you will definitely reduce your risk of illness and death from heart attack.

How Much Will Your Cholesterol Levels Change When You Change Your Diet?

Generally your blood cholesterol level should begin to drop a few weeks after you start eating the heart-healthy way. How much it drops depends on the amount of saturated fat you used to eat, how high your high blood cholesterol is, how much weight you lose if you are overweight, and how your body responds to the changes you make. Over time, you may reduce your cholesterol level by 5 to 35 mg/dL or even more.

How To Find Out More

The National Cholesterol Education Program (NCEP) has other booklets for the public and health professionals on lowering blood

cholesterol. The NCEP has booklets for adults with high blood cholesterol, age-specific booklets for children and adolescents with high blood
cholesterol and their parents, and a pamphlet on physical activity and
how to get started. To order publications on cholesterol, weight and physical activity or request a catalog, write to the address below:

NHLBI Information Center
P.O. Box 30105
Bethesda, MD 20824-0105
301-592-8573
Fax: 301-592-8563
E-mail: NHLBIinfo@rover.nhlbi.nih.gov

Section 41.4

Blood Glucose

This section includes text from "Diagnosing Diabetes," National Institutes of
Health (NIH), Publication No. 97-241, February 10, 1997; and Reprinted with
permission © 1996 "HbA1c Blood Test" from *Managing Type II Diabetes: Your
Invitation to a Healthier Lifestyle* by Arlene Monk, Jan Pearson, Priscilla
Hollander, and Richard M. Bergenstal, IDC Publishing, Minneapolis,
International Diabetes Center.

Diagnosing Diabetes

A doctor can diagnose diabetes by checking for symptoms such as
excessive thirst and frequent urination and by testing for glucose in
blood or urine. When blood glucose rises above a certain point, the
kidneys pass the extra glucose in the urine. However, a urine test
alone is not sufficient to diagnose diabetes.

A second method for testing glucose is a blood test usually done in
the morning before breakfast (fasting glucose test) or after a meal
(postprandial glucose test).

Points to Remember

A doctor will diagnose diabetes by looking for four kinds of evidence:

- risk factors like exercise weight and a family history of diabetes
- symptoms such as thirst and frequent urination
- complications like heart trouble
- signs of excess glucose or sugar in blood and urine tests.

The oral glucose tolerance test is a second type of blood test used to check for diabetes. Sometimes it can detect diabetes when a simple blood test does not. In this test, blood glucose is measured before and after a person has consumed a thick, sweet drink of glucose and other sugars. Normally, the glucose in a person's blood rises quickly after the drink and then falls gradually again as insulin signals the body to metabolize the glucose. In someone with diabetes, blood glucose rises and remains high after consumption of the liquid.

A doctor can decide, based on these tests and a physical exam, whether someone has diabetes. If a blood test is borderline abnormal, the doctor may want to monitor the person's blood glucose regularly. If a person is overweight, he or she probably will be advised to lose weight. The doctor also may monitor the patient's heart, since diabetes increases the risk of heart disease.

HbA1c Blood Test for Blood Glucose

HbA1c is a blood test that measures your average blood glucose level over the past two months, and it is the best indicator of your overall blood glucose control. Along with your blood glucose records, your HbA1c helps you and your diabetes care team determine how well your treatment plan is working.

There is no universal "normal" HbA1c result, because the methods for measuring HbA1c differ from laboratory to laboratory. Check what the normal range is for your lab, then decide with your diabetes care team what a good target HbA1c is for you. In most laboratories, the normal range is 4 percent to 6 percent. It's common to aim for an HbA1c that is, no more than 1.5 percentage points above the laboratory normal.

Section 41.5

Electrolytes: Sodium, Potassium, Chloride, and Carbon Dioxide

In order to function properly, your body needs to maintain specific levels of various chemical and chemical compounds. Four important ones are sodium, potassium, chloride, and carbon dioxide. Their levels are measured in the electrolyte test.

Sodium and chloride are important in determining if your kidneys are working correctly. Sodium is important because a high sodium level may cause high blood pressure in some people. Table salt is sodium chloride, which is why people with high blood pressure sometimes are put on a low-sodium diet. Too much sodium in the body may also cause swelling (or edema) of the ankles.

Common causes of abnormal sodium and chloride levels:

- kidney disease
- prolonged vomiting
- severe dehydration or water loss
- congestive heart failure
- acid-base imbalance (an imbalance of acid and base [alkaline] in the body)

Potassium is important for proper heart function. People taking diuretics tend to lose potassium, so your doctor orders a potassium test to make sure you have enough potassium. People with a low potassium level may have leg cramps.

Common causes of abnormal potassium levels:

- kidney disease
- prolonged vomiting and diarrhea
- heart attack
- people taking certain drugs, such as diuretics

Carbon dioxide (CO_2) is the gas that we exhale when we breathe. People with lung problems may have a high CO_2 level. Too little or too much CO_2 affects the pH (or acidity) of the body, which is a reflection of the acid-base balance in your cells.

Common causes of an abnormal CO_2:

- acid-base disorders (an imbalance of acid and base [alkaline] in the body)
- excessive loss of stomach acid due to severe vomiting
- severe emphysema (lung damage)

—by Jan Hodnett

This content has been medically reviewed by Brian S. Bull, MD, Chairman, Department of Pathology and Laboratory Medicine, and Karen Hay, MS, MT(ASCP) Technical Specialist Hematology Research, Loma Linda University, Loma Linda, Calif.

Section 41.6

Kidney Function Tests

"Medical Tests of Kidney Function," National Institute of Diabetes and Digestive and Kidney Diseases (NIDDK), NIH, February 3, 1998.

Healthy kidneys remove wastes and excess fluid from the blood. Blood tests show whether the kidneys are failing to remove wastes. Urine tests can show how quickly body wastes are being removed and whether the kidneys are also leaking abnormal amounts of protein.

Blood Tests

Serum Creatinine

Creatinine (kree-AT-uh-nin) is a waste product that comes from meat protein in the diet and also comes from the normal wear and tear on muscles of the body. Creatinine levels in the blood can vary, and each laboratory has its own normal range. In many labs the normal range is 0.6 to 1.2 mg/dl. Higher levels may be a sign that the kidneys are not working properly. As kidney disease progresses, the level of creatinine in the blood increases.

Blood Urea Nitrogen (BUN)

Urea nitrogen (yoo-REE-uh NY-truh-jen) also is produced from the breakdown of food protein. A normal BUN level is between 7 and 20 mg/dl. As kidney function decreases, the BUN level increases.

Urine Tests

Some urine tests require only a few ounces of urine. But some tests require collection of all urine produced for a full 24 hours. A 24-hour urine test shows how much urine your kidneys produce in 1 day. The test also can give an accurate measurement of how much protein leaks from the kidney into the urine in 1 day.

Creatinine Clearance

A creatinine clearance test compares the creatinine in a 24-hour sample of urine to the creatinine level in the blood, to show how many milliliters of blood the kidneys are filtering out each minute (ml/min).

More Information Is Available From:

American Kidney Fund
6110 Executive Boulevard, #1010
Rockville, MD 20852
800-638-8299 "Help Line"
301-881-0898
Fax: 301-881-0898
E-mail: helpline@akfinc.org
http://www.akfinc.org

National Kidney Foundation
30 East 33rd Street
New York, NY 10016
800-622-9010
212-889-2210
http://www.kidney.org

Section 41.7

Liver Function Tests

Reprinted with permission © 1998 American Medical Association (AMA).

The liver is a large and important organ in the body. It regulates many blood constituents, including blood glucose. One important function is to help eliminate toxins and chemicals from the body. Liver function tests are routinely ordered during an annual check-up and also are ordered if your skin or eyes are more yellow than normal and you are feeling tired.

ALT (alanine aminotransferase [formerly called SGPT (serum glutamate pyruvate transminase)]) is a type of protein called an enzyme and is found in relatively high concentrations in the liver and kidney. It may also be found in skeletal muscle, the heart, and the pancreas. An ALT test is used to diagnose liver disease.

Common causes of a high ALT level:

- hepatitis
- cirrhosis
- liver disease
- infectious mononucleosis

AST (asparate aminotransferase [formerly called SGOT (serum glutamic-oxaloacetic transaminase)]) is a type of protein called an enzyme and is found primarily in the liver and kidney, but is also found in other parts of the body.

Common causes of a high AST:

- heart attack
- infectious mononucleosis
- strenuous exercise
- liver disease
- hepatitis
- trauma

Gamma GT is a type of protein called an enzyme and is found in the liver and other organs.

Common causes of a high gamma GT level:

- liver disease
- alcohol ingestion
- blocked bile ducts (gallstones)

Bilirubin is a yellow fluid found in the bile as a result of red blood cell destruction. As red blood cells break down, bilirubin collects in the gallbladder. There are two types of bilirubin tests. The total (or indirect) bilirubin level increases in liver disease and in anemia caused by red blood cells being destroyed faster than they should (a process called hemolysis). The direct bilirubin test is increased when the gallbladder is blocked, hampering the flow of bile fluid.

Common causes of a high bilirubin level:

- gallbladder disease

- liver disease

- blood disease with rapid red blood cell breakdown (hemolytic anemia)

- some newborn babies who have a different blood type than their mother.

Chapter 42

Tumor Markers
Including PSA and CA-125

Tumor markers are substances that can often be detected in higher-than-normal amounts in the blood, urine, or body tissues of some patients with certain types of cancer. Tumor markers are produced either by the tumor itself or by the body in response to the presence of cancer or certain benign (noncancerous) conditions. This chapter describes some tumor markers found in the blood.

Measurements of tumor marker levels can be useful-when used along with x-rays or other tests-in the detection and diagnosis of some types of cancer. However, measurements of tumor marker levels alone are not sufficient to diagnose cancer for the following reasons:

- Tumor marker levels can be elevated in people with benign conditions.
- Tumor marker levels are not elevated in every person with cancer-especially in the early stages of the disease.
- Many tumor markers are not specific to a particular type of cancer; the level of a tumor marker can be raised by more than one type of cancer.

In addition to their role in cancer diagnosis, some tumor marker levels are measured before treatment to help doctors plan appropriate therapy. In some types of cancer, tumor marker levels reflect the extent (stage) of the disease and can be useful in predicting how well

"Cancer Facts-Screening," National Cancer Institute (NCI), NIH, April 1998.

the disease will respond to treatment. Tumor marker levels may also be measured during treatment to monitor a patient's response to treatment. A decrease or return to normal in the level of a tumor marker may indicate that the cancer has responded favorably to therapy. If the tumor marker level rises, it may indicate that the cancer is growing. Finally, measurements of tumor marker levels may be used after treatment has ended as a part of follow-up care to check for recurrence.

Currently, the main use of tumor markers is to assess a cancer's response to treatment and to check for recurrence. Scientists continue to study these uses of tumor markers as well as their potential role in the early detection and diagnosis of cancer. The patient's doctor can explain the role of tumor markers in detection, diagnosis, or treatment for that person. Described below are some of the most commonly measured tumor markers.

Prostate-Specific Antigen

Prostate-specific antigen (PSA) is present in low concentrations in the blood of all adult males. It is produced by both normal and abnormal prostate cells. Elevated PSA levels may be found in the blood of men with benign prostate conditions, such as prostatitis (inflammation of the prostate) and benign prostatic hyperplasia (BPH), or with a malignant (cancerous) growth in the prostate. While PSA does not allow doctors to distinguish between benign prostate conditions (which are very common in older men) and cancer, an elevated PSA level may indicate that other tests are necessary to determine whether cancer is present.

PSA levels have been shown to be useful in monitoring the effectiveness of prostate cancer treatment, and in checking for recurrence after treatment has ended. In checking for recurrence, a single test may show a mildly elevated PSA level, which may not be a significant change. Doctors generally look for trends, such as steadily increasing PSA levels in multiple tests over time, rather than focusing on a single elevated result.

Researchers are studying the value of PSA in screening men for prostate cancer (checking for the disease in men who have no symptoms). At this time, it is not known whether using PSA to screen for prostate cancer actually saves lives. The National Cancer Institute-supported Prostate, Lung, Colorectal, and Ovarian Cancer Screening Trial is designed to show whether the use of certain screening tests can reduce the number of deaths caused by those cancers. For prostate cancer, this trial is looking at the usefulness of regular screening using digital rectal exams and PSA level checks in men ages 55 to 74.

Researchers are also working on new ways to increase the accuracy of PSA tests. Improving the accuracy of PSA tests could help doctors distinguish BPH from prostate cancer, and thereby avoid unnecessary follow-up procedures, including biopsies.

Prostatic Acid Phosphatase

Prostatic acid phosphatase (PAP) is normally present only in small amounts in the blood, but may be found at higher levels in some patients with prostate cancer, especially if the cancer has spread beyond the prostate. However, blood levels may also be elevated in patients who have certain benign prostate conditions or early stage cancer.

Although PAP was originally found to be produced by the prostate, elevated PAP levels have since been associated with testicular cancer, leukemia, and non-Hodgkin's lymphoma, as well as noncancerous conditions such as Gaucher's disease, Paget's disease, osteoporosis, cirrhosis of the liver, pulmonary embolism, and hyperparathyroidism.

CA 125

CA 125 is produced by a variety of cells, but particularly by ovarian cancer cells. Studies have shown that many women with ovarian cancer have elevated CA 125 levels. CA 125 is used primarily in the management of treatment for ovarian cancer.

In women with ovarian cancer being treated with chemotherapy, a falling CA 125 level generally indicates that the cancer is responding to treatment. Increasing CA 125 levels during or after treatment, on the other hand, may suggest that the cancer is not responding to therapy or that some cancer cells remain in the body. Doctors may also use CA 125 levels to monitor patients for recurrence of ovarian cancer.

Not all women with elevated CA 125 levels have ovarian cancer. CA 125 levels may also be elevated by cancers of the uterus, cervix, pancreas, liver, colon, breast, lung, and digestive tract. Noncancerous conditions that can cause elevated CA 125 levels include endometriosis, pelvic inflammatory disease, peritonitis, pancreatitis, liver disease, and any condition that inflames the pleura (the tissue that surrounds the lungs and lines the chest cavity). Menstruation and pregnancy can also cause an increase in CA 125.

Carcinoembryonic Antigen

Carcinoembryonic antigen (CEA) is normally found in small amounts in the blood of most healthy people, but may become elevated in people who have cancer or some benign conditions. The primary use of CEA is in monitoring colorectal cancer, especially when the disease has spread (metastasized). CEA is also used after treatment to check for recurrence of colorectal cancer. However, a wide variety of other cancers can produce elevated levels of this tumor marker, including melanoma; lymphoma; and cancers of the breast, lung, pancreas, stomach, cervix, bladder, kidney, thyroid, liver, and ovary.

Elevated CEA levels can also occur in patients with noncancerous conditions, including inflammatory bowel disease, pancreatitis, and liver disease. Tobacco use can also contribute to higher-than-normal levels of CEA.

Alpha-Fetoprotein

Alpha-fetoprotein (AFP) is normally produced by a developing fetus. AFP levels begin to decrease soon after birth and are usually undetectable in the blood of healthy adults (except during pregnancy). An elevated level of AFP strongly suggests the presence of either primary liver cancer or germ cell cancer (cancer that begins in the cells that give rise to eggs or sperm) of the ovary or testicle. Only rarely do patients with other types of cancer (such as stomach cancer) have elevated levels of AFP. Noncancerous conditions that can cause elevated AFP levels include benign liver conditions, such as cirrhosis or hepatitis; ataxia telangiectasia; Wiscott-Aldrich syndrome; and pregnancy.

Human Chorionic Gonadotropin

Human chorionic gonadotropin (HCG) is normally produced by the placenta during pregnancy. In fact, HCG is sometimes used as a pregnancy test because it increases early within the first trimester. It is also used to screen for choriocarcinoma (a rare cancer of the uterus) in women who are at high risk for the disease, and to monitor the treatment of trophoblastic disease (a rare cancer that develops from an abnormally fertilized egg). Elevated HCG levels may also indicate the presence of cancers of the testis, ovary, liver, stomach, pancreas, and lung. Pregnancy and marijuana use can also cause elevated HCG levels.

CA 19-9

Initially found in colorectal cancer patients, CA 19-9 has also been identified in patients with pancreatic, stomach, and bile duct cancer. Researchers have discovered that, in those who have pancreatic cancer, higher levels of CA 19-9 tend to be associated with more advanced disease. Noncancerous conditions that may elevate CA 19-9 levels include gallstones, pancreatitis, cirrhosis of the liver, and cholecystitis.

CA 15-3

CA 15-3 levels are most useful in following the course of treatment in women diagnosed with breast cancer, especially advanced breast cancer. CA 15-3 levels are rarely elevated in women with early stage breast cancer.

Cancers of the ovary, lung, and prostate may also raise CA 15-3 levels. Elevated levels of CA 15-3 may be associated with noncancerous conditions, such as benign breast or ovarian disease, endometriosis, pelvic inflammatory disease, and hepatitis. Pregnancy and lactation can also cause CA 15-3 levels to rise.

CA 27-29

Similar to the CA 15-3 antigen, CA 27-29 is found in the blood of most breast cancer patients. CA 27-29 levels may be used in conjunction with other procedures (such as mammograms and measurements of other tumor marker levels) to check for recurrence in women previously treated for stage II and stage III breast cancer.

CA 27-29 levels can also be elevated by cancers of the colon, stomach, kidney, lung, ovary, pancreas, uterus, and liver. First trimester pregnancy, endometriosis, ovarian cysts, benign breast disease, kidney disease, and liver disease are noncancerous conditions that can also elevate CA 27-29 levels.

Lactate Dehydrogenase

Lactate dehydrogenase is a protein found throughout the body. Nearly every type of cancer, as well as many other diseases, can cause LDH levels to be elevated. Therefore, this marker cannot be used to diagnose a particular type of cancer.

LDH levels can be used to monitor treatment of some cancers, including testicular cancer, Ewing's sarcoma, non-Hodgkin's lymphoma, and some types of leukemia. Elevated LDH levels can be caused by a number of noncancerous conditions, including heart failure, hypothyroidism, anemia, and lung or liver disease.

Neuron-Specific Enolase

Neuron-specific enolase (NSE) has been detected in patients with neuroblastoma; small cell lung cancer; Wilms' tumor; melanoma; and cancers of the thyroid, kidney, testicle, and pancreas. However, studies of NSE as a tumor marker have concentrated primarily on patients with neuroblastoma and small cell lung cancer. Measurement of NSE level in patients with these two diseases can provide information about the extent of the disease and the patient's prognosis, as well as about the patient's response to treatment.

National Cancer Institute Information Resources

You may want more information for yourself, your family, and your doctor. The following National Cancer Institute (NCI) services are available to help you.

Cancer Information Service (CIS)

Provides accurate, up-to-date information on cancer to patients and their families, health professionals, and the general public. Information specialists translate the latest scientific information into understandable language and respond in English, Spanish, or on TTY equipment.

Toll-free: 1-800-4-CANCER (1-800-422-6237)
TTY: 1-800-332-8615

Internet

http://www.nci.nih.gov/

NCI's primary web site—contains information about the Institute and its programs. Also includes news, upcoming events, educational materials, and publications for patients, the public, and the mass media on http://rex.nci.nih.gov/.

http://cancernet.nci.nih.gov/

CancerNet—contains material for health professionals, patients, and the public, including information from PDQ about cancer treatment, screening, prevention, supportive care, and clinical trials, and CAN-CERLIT, a bibliographic database.

http://cancertrials.nci.nih.gov/

cancerTrials—NCI's comprehensive clinical trials information center for patients, health professionals, and the public. Includes information on understanding trials, deciding whether to participate in trials, finding specific trials, plus research news and other resources.

E-mail: CancerMail

Includes NCI information about cancer treatment, screening, prevention, and supportive care. To obtain a contents list, send e-mail to cancermail@icicc.nci.nih.gov with the word "help" in the body of the message.

Fax: CancerFax

Includes NCI information about cancer treatment, screening, prevention, and supportive care. To obtain a contents list, dial 301-402-5874 from a fax machine hand set and follow the recorded instructions.

Chapter 43

Biopsy

If you have a sign or symptom that might mean cancer, the doctor will do a physical exam and ask about your medical history. In addition, the doctor usually orders various tests and exams. These may include imaging procedures, which produce pictures of areas inside the body; endoscopy, which allows the doctor to look directly inside certain organs; and laboratory tests. In most cases, the doctor also orders a biopsy, a procedure in which a sample of tissue is removed.

What Is a Biopsy?

The physical exam, imaging, endoscopy, and lab tests can show that something abnormal is present, but a biopsy is the only sure way to know whether the problem is cancer. In a biopsy, the doctor removes a sample of tissue from the abnormal area or may remove the whole tumor. A pathologist examines the tissue under a microscope. If cancer is present, the pathologist can usually tell what kind of cancer it is and may be able to judge whether the cells are likely to grow slowly or quickly.

Questions to Ask the Doctor

- How much tissue will be removed for the biopsy?
- How long will the biopsy take? Will I be awake? Will it hurt?

Excerpts from "What You Need to Know About Cancer," NIH Publication No. 94-1563, "What You Need to Know About Oral Cancer," NIH Publication No. 97-1574, and "Understanding Breast Changes," National Cancer Institute (NCI), NIH.

- How should I care for the biopsy site afterward?
- How soon will I know the results?
- If I do have cancer, who will talk with me about treatment? When?

Breast Biopsy

The only certain way to learn whether a breast lump or mammographic abnormality is cancerous is by having a biopsy, a procedure in which tissue is removed by a surgeon or other specialist and examined under a microscope by a pathologist. A pathologist is a doctor who specializes in identifying tissue changes that are characteristic of disease, including cancer.

Tissue samples for biopsy can be obtained by either surgery or needle. The doctor's choice of biopsy technique depends on such things as the nature and location of the lump, as well as the woman's general health.

Surgical Biopsy

Surgical biopsies can be either excisional or incisional. An excisional biopsy removes the entire lump or suspicious area. Excisional biopsy is currently the standard procedure for lumps that are smaller than an inch or so in diameter. In effect, it is similar to a lumpectomy, surgery to remove the lump and a margin of surrounding tissue. Lumpectomy is usually used in combination with radiation therapy as the basic treatment for early breast cancer.

An **excisional biopsy** is typically performed in the outpatient department of a hospital. A local anesthetic is injected into the woman's breast. Sometimes she is given a tranquilizer before the procedure. The surgeon makes an incision along the contour of the breast and removes the lump along with a small margin of normal tissue. Because no skin is removed, the biopsy scar is usually small. The procedure typically takes less than an hour. After spending an hour or two in the recovery room, the woman goes home the same day.

An **incisional biopsy** removes only a portion of the tumor (by slicing into it) for the pathologist to examine. Incisional biopsies are generally reserved for tumors that are larger. They too are usually performed under local anesthesia, with the woman going home the same day.

Whether or not a surgical biopsy will change the shape of your breast depends partly on the size of the lump and where it is located in the breast, as well as how much of a margin of healthy tissue the surgeon decides to remove. You should talk with your doctor beforehand, so you understand just how extensive the surgery will be and what the cosmetic result will be.

Needle Biopsy

Needle biopsies can be performed with either a very fine needle or a cutting needle large enough to remove a small nugget of tissue.

- **Fine needle aspiration** uses a very thin needle and syringe to remove either fluid from a cyst or clusters of cells from a solid mass. Accurate fine needle aspiration biopsy of a solid mass takes great skill, gained through experience with numerous cases.

- **Core needle biopsy** uses a somewhat larger needle with a special cutting edge. The needle is inserted, under local anesthesia, through a small incision in the skin, and a small core of tissue is removed. This technique may not work well for lumps that are very hard or very small. Core needle biopsy may cause some bruising, but rarely leaves an external scar, and the procedure is over in a matter of minutes.

At some institutions with extensive experience, aspiration biopsy is considered as reliable as surgical biopsy; it is trusted to confirm the malignancy of a clinically suspicious mass or to confirm a diagnosis that a lump is not cancerous. Should the needle biopsy results be uncertain, the diagnosis is pursued with a surgical biopsy. Some doctors prefer to verify all aspiration biopsy results with a surgical biopsy before proceeding with treatment.

Surgical Biopsy

Localization biopsy (also known as needle localization) is a procedure that uses mammography to locate and a needle to biopsy breast abnormalities that can be seen on a mammogram but cannot be felt (nonpalpable abnormalities). Localization can be used with surgical biopsy, fine needle aspiration, or core needle biopsy.

For a surgical biopsy, the radiologist locates the abnormality on a mammogram (or a sonogram) just prior to surgery. Using the mammogram as a guide, the radiologist inserts a fine needle or wire so the tip rests in the suspicious area—typically, an area of microcalcifications. The needle is anchored with a gauze bandage, and a second mammogram is taken to confirm that the needle is on target.

The woman, along with her mammograms, goes to the operating room, where the surgeon locates and cuts out the needle-targeted area. The more precisely the needle is placed, the less tissue needs to be removed.

Sometimes the surgeon will be able to feel the lump during surgery. In other cases, especially where the mammogram showed only microcalcifications, the abnormality can be neither seen nor felt. To make sure the surgical specimen in fact contains the abnormality, it is x-rayed on the spot. If this specimen x-ray fails to show the mass or the calcifications, the surgeon is able to remove additional tissue.

Stereotactic localization biopsy is a newer approach that relies on a three-dimensional x-ray to guide the needle biopsy of a nonpalpable mass. With one type of equipment, the patient lies face down on an examining table with a hole in it that allows the breast to hang through; the x-ray machine and the maneuverable needle "gun" are set up underneath. Alternatively, specialized stereotactic equipment can be attached to a standard mammography machine.

The breast is x-rayed from two different angles, and a computer plots the exact position of the suspicious area. (Because only a small area of the breast is exposed to the radiation, the doses are similar to those from standard mammography.) Once the target is clearly identified, the radiologist positions the gun and advances the biopsy needle into the lesion.

Tissue Studies

The cells or tissue removed through needle or surgical biopsy are promptly sent (along with the x-ray of the specimen, if one was made) to the pathology lab. If the excised lump is large enough, the pathologist can take a preliminary look by quick-freezing a small portion of the tissue sample. This makes the sample firm enough to slice into razor-thin sections that can be examined under the microscope. A "frozen section" provides an immediate, if provisional, diagnosis, and the surgeon may be able to give you the results before you go home.

The results of a frozen section are not 100 percent certain, however. A more thorough assessment takes several days, while the pathologist processes "permanent sections" of tissue that can be examined in greater detail.

When the biopsy specimen is small as is often the case when the abnormality consists of mammographic calcifications only–many doctors prefer to bypass a frozen section so the tiny specimen can be analyzed in its entirety.

The pathologist looks for abnormal cell shapes and unusual growth patterns. In many cases the diagnosis will be clear-cut. However, the distinctions between benign and cancerous can be subtle, and even experts don't always agree. When in doubt, pathologists readily consult their colleagues. If there is any question about the results of your biopsy, you will want to make sure your biopsy slides have been reviewed by more than one pathologist.

Deciding to Biopsy

Your doctor needs to thoughtfully weigh the findings from your physical exam and mammogram along with your background and your medical history when making a recommendation about a biopsy.

In general, doctors feel it is wise to biopsy
any distinct and persistent lump

Although benign lumps rarely, if ever, turn into cancer, cancerous lumps can develop near benign lumps and can be hidden on a mammogram. Even if you have had a benign lump removed in the past, you cannot be sure any new lump is also benign.

In some cases, the doctor may suggest watching the suspicious area for a month or two. Because many lumps are caused by normal hormonal changes, this waiting period may provide additional information.

Similarly, if the changes on your mammogram show all the signs of benign disease, your doctor may advise waiting several months and then taking another mammogram. This would be followed by more diagnostic mammograms over the next 3 years. If you choose this option, however, you must be strongly committed to regularly scheduled follow-ups.

If you feel uncomfortable about waiting, express your concerns to your doctor. You may also want to get a second opinion, perhaps from a breast specialist or surgeon. Many cities have breast clinics where you can get a second opinion.

Biopsy: One Step or Two?

Not too many years ago, all women undergoing surgery for breast symptoms had a one-step procedure: If the surgical biopsy showed cancer, the surgeon performed a mastectomy immediately. The woman went into surgery not knowing if she had cancer or if her breast would be removed.

Today a woman facing biopsy has a broader range of options. In most cases, biopsy and diagnosis will be separated from any further treatment by an interval of several days or weeks. Such a two-step procedure does not harm the patient, and it has several benefits. It allows time for the tissue sample to be examined in detail and, if cancer is found, it gives the woman time to adjust to the diagnosis. She can review her treatment options, seek a second opinion, receive counseling, and arrange her schedule.

Some women, nonetheless, prefer a one-step procedure. They have decided beforehand that, if the surgical biopsy and frozen section show cancer, they want to go ahead with surgery, either mastectomy or lumpectomy and axillary dissection (removal of the underarm lymph nodes). If, on the other hand, the lump proves to be benign, the incision will be closed. The procedure will have taken less than an hour, and the woman may go home the same day or the next day.

A one-step procedure avoids the physical and psychological stress, as well as the costs in time and money, of two rounds of surgery and anesthesia–a particularly important consideration for women who are ill or frail. Women who have symptoms of breast cancer can find the wait between biopsy and surgery emotionally draining, and they may be relieved to have a one-step procedure to take care of the problem as quickly as possible.

No single solution is right for everyone. Each woman should consult with her doctors and her family, weigh the alternatives, and decide what approach is appropriate. Being involved in the decision-making process can give a woman a sense of control over her body and her life.

Chapter 44

Cultures/Swab Tests

Editor's Note: Although this document on strep screen/throat culture discusses the topic in relation to children, the screening tests are the same for adults.

Strep Screen/Throat Culture

A child's throat can be sore for many reasons, including cheering for a favorite team. When a sore throat is caused by an infection, however, the most common cause is a virus. The soreness goes away as the infection does, almost always with no further problems.

But about 20% of sore throats are caused by a more serious bacterial infection from microbes (or germs) known as group A beta-streptococci, or "beta-strep." These microbes are the ones that cause strep throat, an infection that affects about one in five school-age children who develop a sore throat.

"Strep throat is more serious than the other 80% of sore throats," said Dr. Meier, "because if not treated with antibiotics, it sometimes can cause more serious pus-forming infections." In fact, the scientific name for the strep that causes sore throats is "pyogenes," or "pus-maker." And group A streptococci also produce toxins that can cause circulatory collapse (shock) in streptococcal toxic shock syndrome, or fever and a rash in scarlet fever. Furthermore, strep-caused glomerulonephritis can damage the kidneys. Rheumatic fever can damage the heart, joints, and sometimes the brain. Damage from these still rather mysterious "poststreptococcal diseases" can be life threatening or even permanent.

Timely antibiotic treatment can decrease dramatically the patient's chance of getting rheumatic fever and many of the other possible complications of a strep infection. Whether or not rapid antibiotic treatment affects the damage that strep can do to the kidneys is not so clear.

Although a strep infection may come to a doctor's attention because of a skin infection, such as impetigo, the most common complaint is a sore throat. To treat the one sore throat in five that is caused by beta-strep, without giving antibiotics to all the others, a simple test can be done.

How Is a Strep Screen Done?

The doctor or medical assistant wipes the back of your child's throat with a long cotton swab. In the doctor's laboratory, the swab is placed in a test tube with a chemical mix that removes part of the beta-strep germ from the swab. This "extract" is then combined with antibodies to the group A strep. (Antibodies are natural substances that attach to the group A strep bacteria's surface - just as they would in the body.) When a third substance is added to the tube, the liquid changes color if strep germs are present

A positive test means the child would benefit from taking antibiotics to kill the beta-strep. But it's not always this simple.

"The rapid beta-strep screening test is helpful when it is positive," said Dr. Meier, "but it is sometimes negative, even though the strep germs are present in the throat. In children, the test only picks up about 80 percent of strep throats." In order that the other 20 percent won't be missed, doctors usually collect two swabs at once. If the rapid test is negative, then the second swab is rubbed onto agar, a gelatin-like substance on a flat disk (a "culture plate"). The pattern of growth of group A streptococci is what identifies them as beta-strep.

How Long Does It Take to Get the Results?

A rapid strep screen can give results in minutes. A throat culture may take a day or two. It's important to find out whether strep is the cause of the sore throat since early treatment for strep throat reduces symptoms and decreases the risk of rheumatic fever. Waiting the day or two necessary to get back results still will allow enough time to treat the strep and avoid the serious, preventable complications. Sometimes, depending on how sick the child is and other specific circumstances, the doctor may begin antibiotics while waiting for the culture results.

How Long until the Results Are Ready?

Results usually are reported back within days.

Chapter 45

Pap Test

Questions and Answers About the Pap Smear

What Is a Pap Test?

The Pap test (sometimes called a Pap smear) is a way to examine cells collected from the cervix and vagina. This test can show the presence of infection, inflammation, abnormal cells, or cancer.

What Is a Pelvic Exam?

In a pelvic exam, the uterus, vagina, ovaries, fallopian tubes, bladder, and rectum are felt to find any abnormality in their shape or size. During a pelvic exam, an instrument called a speculum is used to widen the vagina so that the upper portion of the vagina and the cervix can be seen.

Why Are a Pap Smear and Pelvic Exam Important?

A Pap test and pelvic exam are important parts of a woman's routine health care because they can detect abnormalities that may lead to invasive cancer. These abnormalities can be treated before cancer develops. Most invasive cancers of the cervix can be prevented if women have Pap tests and pelvic exams regularly. Also, as with many types of cancer, cancer of the cervix is more likely to be treated successfully if it is detected early.

"Cancer Facts 5.16," National Cancer Institute (NCI), NIH.

Who Performs a Pap Test?

Doctors and other specially trained health care professionals, such as physician assistants, nurse midwives, and nurse practitioners, may perform Pap tests and pelvic exams. These individuals are often called clinicians.

How Is a Pap Test Done?

A Pap test is simple, quick, and painless; it can be done in a doctor's office, a clinic, or a hospital. While a woman lies on an exam table, the clinician inserts a speculum into her vagina to open it. To do the test, a sample of cells is taken from in and around the cervix with a wooden scraper or a small cervical brush or broom. The specimen (or smear) is placed on a glass slide or rinsed in liquid fixative and sent to a laboratory for examination.

Who Should Have Pap Tests?

Women who are or have been sexually active, or have reached age 18, should have Pap tests and physical exams regularly. Women may want to discuss with their doctor how often to have the test. There is no known upper age at which Pap tests cease to be effective. Older women should continue to have regular physical exams, including pelvic exams and Pap tests. Women who have had consistently normal Pap test results may want to ask the doctor how often they need to have a Pap test. Women who have had a hysterectomy (surgery to remove the uterus, including the cervix) should talk with their doctor about whether to continue to have regular Pap tests. If the hysterectomy was performed for treatment of a precancerous or cancerous condition, the end of the vaginal canal still needs to be sampled for abnormal changes. If the uterus (including the cervix) was removed because of a noncancerous condition such as fibroids, routine Pap tests may not be necessary. However, it is still important for a woman to have regular gynecologic examinations as part of her health care.

When Should the Pap Test Be Done?

A woman should have this test when she is not menstruating; the best time is between 10 and 20 days after the first day of the menstrual period. For about 2 days before a Pap test, she should avoid douching, or using vaginal medicines or spermicidal foams, creams, or jellies (except as directed by a physician). These may wash away or hide abnormal cells.

How Are the Results of a Pap Test Reported?

The way of reporting Pap test results has sometimes been confusing. A new reporting method, called the Bethesda System, was developed following a 1988 National Cancer Institute-sponsored workshop. The Bethesda System uses descriptive diagnostic terms rather than class numbers, which were used to report Pap test results in the past. This system of reporting includes an evaluation of specimen adequacy.

What Do Abnormal Test Results Mean?

A physician may simply describe Pap test results to a patient as "abnormal." Cells on the surface of the cervix sometimes appear abnormal but are not cancerous. It is important to remember that abnormal conditions do not always become cancerous, and some conditions are more of a threat than others. A woman may want to ask her doctor for specific information about her Pap test result and what the result means.

There are several terms that may be used to describe abnormal results.

- Dysplasia is a term used to describe abnormal cells. Dysplasia is not cancer, although it may develop into very early cancer of the cervix. In dysplasia, cervical cells undergo a series of changes in their appearance. The cells look abnormal under the microscope, but they do not invade nearby healthy tissue. There are three degrees of dysplasia, classified as mild, moderate, or severe, depending on how abnormal the cells appear under the microscope.

- Squamous intraepithelial lesion (SIL) is another term that is used to describe abnormal changes in the cells on the surface of the cervix. The word squamous describes cells which are thin, flat, and lie on the outer surface of the cervix. The word lesion refers to abnormal tissue. An intraepithelial lesion means that the abnormal cells are present only in the surface layers of the cells. A doctor may describe SIL as being low-grade (early changes in the size, shape, and number of cells) or high-grade (a large number of precancerous cells that look very different from normal cells).

- Cervical intraepithelial neoplasia (CIN) is another term that is sometimes used to describe abnormal cells. Neoplasia means a new abnormal growth of cells. Intraepithelial refers to the surface layers of the cells. The term CIN, along with a number (1 to 3), describes how much of the cervix contains abnormal cells.

- Carcinoma in situ describes a pre-invasive cancer that involves only the surface cells and has not spread into deeper tissues. Cervical cancer, or invasive cervical cancer, occurs when abnormal cells spread deeper into the cervix or to other tissues or organs.

How Do these Terms Compare?

- Mild dysplasia may also be classified as low-grade SIL or CIN 1.

- Moderate dysplasia may also be classified as high-grade SIL or CIN 2.

- Severe dysplasia may also be classified as high-grade SIL or CIN 3.

- Carcinoma in situ may also be classified as high-grade SIL or CIN 3.

What Are Atypical Squamous Cells of Undetermined Significance (ASCUS)?

Abnormalities that do not fulfill the criteria that define SIL, CIN, or dysplasia are termed atypical squamous cells of undetermined significance (ASCUS). Persistent abnormal smears are often further evaluated by a physician.

Is the Human Papillomavirus Associated with the Development of Cervical Cancer?

Human papillomaviruses (HPV) are viruses that can cause warts. Some HPVs are sexually transmitted and cause wart-like growths on the genitals. Scientists have identified more than 70 types of HPV; 30 types infect the cervix, and about 15 types are associated with cervical cancer. HPV is a major risk factor for cervical cancer. In fact, nearly all cervical cancers show evidence of HPV. However, not all cases of HPV develop into cervical cancer. A woman with HPV may want to discuss any concerns with her doctor.

Who Is at Risk for HPV Infection?

HPV infection is more common in younger age groups, particularly in women in their late teens and twenties. Because HPV is spread mainly through sexual contact, risk increases with number of sexual partners. Women who become sexually active at a young age, who have multiple sexual partners, and whose sexual partners have other partners are at increased risk. Nonsexual transmission is also possible. The virus often disappears but may remain detectable for years after infection.

Does Infection with a Cancer-Associated Type of HPV Always Lead to a Precancerous Condition or Cancer?

No. Most infections appear to go away on their own without causing any kind of abnormality. However, infection with cancer-associated HPV types may increase the risk that mild abnormalities will progress to more severe abnormalities or cervical cancer. With regular follow-up care by trained clinicians, women with precancerous cervical abnormalities should not develop invasive cervical cancer.

What Are False Positive and False Negative Results?

Unfortunately, there are occasions when Pap test results are not accurate. Although these errors do not occur very often, they can cause anxiety and can affect a woman's health. A false positive Pap test occurs when a patient is told she has abnormal cells when the cells are actually normal. A false negative Pap test result occurs when a specimen is called normal, but the woman has a lesion. A variety of factors may contribute to a false negative result. A false negative Pap test may delay the diagnosis and treatment of a precancerous condition. However, regular screening helps to compensate for the false negatives because if abnormal cells are missed at one time, chances are good that the cells will be detected next time. The Food and Drug Administration has recently approved two computerized systems for rescreening of samples to detect abnormal cells from a Pap test. These systems are beginning to be used in laboratories across the country. Rescreening may also be done manually. It is important for a woman to discuss the results of her Pap test with her physician and to inquire about the quality control measures that are taken in the laboratory in which the tissue sample is evaluated.

What if Pap Test Results Are Abnormal?

If the Pap test shows an ambiguous or minor abnormality, the physician may repeat the test to ensure accuracy. If the Pap test shows a significant abnormality, the physician may then perform a colposcopy using an instrument much like a microscope (called a colposcope) to examine the vagina and the cervix. The colposcope does not enter the body. A Schiller test may also be performed. For this test, the doctor coats the cervix with an iodine solution. Healthy cells turn brown and abnormal cells turn white or yellow. Both of these procedures can be done in the doctor's office.

The doctor may also remove a small amount of cervical tissue for examination by a pathologist. This procedure is called a biopsy and is the only sure way to know whether the abnormal cells indicate cancer.

For the Most Up to Date Information

Call the Cancer Information Service (CIS). The CIS, a program of the National Cancer Institute, is a nationwide telephone service for cancer patients and their families, the public, and health care professionals. CIS information specialists have extensive training in providing up-to-date and understandable information about cancer. They can answer questions in English and Spanish and can send free printed material. In addition, CIS offices serve specific geographic areas and have information about cancer-related services and resources in their region. The toll-free number of the CIS is

1-800-4-CANCER (1-800-422-6237).

Chapter 46

Spinal Tap

Lumbar Puncture (Spinal Tap)

Editor's Note: This article discusses fluid sample tests for children; however, the screening tests are the same for adults.

A lumbar puncture (LP) is done when physicians need to examine the spinal fluid that bathes the brain and spinal cord. While there are a number of reasons that a lumbar puncture may be needed, the most common reason is if meningitis is suspected. Meningitis is an infection of the coverings of the brain and spinal cord (the meninges).

When a lumbar puncture is performed, fluid pressure can be measured and a small amount of spinal fluid removed to be analyzed for blood cells, protein, and glucose. In meningitis, the number of white blood cells and protein level are usually elevated. In bacterial meningitis, the spinal fluid glucose level is frequently decreased. Spinal fluid is also cultured to find the type of bacterium (or virus or fungus) that might be the cause of the infection

Some of the fluid that has been collected is examined under a microscope for red and white blood cells and for bacteria and other infectious agents. Some is sent for culture. Some is sent for chemical analysis looking for, among other things, protein and glucose.

"Fluid Sample Tests," used with permission © 1998, The Nemours Foundation.

How Is a Lumbar Puncture Done?

A small, hollow needle is inserted carefully through the space between the vertebrae in the lower ("lumbar") part of the spine. The skin over the chosen spot will have been cleansed carefully with an antibacterial solution. Sometimes the area is numbed slightly. Then the very narrow needle is carefully inserted until it enters the space where the spinal fluid is. The needle does not enter the nerves of the spinal cord. A small sample of this fluid drips into the sample tubes held by the physician. After the sample is collected (usually this takes a minute or so), the needle is withdrawn and a band-aid placed. During the procedure, the physician can measure the pressure of the spinal fluid, although this is not routinely done in children.

During the lumbar puncture, the patient lies curled up in the "fetal" position, with knees and thighs bent. A sick or young child may need to be held in this position, which opens the spaces between the lumbar vertebrae. Sometimes, in the case of small infants, the child may be placed in a sitting position with the head slightly flexed or supported with a pillow propped between arms and legs.

Despite the careful efforts of the medical team and parents, the child frequently is frightened by this procedure. A child undergoing a lumbar puncture is often quite ill and irritable. The emergency room with its noise, bright lights, and unfamiliar faces is a "scary" place, even under the best of circumstances. Parents are understandably upset about their child and the thought of a lumbar puncture is further upsetting.

The lumbar puncture itself takes only minutes. Preparing the child for the procedure—proper positioning, cleaning and draping the area, and the other details required to make everything run smoothly—takes more time. And while it all may be over in a matter of 15-20 minutes or so, it can seem like an eternity to a worried family.

Yet, the lumbar puncture itself is generally quite safe and not nearly as uncomfortable as you might imagine. "Extreme care and cleanliness are always used when doing a lumbar puncture," Dr. Meier pointed out. "And the procedure is done as rapidly as possible to minimize discomfort. "CT scans and x-rays cannot tell the cause of an infection and therefore cannot substitute for a lumbar puncture.

How Long Does It Take to Get the Results Back?

Fluid collected from a lumbar puncture must be rushed to the laboratory immediately. This is not only because it is usually important to get the results as soon as possible, but also because rapid process-ing of the fluid is required for best accuracy. Some of the results—such as cell counts—will be ready within minutes to hours. Cultures will take 48-72 hours, and occasionally longer, depending on how slow-growing the organism might be.

Sweat Test

Since this test helps diagnose cystic fibrosis (CF), it can be a wor-risome test for parents and child. This test may be ordered if a doc-tor is considering the diagnosis of CF; most of the time, the test is normal. Cystic fibrosis is an inherited disease that causes sweat glands and other glands, especially in the pancreas and the air pas-sages of the lungs, to produce abnormally thick mucus that has a clog-ging effect. This clogging causes many problems for the patient, especially in the lungs. Though there are some promising new devel-opments, there currently is no cure for cystic fibrosis, so early diag-nosis and proper treatments are essential to improve the patient's quality of life and lifespan.

How Is a Sweat Test Done?

A device for collecting sweat is placed on a patch of the child's skin, and the skin is forced to perspire through chemical means. Sweat is collected for about one-half to one hour on filter paper. Assuming enough sweat is collected (sometimes that's difficult), the sweat is analyzed for sodium and chloride. These same components of table salt also are in blood, sweat, and tears. When chloride is elevated beyond a certain point, using two consecutive tests, the diagnosis of cystic fibrosis needs to be considered. There are, however, a number of other conditions that can give elevated sweat electrolytes.

How Long Does a Sweat Test Take?

The sweat collection takes about 30 minutes to one hour once it begins. If the collection is found to be inadequate, it may need to be repeated another time. The diagnosis of cystic fibrosis requires two (or more) abnormal sweat tests, and is not made on the basis of just one test. Afterwards, further genetic testing can help physicians de-termine which subtype of cystic fibrosis is present.

Chapter 47

Stool Test

Stool Collection and Testing

A physician will order a stool collection to test for a variety of conditions. We usually think of stool (feces) as nothing but waste—something to quickly flush away. But since ancient times it has been recognized that bowel movements can contain valuable information. One of the many substances that can be analyzed in a stool specimen is fat. Normally, fat is completely absorbed from the intestine, and the stool contains virtually no fat. In certain types of digestive disorders, however, fat is incompletely absorbed ("malabsorbed") and can be a key to diagnosis.

In today's world, the most common reason to collect stool is to determine which bacteria or, less often, parasite, may be infecting the intestine. An incredible variety of microscopic organisms (mostly billions of harmless bacteria) live in the intestine. In fact, they are necessary for normal digestion. Sometimes, however, the intestine may become infected with harmful bacteria or parasites which cause a variety of conditions, such as certain types of diarrhea. It may then be necessary to examine the stool under a microscope, culture the stool, and perform other tests to help find the cause of the problem.

This chapter contains text from "Stool Tests," Used with permission © 1998, The Nemours Foundation, and from *Cancer Facts 5.15*, National Cancer Institute, NIH, March 1994.

How Is a Stool Collection Done?

Unlike most other lab tests, stool is often collected by the patient or their family at home, not by a health-care professional. Studies have shown that liquid stool is of the most value in looking for a diagnosis. Such collections are messy. **(Be sure to wear latex gloves.)**

Many patients with diarrhea, especially young children, can't always let their parent know in advance when a bowel movement is coming. Sometimes a curious-looking, hat-shaped plastic lid is used to collect the bowel movement. This "catching" device can be quickly placed over the toilet bowl or child's rear end to collect the specimen. Its use can prevent contamination of the stool by water and dirt. Sometimes, however, urine contaminates the stool sample. Then the frustrated parent or caregiver must try again. "Fishing" the bowel movements out of the toilet is not useful.

The stool should be collected into clean, dry plastic jars with screw cap lids. These containers can be obtained through the hospital laboratories or pharmacies, although any clean, sealable container could do the job. For best results, the stool should then be brought to the laboratory immediately, if there is somebody at the laboratory to start analysis.

If it is impossible to get the sample to the laboratory right away, the stool should be refrigerated, then taken to the laboratory to be cultured within one to four hours after collection. When the sample arrives at the laboratory, it is either examined and cultured immediately or placed in a special liquid medium that attempts to preserve potential bacteria or parasites.

The physician or the hospital laboratory usually gives patients or their parents written directions on how to successfully collect a stool sample.

Most of the time, pathogenic (disease-causing) bacteria or parasites can be identified from just one stool specimen. Sometimes, however, up to three samples must be taken. The three samples are taken on three consecutive days.

How Long Until the Results Are Ready?

This varies, but results usually are reported back within days.

Stool for Blood

Stool (bowel movement) is sometimes examined for blood. Blood in the stool might be found with certain kinds of diarrhea, with ulcers, or with a variety of other conditions. Of course, one of the most common causes in an infant or toddler is not the result of infection. It's due to a slight rectal tear from straining against a hard stool. Hemorrhoids can also result in blood in the stool.

How Is the Test for Blood in the Stool Done?

If a stool collection (as described above) is performed, some of the stool usually will be tested for blood. Stool in a diaper or obtained by a rectal examination can also be tested.

How Long until the Test for Stool Blood Is Ready?

Some of the tests are performed with a strip of paper that can give the answer virtually immediately. Most of the time, a laboratory result will be reported within days.

Stool for Culture

Stool can be cultured for disease-causing bacteria. Not all bacteria in the stool cause problems; in fact, over 80% of stool is bacteria, most of which are fine and dandy. Cultures of stool are only looking for those bacteria that may be causing disease.

How Is the Stool Culture Done?

Stool is collected (as described above). The lab will need two or three specimens collected at different times. The stool should be loose and "fresh." Well-formed stool is rarely positive for disease-causing bacteria.

How Long until the Stool Culture Is Ready?

Stool cultures take five or more days until a result is known.

Stool for Ova and Parasites

Stool may be tested for the presence of parasites and ova (the egg stage) if a child has prolonged diarrhea or other intestinal symptoms. If parasites or their eggs are seen when a smear of stool is examined under the microscope, the patient will be treated for a parasitic infestation.

What Is a Fecal Occult Blood Test?

The fecal occult blood test (FOBT) is a chemical test for hidden blood in a stool sample. It is only a test for blood, not a test that directly detects cancer.

Does Blood in the Stool Always Mean Cancer?
Are there False Positives on the FOBT?
Are there False Negatives on the FOBT?

A positive test can be caused by bleeding due to conditions other than cancer. In a number of screening programs, less than 10 percent of all positive occult blood tests were caused by cancer.

A positive test can be caused by bleeding from hemorrhoids, ulcers, noncancerous growths called polyps, or other noncancerous conditions. In addition, some foods and medications may cause a positive FOBT.

The FOBT is negative in many patients known to have colon cancer. False negative test results may occur because some cancers bleed intermittently, some bleed too little to be detected, and some do not bleed at all.

The results of the FOBT can be influenced by a variety of factors, including how a patient prepares for the test and how the stool specimen is processed.

What Are the Symptoms of Colorectal Cancer?

The most common warning signs are changes in bowel habits, such as constipation or diarrhea; very dark, mahogany red, or bright red blood in or on the stool; and abdominal discomfort.

Who Should Have an FOBT?

People who have no symptoms of colon or rectal cancer should have an FOBT every year, beginning at age 50.

Why Should an FOBT Be Done Every Year?

Colorectal tumors may bleed only intermittently, so an FOBT will miss some cancers. By testing every year, tumors missed one year may be detected the next year. Because colorectal cancer appears to be relatively slow growing, chances are good that these cancers may still be found at an early stage when they are curable. A recent NCI-sponsored study confirmed the effectiveness of annual screening.

Chapter 48

Urine Tests

Contents

Section 48.1

Urinalysis

Urinalysis

Examining urine for signs of disease has been recommended since at least the time of Hippocrates, the father of Western medicine, who told his followers to check its colors in those who were sick.

Kidneys act as filters for the bloodstream, purifying all the blood as it passes through them. The kidneys filter the equivalent of about 150 quarts of blood that recycles daily. The kidneys remove wastes and ensure needed substances are left in the blood. Urine is produced by the kidneys when they remove soluble waste products from the body. Kidneys, like most of the organs of the body, perform a number of functions. Among their roles, kidneys help control blood pressure and synthesize an active form of vitamin D.

A urinalysis is most often ordered if a urinary tract infection is suspected, although there are other reasons why such a test could be useful. Like the complete blood count, a urinalysis can check on several different things:

- The number and kind of cells from the lining of the kidneys and bladder that have appeared in the urine;

- The number and variety of both red (RBCs) and white blood cells (WBCs);

- The presence of bacteria or other organisms;

- A variety of chemicals that the kidneys filter (when healthy or sick), such as glucose;

- The pH, measuring how acidic or basic the urine is;

- The concentration of the urine.

Sometimes results that may seem abnormal, such as the presence of white or red cells in the urine, may be the result of how or when the urine was collected rather than disease. For example, a dehydrated, crying child may have a few RBCs or WBCs in the urine. Once she is rehydrated, these "abnormal" results may disappear.

How Is a Urinalysis Done?

Urine is collected in a clean container. The first part of the test is the urine dipstick. Here, a plastic stick that has patches of chemical indicators on it (the dipstick) is placed in the urine. Depending on the color changes of the patches, various things will be revealed. These include the presence or absence of hemoglobin (found in red blood cells), white blood cells, sugar, and pH (whether the urine is acid or base).

The urine also is examined under a microscope. In addition to looking for red and white cells, the doctor or laboratory technologist can check for crystals, measure how concentrated the urine is, and perform other useful measures. In order to be accurate, the urine must be "fresh" when tested, and there needs to be enough collected.

How Long Will It Take to Get Results?

Some of the tests can be done rapidly. Some of the tests may take minutes to hours. As with all tests, it also depends on how busy the laboratory is. Most urinalyses are reported back within a few days.

Urine Culture

If a urinalysis shows white blood cells and bacteria, which may indicate infection in the kidneys or bladder, the doctor may decide to culture the urine. This will identify the kind of bacteria present.

It is hard to get a good urine sample from children," Dr. Meier said, and it's easy to understand why. The skin around the urinary opening normally is home to the same bacteria that cause infection inside the body. Contamination with these bacteria can make the sample inaccurate or unusable. To avoid this, the skin surrounding the urinary opening must either be cleaned and rinsed immediately before the urine is collected, or bypassed through use of a catheter—a narrow, soft tube inserted gently through the urinary tract opening (urethra) into the bladder.

How Is a Urine Culture Done?

In the "clean-catch" method, the patient (or parent) cleans the skin around the urethra, urinates, stops urination, and then urinates again

417

into the collection container. Catching urine in "midstream" is the goal. "Understandably, this is difficult for young children to do," said Dr. Meier. The "clean-catch" method may be difficult for girls under four or five, who have most of the urinary infections. Very young children who need a urine culture may be catheterized to obtain an accurate specimen.

How Long Does It Take until the Culture Is Done?

About 48-72 hours.

Section 48.2

Urodynamic Tests

Excerpts from *Your Urinary System and How It Works*, National Kidney and Urologic Diseases Information Clearinghouse (NKUDIC), NIH Publication No. 98-3195, April 1998.

What Causes Problems in the Urinary System?

Problems in the urinary system can be caused by aging, illness, or injury. As you get older, changes in the kidneys' structure cause them to lose some of their ability to remove wastes from the blood. Also, the muscles in your ureters, bladder, and urethra tend to lose some of their strength. You may have more urinary infections because the bladder muscles do not tighten enough to empty your bladder completely. A decrease in strength of muscles of the sphincters and the pelvis can also cause incontinence, the unwanted leakage of urine. Illness or injury can also prevent the kidneys from filtering the blood completely or block the passage of urine.

How Are Problems in the Urinary System Detected?

Urinalysis is a test that studies the content of urine for abnormal substances such as protein or signs of infection. This test involves urinating into a special container and leaving the sample to be studied.

Urodynamic tests evaluate the storage of urine in the bladder and the flow of urine from the bladder through the urethra. Your doctor may want to do a urodynamic test if you are having symptoms that suggest problems with the muscles or nerves of your lower urinary system and pelvis (ureters, bladder, urethra, and sphincter muscles).

Urodynamic tests measure the contraction of the bladder muscle as it fills and empties. The test is done by inserting a small tube called a catheter through your urethra into your bladder to fill it either with water or a gas. Another small tube is inserted into your rectum to measure the pressure put on your bladder when you strain or cough. Other bladder tests use x-ray dye instead of water so that x-ray pictures can be taken when the bladder fills and empties to detect any abnormalities in the shape and function of the bladder. These tests take about an hour.

Section 48.3.

Bladder Cancer Urine Test

News, Journal of the National Cancer Institute, Issue 3/4, Vol. 88, February 21, 1996.

DNA Test for Bladder Cancer Hits a High Mark

A bladder cancer urine test based on DNA markers called microsatellites has proved accurate in a stunning 95% of cases in a small pilot study. The high sensitivity of the test, reported in February 1996 *Science*, makes microsatellite analysis a solid contender in the increasingly crowded race to detect cancers via tumor markers in blood and urine.

"It sounds good, very good," said Dan Theodorescu, M.D., a urologic oncologist who is not connected with the study. "The big issue in diagnosis is the stage of the cancer," said Theodorescu, who studies bladder cancer at the University of Virginia Cancer Center, Charlottesville. "Anything that could improve sensitivity in the early stages would be a significant advance."

Although the numbers are small, the microsatellite test detected all grades and stages of bladder cancer in 19 of 20 patients with biopsied tumors, according to the report by David Sidransky, M.D., and his colleagues at the Johns Hopkins University, Baltimore. The test was almost twice as accurate as urine cytology—the visual inspection of urine cells under a microscope—which spotted only 50% of the cancers in these patients.

Whether the high accuracy rate will hold in larger studies is, of course, a major question. Plans are still at a very early stage, said Mark Schoenberg, M.D., one of the Hopkins investigators. But a priority is a multi-institutional trial with patients who have had bladder cancer and thus are at risk for recurrence.

"We don't want to be less than definitive, so we're going to ask a small question first," Schoenberg said. "Can this assay replace cystoscopy in the follow-up of patients who have already had bladder cancer?"

Most bladder cancer patients have polyps that can be removed surgically. Although the polyps have a low likelihood of developing into invasive cancer, they do often recur, so patients must be followed carefully. Right now, the most sensitive method of follow-up is cystoscopy, an outpatient procedure in which a physician looks for lesions via a tube threaded through the urethra. Imaging and urine cytology are other possibilities. All the current options have a range of disadvantages, including expense.

Inexpensive Test

Microsatellite analysis, which uses the polymerase chain reaction to detect the DNA abnormalities in urine, will be cheap—about $25 to $50 for each test, Sidransky said. Cytology costs about $150 and cystoscopy about $600 at Hopkins.

Microsatellite disruption is one of numerous tumor markers that have entered the research pipeline in recent years, part of what Theodorescu calls the "leap from microscopic to molecular pathology." Unlike microsatellites, most of these markers are genes or their protein products, like HER-2/neu or p53.

In bladder cancer, one marker nearing approval by the U.S. Food and Drug Administration is a nuclear matrix protein called NMP22. Matritech, a company in Cambridge, Mass., has applied for FDA approval to use the test after surgery to predict which patients need cystoscopy on follow- up. Matritech's findings have yet to be published, but the company says the test has also proved nearly twice as accurate as cystology.

Other protein markers for bladder cancer may also be on the horizon. Compared to such protein-based assays, microsatellite analysis is "a big departure," said Sidransky.

Microsatellites are neither proteins nor genes, but strings of DNA with short, repetitive sequences of bases—for instance, CTA, CTA, CTA—that occur in so-called junk DNA, the non-gene segments that do not encode proteins. In almost all human cancers, microsatellites alter, growing longer or shorter than normal. These alterations show up early in the process of carcinogenesis, as cancer cells are cloned and some shed into body fluids.

Highly Cancer Specific

Microsatellite alterations do not show up in healthy tissue, a fact that should make the Hopkins/Oncor assay highly specific for cancer. In the pilot study, none of the control group—five people without bladder cancer symptoms—had microsatellite alterations.

The high sensitivity in the latest study was unexpected, the researchers said. In 1995 at a meeting sponsored by the General Motors Cancer Research Foundation, Sidransky reported that the Hopkins team had identified about 66% of bladder cancers by looking for 15 different microsatellite alterations that they had found in bladder tumors.

The jump from 66% to 95% sensitivity in this study came when the investigators looked not only for microsatellite alterations but also for another abnormality: the loss of heterozygosity in genes. LOH, in which a gene exists in only one version instead of the normal two, is a common characteristic of cancer cells and one that microsatellite analysis can easily detect.

Still ahead is the possibility of microsatellite analysis in other cancers. Kaiser Permanente in Oakland, Calif., is discussing plans to test the assay with cervical cancer, using Pap smears. And there is talk of using microsatellites to test for prostate cancer in ejaculate, Sidransky said. Other possibilities are lung, breast, and colon cancer.

—Caroline McNeil

Part Seven

Scope Tests

Chapter 49

Digestive System Scope Tests:

Colonoscopy, Sigmoidoscopy, Upper Endoscopy (EGD), Endoscopic Retrograde Cholangiopancreatography (ERCP), Upper Gastrointestinal (GI) Series, and Lower Gastrointestinal (GI) Series

Your Digestive System and How It Works

The digestive system is a series of hollow organs joined in a long, twisting tube from the mouth to the anus. Inside this tube is a lining called the mucosa. In the mouth, stomach, and small intestine, the mucosa contains tiny glands that produce juices to help digest food.

There are also two solid digestive organs, the liver and the pancreas, which produce juices that reach the intestine through small tubes. In addition, parts of other organ systems (for instance, nerves and blood) play a major role in the digestive system.

Why Is Digestion Important?

When we eat such things as bread, meat, and vegetables, they are not in a form that the body can use as nourishment. Our food and drink must be changed into smaller molecules of nutrients before they can be absorbed into the blood and carried to cells throughout the body. Digestion is the process by which food and drink are broken

---

This chapter contains text from the following National Institute of Diabetes and Digestive and Kidney Diseases (NIDDK) publications: "Your Digestive System and How It Works", NIH Pub. No. 97-2681, August 1992; "Colonoscopy," NIH Pub. No. 98-4331, June 1998; "Sigmoidoscopy", NIH Pub. No. 98-4332, 1998; "Upper Endoscopy," NIH Pub. No. 98-4333, 1998; "ERCP," NIH Pub. No. 98-4336, 1998; "Upper GI Series," NIH Pub. No. 98-4335, 1998; and "Lower GI Series," NIH Pub. No. 98-4331, 1998.

down into their smallest parts so that the body can use them to build and nourish cells and to provide energy.

How Is Food Digested?

Digestion involves the mixing of food, its movement through the digestive tract, and chemical breakdown of the large molecules of food into smaller molecules. Digestion begins in the mouth, when we chew and swallow, and is completed in the small intestine. The chemical process varies somewhat for different kinds of food.

Movement of Food Through the System

The large, hollow organs of the digestive system contain muscle that enables their walls to move. The movement of organ walls can propel food and liquid and also can mix the contents within each organ.

Figure 49.1. *The Digestive System*

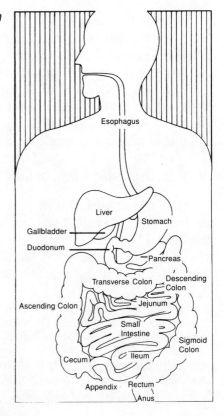

Typical movement of the esophagus, stomach, and intestine is called peristalsis. The action of peristalsis looks like an ocean wave moving through the muscle. The muscle of the organ produces a narrowing and then propels the narrowed portion slowly down the length of the organ. These waves of narrowing push the food and fluid in front of them through each hollow organ.

The first major muscle movement occurs when food or liquid is swallowed. Although we are able to start swallowing by choice, once the swallow begins, it becomes involuntary and proceeds under the control of the nerves.

The esophagus is the organ into which the swallowed food is pushed. It connects the throat above with the stomach below. At the junction of the esophagus and stomach, there is a ring-like valve closing the passage between the two organs. However, as the food approaches the closed ring, the surrounding muscles relax and allow the food to pass.

The food then enters the stomach, which has three mechanical tasks to do. First, the stomach must store the swallowed food and liquid. This requires the muscle of the upper part of the stomach to relax and accept large volumes of swallowed material. The second job is to mix up the food, liquid, and digestive juice produced by the stomach. The lower part of the stomach mixes these materials by its muscle action. The third task of the stomach is to empty its contents slowly into the small intestine.

Several factors affect emptying of the stomach, including the nature of the food (mainly its fat and protein content) and the degree of muscle action of the emptying stomach and the next organ to receive the stomach contents (the small intestine). As the food is digested in the small intestine and dissolved into the juices from the pancreas, liver, and intestine, the contents of the intestine are mixed and pushed forward to allow further digestion.

Finally, all of the digested nutrients are absorbed through the intestinal walls. The waste products of this process include undigested parts of the food, known as fiber, and older cells that have been shed from the mucosa. These materials are propelled into the colon, where they remain, usually for a day or two, until the feces are expelled by a bowel movement

Production of Digestive Juices

Glands of the digestive system are crucial to the process of digestion. They produce both the juices that break down the food and the hormones that help to control the process.

The glands that act first are in the mouth—the salivary glands. Saliva produced by these glands contains an enzyme that begins to digest the starch from food into smaller molecules.

The next set of digestive glands is in the stomach lining. They produce stomach acid and an enzyme that digests protein. One of the unsolved puzzles of the digestive system is why the acid juice of the stomach does not dissolve the tissue of the stomach itself. In most people, the stomach mucosa is able to resist the juice, although food and other tissues of the body cannot.

After the stomach empties the food and its juice into the small intestine, the juices of two other digestive organs mix with the food to continue the process of digestion. One of these organs is the pancreas. It produces a juice that contains a wide array of enzymes to break down the carbohydrates, fat, and protein in our food. Other enzymes that are active in the process come from glands in the wall of the intestine or even a part of that wall.

The liver produces yet another digestive juice—bile. The bile is stored between meals in the gallbladder. At mealtime, it is squeezed out of the gallbladder into the bile ducts to reach the intestine and mix with the fat in our food. The bile acids dissolve the fat into the watery contents of the intestine, much like detergents that dissolve grease from a frying pan. After the fat is dissolved, it is digested by enzymes from the pancreas and the lining of the intestine.

Absorption and Transport of Nutrients

Digested molecules of food, as well as water and minerals from the diet, are absorbed from the cavity of the upper small intestine. The absorbed materials cross the mucosa into the blood, mainly, and are carried off in the bloodstream to other parts of the body for storage or further chemical change. As noted earlier, this part of the process varies with different types of nutrients.

Carbohydrates—An average American adult eats about half a pound of carbohydrate each day. Some of our most common foods contain mostly carbohydrates. Examples are bread, potatoes, pastries, candy, rice, spaghetti, fruits, and vegetables. Many of these foods contain both starch, which can be digested, and fiber, which the body cannot digest.

The digestible carbohydrates are broken into simpler molecules by enzymes in the saliva, in juice produced by the pancreas, and in the lining of the small intestine. Starch is digested in two steps: First, an enzyme in the saliva and pancreatic juice breaks the starch into molecules called maltose; then an enzyme in the lining of the small intestine (maltase) splits the maltose into glucose molecules that can be absorbed into the blood. Glucose is carried through the bloodstream to the liver, where it is stored or used to provide energy for the work of the body.

Table sugar is another carbohydrate that must be digested to be useful. An enzyme in the lining of the small intestine digests table sugar into glucose and fructose, each of which can be absorbed from the intestinal cavity into the blood. Milk contains yet another type of sugar, lactose, which is changed into absorbable molecules by an enzyme called lactase, also found in the intestinal lining.

Protein—Foods such as meat, eggs, and beans consist of giant molecules of protein that must be digested by enzymes before they can be used to build and repair body tissues. An enzyme in the juice of the stomach starts the digestion of swallowed protein. Further digestion of the protein is completed in the small intestine. Here, several enzymes from the pancreatic juice and the lining of the intestine carry out the breakdown of huge protein molecules into small molecules called amino acids. These small molecules can be absorbed from the hollow of the small intestine into the blood and then be carried to all parts of the body to build the walls and other parts of cells.

Fats—Fat molecules are a rich source of energy for the body. The first step in digestion of a fat such as butter is to dissolve it into the watery content of the intestinal cavity. The bile acids produced by the liver act as natural detergents to dissolve fat in water and allow the enzymes to break the large fat molecules into smaller molecules, some of which are fatty acids and cholesterol. The bile acids combine with the fatty acids and cholesterol and help these molecules to move into the cells of the mucosa. In these cells the small molecules are formed back into large molecules, most of which pass into vessels (called lymphatics) near the intestine. These small vessels carry the reformed fat to the veins of the chest, and the blood carries the fat to storage depots in different parts of the body.

Vitamins—Another vital part of our food that is absorbed from the small intestine is the class of chemicals we call vitamins. There are two different types of vitamins, classified by the fluid in which they can be dissolved: water-soluble vitamins (all the B vitamins and vitamin C) and fat-soluble vitamins (vitamins A, D, and K).

Water and Salt—Most of the material absorbed from the cavity of the small intestine is water in which salt is dissolved. The salt and water come from the food and liquid we swallow and the juices secreted by the many digestive glands. In a healthy adult, more than a gallon of water containing over an ounce of salt is absorbed from the intestine every 24 hours.

How Is the Digestive Process Controlled?

Hormone Regulators

A fascinating feature of the digestive system is that it contains its own regulators. The major hormones that control the functions of the digestive system are produced and released by cells in the mucosa of the stomach and small intestine. These hormones are released into the blood of the digestive tract, travel back to the heart and through the arteries, and return to the digestive system, where they stimulate digestive juices and cause organ movement. The hormones that control digestion are gastrin, secretin, and cholecystokinin (CCK):

- Gastrin causes the stomach to produce an acid for dissolving and digesting some foods. It is also necessary for the normal growth of the lining of the stomach, small intestine, and colon.

- Secretin causes the pancreas to send out a digestive juice that is rich in bicarbonate. It stimulates the stomach to produce pepsin, an enzyme that digests protein, and it also stimulates the liver to produce bile.

- CCK causes the pancreas to grow and to produce the enzymes of pancreatic juice, and it causes the gallbladder to empty.

Nerve Regulators

Two types of nerves help to control the action of the digestive system. Extrinsic (outside) nerves come to the digestive organs from the unconscious part of the brain or from the spinal cord. They release a chemical called acetylcholine and another called adrenaline. Acetylcholine causes the muscle of the digestive organs to squeeze with more force and increase the "push" of food and juice through the digestive tract. Acetylcholine also causes the stomach and pancreas to produce more digestive juice. Adrenaline relaxes the muscle of the stomach and intestine and decreases the flow of blood to these organs.

Even more important, though, are the intrinsic (inside) nerves, which make up a very dense network embedded in the walls of the esophagus, stomach, small intestine, and colon. The intrinsic nerves are triggered to act when the walls of the hollow organs are stretched by food. They release many different substances that speed up or delay the movement of food and the production of juices by the digestive organs.

Diagnostic Tests of the Digestive System

Colonoscopy

Colonoscopy (koh-luh-NAH-skuh-pee) lets the physician look inside your entire large intestine, from the lowest part, the rectum all the way up through the colon to the lower end of the small intestine. The procedure is used to diagnose the causes of unexplained changes in bowel habits. It is also used to look for early signs of cancer in the

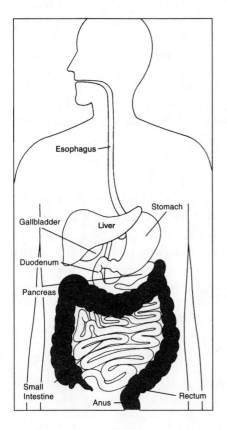

Figure 49.2. The Digestive System: Large Intestine and Rectum

colon and rectum. Colonoscopy enables the physician to see inflamed tissue, abnormal growths, ulcers, bleeding, and muscle spasms.

For the procedure, you will lie on your left side on the examining table. You will probably be given pain medication and a mild sedative to keep you comfortable and to help you relax during the exam. The physician will insert a long, flexible, lighted tube into your rectum and slowly guide it into your colon. The tube is called a colonoscope (koh-LON-oh-skope). The scope transmits an image of the inside of the colon, so the physician can carefully examine the lining of the colon. The scope bends, so the physician can move it around the curves of your colon. You may be asked to change position occasionally to help the physician move the scope. The scope also blows air into your colon, which inflates the colon and helps the physician see better.

If anything unusual is in your colon, like a polyp or inflamed tissue, the physician can remove a piece of it using tiny instruments passed through the scope. That tissue (biopsy) is then sent to a lab for testing. If there is bleeding in the colon, the physician can pass a laser, heater probe, or electrical probe, or inject special medicines, through the scope and use it to stop the bleeding.

Bleeding and puncture of the colon are possible complications of colonoscopy. However, such complications are uncommon.

Colonoscopy takes 30 to 60 minutes. The sedative and pain medicine should keep you from feeling much discomfort during the exam. You will need to remain at the physician's office for 1 to 2 hours until the sedative wears off.

Preparation

Your colon must be completely empty for the colonoscopy to be thorough and safe. To prepare for the procedure you may have to follow a liquid diet for 1 to 3 days beforehand. A liquid diet means fat-free bouillon or broth, gelatin, strained fruit juice, water, plain coffee, plain tea, or diet soda. You may need to take laxatives or an enema before the procedure. Also, you must arrange for someone to take you home afterward. You will not be allowed to drive because of the sedatives. Your physician may give you other special instructions.

Sigmoidoscopy

Sigmoidoscopy (SIG-moy-DAH-skuh-pee) enables the physician to look at the inside of the large intestine from the rectum through the last part of the colon, called the sigmoid colon. Physicians may use this procedure to find the cause of diarrhea, abdominal pain, or constipation. They also use sigmoidoscopy to look for early signs of cancer in the colon and rectum. With sigmoidoscopy, the physician can see bleeding, inflammation, abnormal growths, and ulcers.

For the procedure, you will lie on your left side on the examining table. The physician will insert a short, flexible, lighted tube into your rectum and slowly guide it into your colon. The tube is called a sigmoidoscope (sig-MOY-duh-skope). The scope transmits an image of the inside of the rectum and colon, so the physician can carefully examine the lining of these organs. The scope also blows air into these organs, which inflates them and helps the physician see better.

If anything unusual is in your rectum or colon, like a polyp or inflamed tissue, the physician can remove a piece of it using instruments inserted into the scope. The physician will send that piece of tissue (biopsy) to the lab for testing.

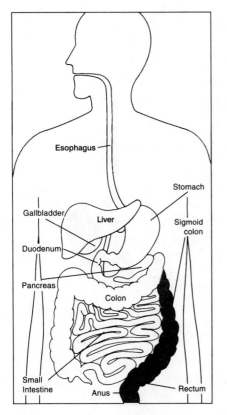

Figure 49.3. *The Digestive System: Sigmoid Colon and Rectum*

Bleeding and puncture of the colon are possible complications of sigmoidoscopy. However, such complications are uncommon.

Sigmoidoscopy takes 10 to 20 minutes. During the procedure, you might feel pressure and slight cramping in your lower abdomen. You win feel better afterwards when the air leaves your colon.

Preparation

The colon and rectum must be completely empty for sigmoidoscopy to be thorough and safe, so the physician will probably tell you to drink only clear liquids for 12 to 24 hours beforehand. A liquid diet means fat-free bouillon or broth, gelatin, strained fruit juice, water, plain coffee, plain tea, or diet soda. The night before or right before the procedure, you may also be given an enema, which is a liquid solution that washes out the intestines. Your physician may give you other special instructions.

Figure 49.4. The Digestive System: Esophagus, Stomach, and Duodenum

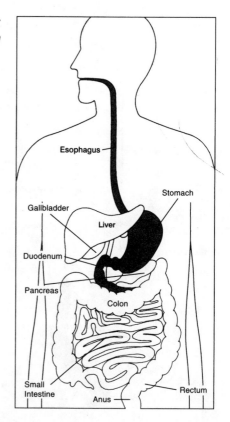

434

Upper Endoscopy

Upper endoscopy enables the physician to look inside the esophagus, stomach, and duodenum (first part of the small intestine). The procedure might be used to discover the reason for swallowing difficulties, nausea, vomiting, reflux, bleeding, indigestion, abdominal pain, or chest pain. Upper endoscopy is also called EGD, which stands for esophagogastroduodenoscopy (eh-SAH-fuh-goh-GAS-troh-doo-AH-duhNAH-skuh-pee).

For the procedure you will swallow a thin, flexible, lighted tube called an endoscope (EN-doh-skope). Right before the procedure the physician will spray your throat with a numbing agent that may help prevent gagging. You may also receive pain medicine and a sedative to help you relax during the exam. The endoscope transmits an image of the inside of the esophagus, stomach, and duodenum, so the physician can carefully examine the lining of these organs. The scope also blows air into the stomach; this expands the folds of tissue and makes it easier for the physician to examine the stomach.

The physician can see abnormalities, like ulcers, through the endoscope that don't show up well on x-rays. The physician can also insert instruments into the scope to remove samples of tissue (biopsy) for further tests.

Possible complications of upper endoscopy include bleeding and puncture of the stomach lining. However, such complications are rare. Most people will probably have nothing more than a mild sore throat after the procedure.

The procedure takes 20 to 30 minutes. Because you will be sedated, you will need to rest at the physician's office for 1 to 2 hours until the medication wears off.

Preparation

Your stomach and duodenum must be empty for the procedure to be thorough and safe, so you will not be able to eat or drink anything for at least 6 hours beforehand. Also, you must arrange for someone to take you home. You will not be allowed to drive because of the sedatives. Your physician may give you other special instructions.

ERCP (Endoscopic Retrograde Cholangiopancreatography)

Endoscopic retrograde cholangiopancreatography (en-doh-SKAH-pik REH-troh-grayd koh-LAN-jee-oh-PANG-kree-uh-TAH-gruh-fee) (ERCP) enables the physician to diagnose problems in the liver, gallbladder, bile ducts, and pancreas. The liver is a large organ that, among other things, makes a liquid called bile that helps with digestion. The gallbladder is a small, pear-shaped organ that stores bile until it is needed for digestion. The bile ducts are tubes that carry bile from the liver to the gallbladder and small intestine. These ducts are sometimes called the biliary tree. The pancreas is a large gland that produces chemicals that help with digestion.

ERCP may be used to discover the reason for jaundice, upper abdominal pain, and unexplained weight loss. ERCP combines the use of x-rays and an endoscope, which is a long, flexible, lighted tube. Through it, the physician can see the inside of the stomach, duodenum, and ducts in the biliary tree and pancreas.

For the procedure, you will lie on your left side on an examining table in a x-ray room. You will be given medication to help numb the back of your throat and a sedative to help you relax during the exam.

Figure 49.5. The Digestive System: Liver, Gallbladder, and Pancreas

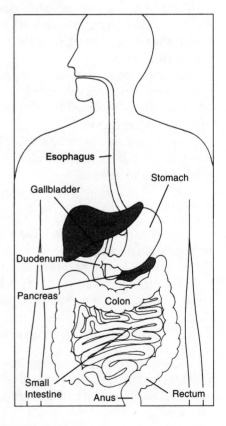

You will swallow the endoscope, and the physician will then guide the scope through your esophagus, stomach, and duodenum until it reaches the spot where the ducts of the biliary tree and pancreas open into the duodenum. At this time, you will be turned to lie flat on your stomach, and the physician will pass a small plastic tube through the scope. Through the tube, the physician will inject a dye into the ducts to make them show up clearly on x-rays. A radiographer will begin taking x-rays as soon as the dye is injected.

If the exam shows a gallstone or narrowing of the ducts, the physician can insert instruments into the scope to remove or work around the obstruction. Also, tissue samples (biopsy) can be taken for further testing.

Possible complications of ERCP include pancreatitis (inflammation of the pancreas), infection, bleeding, and perforation of the duodenum. However, such problems are uncommon. You may have tenderness or a lump where the sedative was injected, but that should go away in a few days or weeks.

ERCP takes 30 minutes to 2 hours. You may have some discomfort when the physician blows air into the duodenum and injects the dye into the ducts. However, the pain medicine and sedative should keep you from feeling too much discomfort. After the procedure, you will need to stay at the physician's office for 1 to 2 hours until the sedative wears off. The physician will make sure you do not have signs of complications before you leave. If any kind of treatment is done during ERCP, such as removing a gallstone, you may need to stay in the hospital overnight.

Preparation

Your stomach and duodenum must be empty for the procedure to be accurate and safe. You will not be able to eat or drink anything after midnight the night before the procedure, or for 6 to 8 hours beforehand, depending on the time of your procedure. Also, the physician will need to know whether you have any allergies, especially to iodine, which is in the dye. You must also arrange for someone to take you home. You will not be allowed to drive because of the sedatives. The physician may give you other special instructions.

Upper GI Series

The upper gastrointestinal (GI) series uses x-rays to diagnose problems in the esophagus, stomach, and duodenum (first part of the small intestine). It may also be used to examine the small intestine. The upper GI series can show a blockage, abnormal growth, ulcer, or a problem with the way an organ is working.

During the procedure, you will drink barium, a thick, white, milkshake-like liquid. Barium coats the inside lining of the esophagus, stomach, and duodenum and makes them show up more clearly on x-rays. The radiologist can also see ulcers, scar tissue, abnormal growths, hernias, or areas where something is blocking the normal path of food through the digestive system. Using a machine called a fluoroscope, the radiologist is also able to watch your digestive system work as the barium moves through it. This part of the procedure shows any problems in how the digestive system functions, for example, whether the muscles that control swallowing are working properly. As the barium moves into the small intestine, the radiologist can take x-rays of it as well.

An upper GI series takes 1 to 2 hours. It is not uncomfortable. The barium may cause constipation and white-colored stool for a few days after the procedure.

Figure 49.6. The Digestive System: Esophagus, Stomach, Duodenum, and Small Intestine

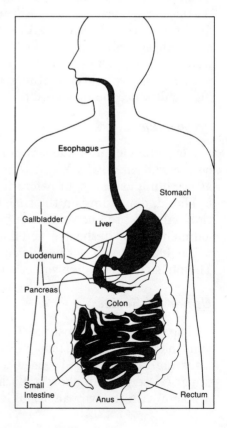

Preparation

Your stomach and small intestine must be empty for the procedure to be accurate, so the night before you will not be able to eat or drink anything after midnight. Your physician may give you other specific instructions.

Lower Gastrointestinal (GI) Series

A lower gastrointestinal (GI) series uses x-rays to diagnose problems in the large intestine, which includes the colon and rectum. The lower GI series may show problems like abnormal growths, ulcers, polyps, and diverticuli.

Before taking x-rays of your colon and rectum, the radiologist will put a thick liquid called barium into your colon. This is why a lower GI series is sometimes called a barium enema. The barium coats the

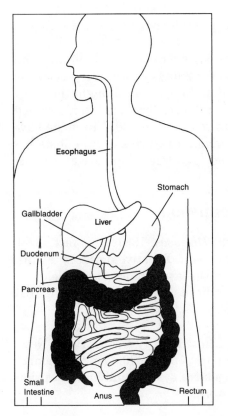

Figure 49.7. The Digestive System: Colon and Rectum

lining of the colon and rectum and makes these organs, and any signs of disease in them, show up more clearly on x-rays. It also helps the radiologist see the size and shape of the colon and rectum.

You may be uncomfortable during the lower GI series. The barium will cause fullness and pressure in your abdomen and will make you feel the urge to have a bowel movement. However, that rarely happens because the tube the physician uses to inject the barium has a balloon on the end of it that prevents the liquid from coming back out.

You may be asked to change positions while x-rays are taken. Different positions give different views of the intestines. After the radiologist is finished taking x-rays, you will be able to go to the bathroom. The radiologist may also take an x-ray of the empty colon afterwards.

A lower GI series takes about 1 to 2 hours. The barium may cause constipation and make your stool turn gray or white for a few days after the procedure.

Preparation

Your colon must be empty for the procedure to be accurate. To prepare for the procedure you will have to restrict your diet for a few days beforehand. For example, you might be able to drink only liquids and eat only non-sugar, non-dairy foods for 2 days before the procedure; only clear liquids the day before; and nothing after midnight the night before. A liquid diet means fat-free bouillon or broth, gelatin, strained fruit juice, water, plain coffee, plain tea, or diet soda. To make sure your colon is empty, you might be given a laxative or an enema before the procedure. Your physician may give you other special instructions.

Additional Readings and Information

Facts and Fallacies About Digestive Diseases. 1991. This fact sheet discusses commonly held beliefs about digestive diseases. Available from the National Digestive Diseases Information Clearinghouse, 2 Information Way, Bethesda, MD 20892-3570. (310) 654-3810.

Larson DE, Editor-in-chief. *Mayo Clinic Family Health Book*. New York: William Morrow and Company, Inc., 1990. General medical guide with section on the digestive system and how it works. Available in libraries and bookstores.

Tapley DF, et al., eds. *The Columbia University College of Physicians and Surgeons Complete Home Medical Guide*, revised edition. New York: Crown Publishers, Inc., 1990. General medical guide with section on the digestive system and how it works. Available in libraries and bookstores.

The National Digestive Diseases Information Clearinghouse (NDDIC) is a service of the National Institute of Diabetes and Digestive and Kidney Diseases (NIDDK). The NIDDK is part of the National Institutes of Health under the U.S. Department of Health and Human Services. Established in 1980, the clearinghouse provides information about digestive diseases to people with digestive disorders and to their families, health care professionals, and the public. NDDIC answers inquiries; develops, reviews, and distributes publications; and works closely with professional and patient organizations and Government agencies to coordinate resources about digestive diseases. Contact NIDDK at:

National Digestive Diseases Information Clearinghouse
2 Information Way
Bethesda, MD 20892-3570
Tel: (301) 654-3810
Fax: (301) 907-8906
E-mail: nddic@aerie.com

Chapter 50

Cardiac Catheterization

Cardiac catheterization is a diagnostic procedure, a test that can measure blood pressure and blood flow in the heart's chambers, examine the arteries of the heart (coronary arteries), and provide information about the pumping ability of the heart muscle. It is not surgery.

In this procedure, long, flexible tubes called catheters are used to both take measurements and to inject dye into your blood vessels and into your heart. The dye enables the doctor to take X-ray pictures (angiograms) of the heart and coronary arteries.

Cardiac catheterization is also performed to evaluate heart valve disease and congenital heart abnormalities.

Why Does My Doctor Want Me to Undergo This Test?

Cardiac catheterization is performed for a variety of reasons. You may have presented to your physician with one or more of the following symptoms: shortness of breath, dizziness, palpitations or angina (pain or discomfort in the chest, arm or jaw).

You may have been taking nitroglycerin to relieve your angina, and recently your doctor has had to increase the dosage. Cardiac catheterization may be ordered to create pictures of your arteries (angiograms), which will help your doctor diagnose the existence and severity of coronary artery disease.

Sometimes your doctor wants information about the left lower chamber of your heart (left ventricle). In that case, cardiac catheterization may be used to create pictures of that chamber (ventriculograms). Ventriculograms enable your doctor to visualize your left ventricle from many angles. They reveal much information about the ventricle's structure and functioning.

You might have already taken other, less invasive, diagnostic tests such a treadmill test, an echocardiogram or a nuclear scan. Based upon the results of those tests, your history, physical examination and symptoms, your doctor has determined that additional information is required. Cardiac catheterization can provide that information.

Finally, you may be scheduled to undergo surgery on another part or system of your body. Your doctor has ordered a cardiac catheterization test to determine whether you have severe coronary artery disease. If so, he may want you to undergo one of two corrective procedures first. These are coronary artery bypass surgery (CABG) or percutaneous transluminal coronary angioplasty (PTCA).

What Are the Risks of This Test?

The risks associated with cardiac catheterization include abnormal heart rhythms, perforation of a blood vessel, low blood pressure, infection, blood clots, allergic reaction to the dye, bleeding, kidney damage or failure, stroke and heart attack. These events are rare.

What Preparations Should I Make before This Procedure?

Discuss your current medications with your physician. He may ask you to discontinue certain medicines, such as anticoagulants, prior to the catheterization. If you are taking insulin, your doctor will most likely recommend that you take a half dose prior to the procedure.

Shower the night before. Do not eat or drink after midnight. If you have diabetes, consult your physician about eating. You may take approved medications with small sips of water.

Leave all valuables and money at home or with a relative. Do not wear any jewelry to the hospital. You may be allowed to wear eyeglasses, dentures or dental bridges. This varies from place to place.

Bring something to read. There may be periods of waiting before the actual procedure commences.

What Happens on the Day of the Procedure?

Before the catheterization, a heart doctor (cardiologist), will examine you and review your medical history and diagnostic tests. He will explain the procedure and its risks and benefits, and will ask you to sign a consent form. Do not hesitate to ask questions and voice your concerns. Tell the doctor if you are pregnant or think you may be.

During your discussion with the doctor, he will ask you if you have any allergies, particularly to certain food or dyes. If you have allergic reactions to shellfish, and/or iodine-containing X-ray contrast liquid, you may be given medication to prevent an allergic reaction during the procedure.

You will also discuss your current medications. It is always a good idea to bring all your medicines with you whenever you visit a doctor or have a procedure performed. This enables the doctor to learn the exact dosages you are taking. Make sure to tell this doctor if you are taking nitroglycerin medicine.

Usually, you will have blood tests, an electrocardiogram, and a chest X-ray taken prior to the procedure.

Will I Be Given Local or General Anesthesia?

You may be given a mild sedative about half an hour before the procedure to help you relax. You will stay awake throughout the procedure and will be asked to perform some simple tasks. At times you will be asked to take a deep breath, cough, turn your head to one side, or refrain from speaking for a few minutes while pressures are being measured.

You will be given a local anesthetic during the catheterization.

What Happens during the Procedure?

In most cases, the procedure takes place in the catheterization laboratory, which is usually cold and dimly lit. The dimmed lights will make the TV screens that monitor the procedure appear brighter to the catheterization team. In addition to the television screens, you will see heart monitors, a blood pressure machine and other various instruments and devices in the laboratory. You will lie on a bed near an X-ray camera. The camera will move across you on an arm over the bed.

Electrodes will be applied to your chest and back to monitor your heart rhythm at all times. A blood pressure cuff will be placed on your arm to monitor your blood pressure. You will be shaved and cleansed with antiseptic solution in the area of your groin where the catheter will be inserted. These steps are taken to prevent infection.

An intravenous line will be started in your arm to allow for the administration of medication during the procedure.

A local anesthetic will be injected into the skin to numb the catheter insertion site. This stings a little bit. Then a small incision will be made in the skin. The doctors will use a special needle to puncture the blood vessel (vein or artery), into which the catheter will be introduced. A radiologist or cardiologist will insert the catheter through a small incision in an artery or vein in your arm or groin. You will feel some pressure but no pain. If you do feel pain, let the doctor know, so more numbing medication can be given to you.

If the doctors want to view your left ventricle, the catheter will then be carefully threaded into your heart using X-ray images called fluoroscopy, to guide the insertion. When the catheter is in place, dye is injected to visualize the structures and vessels within the heart. The structures, vessels and blood flow are recorded immediately on the television screens. A permanent record is also produced.

If the doctors want to view your coronary arteries, the catheter is guided into each of the coronary artery openings. Dye is pumped into the arteries a few times. This flow of dye is also recorded on the television screens.

While the dye is moving through your blood vessels, you may feel hot or flushed for up to 30 seconds. Some people experience slight nausea or extra heartbeats.

How Long Does the Procedure Last?

The procedure takes from 20 to 40 minutes from the time of catheter insertion. The total procedure lasts about an hour to an hour and a half.

What Will Happen after the Tests?

When the tests are finished, the catheter will be removed. If the femoral artery in the groin was used, firm pressure will be applied to the site for 10 to 20 minutes. Then bandages will be applied. Sometimes a five-pound sandbag will be placed on top of the bandages for four to six hours. This additional pressure helps to stop bleeding.

You will leave the catheterization laboratory and go to another room where you will have bed rest for up to six hours. You must lie straight, with your head slightly raised. Depending on the insertion site, you should not bend your knee or arm. You may wiggle your foot and toes to prevent stiffness.

A nurse will check your insertion site. and vital signs. If you are in pain, ask her for medicine to relieve it. You may feel drowsy. Notify the nurse if you experience a sudden pain at the insertion site or if you have a warm, sticky or wet feeling around the site.

It's a good idea to drink a lot of fluids. This will hasten the removal of dye from your body.

You will be able to go home after the period of bed rest.

What Happens When I Get Home?

Your doctor will tell you when you will be able to shower. It's usually after 24 to 36 hours. The bruise at the insertion site may take up to two weeks to heal. Call your doctor if pain or the size of the bruise increases.

What Happens Next?

The tests will provide your doctor with valuable information regarding your coronary arteries, the heart valves, your heart's electrical function, blood flow and the presence of any blockages of blood flow. Based on this information your doctor will be better able to diagnose your heart problem and advise you.

Chapter 51

Bronchoscopy

Note: This information may not apply to all patients.

What Is a Bronchoscopy?

Bronchoscopy is a routine diagnostic procedure that lets your doctor see inside your lungs and get tissue to examine. The procedure uses a bronchoscope: a small, narrow, tube with a light and lens at the tip.

Who Might Have a Bronchoscopy?

People who have symptoms of a lung problem may have a bronchoscopy to help make an exact diagnosis. Patients with known lung disease may need this test to check the status of their disease. A bronchoscopy may also be done on people with normal lungs, so that researchers can get tissue samples for comparison.

How Do I Prepare for It?

Before the procedure, you will have a chest x-ray, pulmonary function test, physical exam, blood work, and an electrocardiogram. Also, you will be asked to sign an informed consent, which will be signed by your doctor.

"Information for Clinical Center Patients," Warren Grant Magnuson Clinical Center, National Institutes of Health (NIH), May 1998.

449

Do not eat or drink anything 8 hours before the procedure.

The morning of the procedure, a small, intravenous tube (catheter) will be put into one of your arm veins. This will be used to give you fluids and medication to help you relax. You may get an injection of medications into your muscle to help control coughing and secretions in your mouth.

After this, you will breathe a mist of topical anesthesia (numbing medication) through your mouth. You will breathe this mist from a tube attached to an oxygen flowmeter. You will be asked to breathe through your mouth until this mist is gone.

What Happens during a Bronchoscopy?

When you are in the bronchoscopy suite, the nurse will attach three patches to your chest to monitor your heart, a blood pressure cuff to monitor your blood pressure, and a clip on your finger to check how much oxygen is in your blood.

The nurse will give you a topical anesthetic to gargle, and the back of your throat will also be sprayed with anesthetic. A small amount of Lidocaine (numbing medication) will be put into one of your nostrils to let the bronchoscopy tube pass through.

What Are the Side Effects?

Because of the sedatives you may have received, you may feel groggy for several hours. Your mouth may feel dry during, and shortly after, the procedure. Some people also have a slight sore throat, blood-tinged saliva, or a low fever.

What Happens Afterwards?

When the procedure is over, the nurse will take you back to your room. Your vital signs (temperature, heartbeat, blood pressure) will be monitored. Your nurse will also ask you to take deep breaths and cough gently. This helps clear your lungs of the fluid used during the procedure.

Because your throat and gag reflex will be numb, do not eat or drink for at least 2 hours after the bronchoscopy. In 2 hours, your nurse will check your gag reflex. If it has returned, you may try to drink; then eat.

Are there Special Instructions to Follow after the Procedure?

If you develop a fever higher than 100 degrees Fahrenheit, take Tylenol every 4 hours as recommended by your NIH doctor or nurse practitioner. If your fever lasts longer than 24 hours, call the doctor. If you have a sore throat, take throat lozenges as needed. If you have any of the following, go to the nearest emergency room:

- difficulty catching your breath
- bleeding from your nose
- coughing up blood
- chest pain or chest discomfort.

Chapter 52

Cystoscopy, Arthroscopy, and Laparoscopy

Cytoscopy

Interstitial Cystitis: A Bladder Disorder

People with interstitial cystitis (IC) have an enflamed, or irritated, bladder wall. This inflammation can lead to scarring and stiffening of the bladder, decreased bladder capacity, glomerulations (pinpoint bleeding) and, in rare cases, ulcers in the bladder lining.

The diagnosis of IC in the general population is based on:

- presence of urgency, frequency or pelvic/bladder pain,
- cyctoscopic evidence (under anesthesia) of bladder wall inflammation and glomerulations or Hunner's ulcers,
- absence of other diseases that may cause the symptoms.

Cystoscopy Under Anesthesia with Bladder Distension

During cystoscopy to diagnose IC, the doctor uses a cystoscope— an instrument made of a hollow tube about the diameter of a drink-

This chapter contains text from, "Prostate Enlargement: Benign Prostatic Hyperplasia," National Kidney and Urologic Diseases Information Clearinghouse (NIDDK); "Interstitial Cystitis," National Kidney and Urologic Diseases Information Clearinghouse, NIH Publication No. 94-3220, 1994; "Facts About Endometriosis," National Institute of Child Health and Human Development, NIH Publication No. 91-2413, 1991; and "Questions and Answers About Knee Problems," National Institute of Arthritis and Musculoskeletal and Skin Diseases (NIAMS), NIH Fact Sheet.

ing straw with several lenses and a light—to see inside the bladder and urethra. The doctor will also distend or stretch the bladder to its capacity by filling it with a liquid or gas. Because bladder distension is painful in IC patients, before the doctor inserts the cystoscope through the urethra into the bladder, the patient must be given either regional or general anesthesia. These tests can detect inflammation; a thick, stiff bladder wall; Hunner's ulcers; and glomerulations (pinpoint bleeding) that may be seen only after the bladder is stretched.

The doctor may also test the patient's maximum bladder capacity, the amount of liquid or gas the bladder can hold under anesthesia. Without anesthesia, capacity is limited by either pain or a sever urge to urinate. Many people with IC have normal or large maximum bladder capacities under anesthesia., However, a small bladder capacity under anesthesia helps to support the diagnosis of IC.

Biopsy

A biopsy is a microscopic examination of tissue. Samples of the bladder and urethra may be removed during a cystoscopy and examined with a microscope later. A biopsy helps rule out bladder cancer and confirm bladder wall inflammation.

Benign Prostatic Hyperplasia (BPH)

You may first notice symptoms of Benign Prostatic Hyperplasia (BPH) yourself, or your doctor may find that your prostate is enlarged during a routine checkup. When BPH is suspected, you may be referred to a urologist, a doctor who specializes in problems of the urinary tract and the male reproductive system. Several tests help the doctor identify the problem and decide whether surgery is needed. The tests vary from patient to patient, but the most common ones include a rectal exam, ultrasound, urine flow study, intravenous pyelogram, and cytoscopy.

In cytoscopy, the doctor inserts a small tube through the opening of the urethra in the penis. This procedure is done after a solution numbs the inside of the penis so all sensation is lost. The tube, called a cystoscope, contains a lens and a light system, which help the doctor see the inside of the urethra and the bladder. This test allows the doctor to determine the size of the gland and identify the location and degree of the obstruction.

Arthroscopy

Arthroscopy is one method used by doctors to diagnose knee problems. The doctor manipulates a small, lighted optic tube (arthroscope) that has been inserted into the joint through a small incision in the knee. Images of the inside of the knee joint are projected onto a television screen. This procedure is used both to diagnose and to surgically repair the knee.

Laparoscope

Editor's Note: This procedure is also used to diagnose diseases other than endometriosis.

Endometriosis is a common yet poorly understood disease. It can strike women of any socioeconomic class, age, or race. It is estimated that between 10 and 20 percent of American women of childbearing age have endometriosis.

Diagnosis of endometriosis begins with a gynecologist evaluating the patient's medical history. A complete physical exam, including a pelvic examination, is also necessary. However, diagnosis of endometriosis is only complete when proven by a laraoscopy, a minor surgical procedure in which a laparoscope (a tube with a light in it) is inserted into a small incision in the abdomen. The laparoscope is moved around the abdomen, which has been distended with carbon dioxide gas to make the organs easier to see. The surgeon can then check the condition of the abdominal organs and see the endometrial implants.

The laparoscopy will show the locations, extent, and size of the growths and will help the patient and her doctor make informed decisions about treatment.

Part Eight

Lung (Pulmonary) Tests

Chapter 53

Diagnosing Lung Disease

When a person's symptoms suggest lung disease, a chest x-ray is usually the first examination the doctor orders. Then various tests are performed to identify the disease and to determine how severe it is. These tests include:

- pulmonary function tests;

- microscopic examination of lung tissue, cells, and fluids using a light microscope and an electron microscope; and

- biochemical and cellular studies of respiratory fluids removed from the lung by lavage (washing).

To determine how well the lungs are working, doctors can measure respiratory or gas exchange functions, airway or bronchial activity, particle clearance rates, and permeability of the blood air barrier.

Spirometry

Spirometry, like the measurement of blood pressure, is useful for assessing lung function as well as general health. It is the simplest and most common of the lung function tests.

Spirometry measures how much and how quickly air can be expelled following a deep breath. It is performed by having the patient

Excerpts from "The Lungs in Health and Disease", National Heart, Lung, and Blood Institute (NHLBI), NIH Publication No. 97-3279, August 1997.

breathe out forcefully into a device called a spirometer. At the same time a machine makes a tracing of the rate at which the air leaves the lung. Diseases of airflow obstruction and of lung stiffening give characteristic tracings with spirometry.

Measures of the amount of air that can be expelled following a deep breath, forced vital capacity (FVC), and the amount of air that can be forcibly exhaled in 1 second, forced expiratory volume in 1 second (FEV_1), are the most useful numbers derived from spirometry. The ratio of FEV_1 to FVC is often used to assess patients for airflow obstruction. It is normally 75 to 85 percent, depending on the patient's age. The ratio is reduced in obstructive diseases, while it is preserved or even increased in restrictive disorders. A lower than normal FEV_1 is a sign that a person's lung disease is getting worse.

The "normal" values for FVC and FEV_1 for a patient depend on the individual's age, gender, height, and race. They are higher for younger than for older people, higher for tall than for short individuals, higher for men than for women, and higher for whites than blacks or Asians. Therefore, the numbers are presented as percentages of the average expected in someone of the same age, height, sex, and race. This is called percent predicted. Any number smaller than 85 percent of predicted is considered abnormal.

If these numbers are abnormal, the patient is referred for additional pulmonary function tests to find out why. These may include checking the patient's response to bronchodilators, absolute lung volumes, and blood levels of oxygen and carbon dioxide which tell how well gas exchange is occurring. Other important measures of lung function are arterial blood gas tensions (PaO_2 and $PaCO_2$) and the diffusing capacity of the lung for carbon monoxide (DLCO).

Some doctors recommend having spirometry before age 25 to get baseline numbers. However, if you are a smoker, are occupationally exposed to irritants, or have symptoms of cough, wheeze, or shortness of breath, you should be checked with a spirometer at intervals of 3 to 5 years or more frequently if your doctor recommends it.

Abnormal spirometry numbers at any age means that you are at risk for early lung disease and even potentially fatal lung cancer, heart disease, or stroke. You should immediately stop smoking if you still smoke, and talk to your doctor about other measures you may need to take depending on the reasons for your abnormal numbers.

For More Information

The NHLBI Information Center is a service of the National Heart, Lung, and Blood Institute (NHLBI) of the National Institutes of Health. The Information Center provides information to health professionals, patients, and the public about the treatment, diagnosis, and prevention of heart, lung, and blood diseases.

NHLBI Information Center
P.O. Box 30105
Bethesda, MD 20824-0105
Telephone: 301-592-8573
Fax: 301-592-8563
http://www.nhlbi.nih.gov/nhlbi/nhlbi.htm

Chapter 54

Asthma Diagnosis

Diagnosis of Asthma in Adults and Children over 5 Years of Age

Recurrent episodes of coughing or wheezing are almost always due to asthma in both children and adults. Cough can be the sole symptom.

Findings that increase the probability of asthma include:

Medical History:

- Episodic wheeze, chest tightness, shortness of breath, or cough.
- Symptoms worsen in presence of aeroallergens, irritants, or exercise.
- Symptoms occur or worsen at night, awakening the patient.
- Patient has allergic rhinitis or atopic dermatitis.
- Close relatives have asthma, allergy, sinusitis, or rhinitis.

Physical Examination of the Upper Respiratory Tract, Chest, and Skin:

- Hyperexpansion of the thorax
- Sounds of wheezing during normal breathing or prolonged phase of forced exhalation

---

Excerpts from "Practical Guide for the Diagnosis and Management of Asthma," NIH Publication No. 97-4053, October 1997.

- Increased nasal secretions, mucosal swelling, sinusitis, rhinitis, or nasal polyps

- Atopic dermatitis/eczema or other signs of allergic skin problems

To Establish an Asthma Diagnosis, Determine the Following:

1. **History or presence of episodic symptoms of airflow obstruction** (i.e., wheeze, shortness of breath, tightness in the chest, or cough). Asthma symptoms vary throughout the day; absence of symptoms at the time of the examination does not exclude the diagnosis of asthma.

2. **Airflow obstruction is at least partially reversible**. Use spirometry to:

    Establish airflow obstruction: FEV_1 (forced expiratory volume in 1 second) <80 percent predicted; FEV_1/FVC (forced vital capacity) <65 percent or below the lower limit of normal.

    Establish reversibility: FEV_1 increases ≥12 percent and at least 200 ml. After using a short-acting inhaled beta$_2$-agonist (e.g., albuterol, terbutaline).

    Note: Older adults may need to take oral steroids for 2 to 3 weeks and then take the spirometry test to measure the degrees of reversibility achieved. Chronic bronchitis and emphysema may coexist with asthma in adults. The degree of reversibility indicates the degree to which asthma therapy may be beneficial.

3. **Alternative diagnoses are excluded** (e.g., vocal cord dysfunction, vascular rings, foreign bodies, or other pulmonary diseases).

In general, FEV_1 predicted norms or reference values used for children should also be used for adolescents.

Diagnosis in Infants and Children Younger than 5 Years of Age

Because children with asthma are often mislabeled as having bronchiolitis, bronchitis, or pneumonia, many do not receive adequate therapy.

- The diagnostic steps listed previously are the same for this age group except that spirometry is not possible. A trial of asthma medications may aid in the eventual diagnosis.

- Diagnosis is not needed to begin to treat wheezing associated with an upper respiratory viral infection, which is the most

Table 54.1. Additional Tests for Adults and Children

Reasons for Additional Tests	The Tests
Additional tests may be needed when asthma is suspected but spirometry is normal, when coexisting conditions are suspected, or for other reasons.	These tests can aid diagnosis or confirm suspected contributors to asthma morbidity (e.g., allergens and irritants).
• Patient has symptoms but spirometry is normal or near normal	• Assess diurnal variation of peak flow over 1 to 2 weeks. • Refer to a specialist for broncho-provocation with methacholine, histamine, or exercise; negative test may help rule out asthma.
• Suspect infection, large airway lesions, heart disease, or obstruction by foreign object	• Chest x-ray
• Suspect coexisting chronic obstructive pulmonary disease, restrictive defect, or central airway obstruction	• Additional pulmonary function studies • Diffusing capacity test
• Suspect other factors contribute to asthma (These are not diagnostic tests for asthma.)	• Allergy tests—skin or in vitro • Nasal examination • Gastroesophageal reflux assessment

common precipitant of wheezing in this age group. Patients should be monitored carefully.

- There are two general patterns of illness in infants and children who have wheezing with acute viral upper respiratory infections: a remission of symptoms in the preschool years and persistence of asthma throughout childhood. The factors associated with continuing asthma are allergies, a family history of asthma, and perinatal exposure to aeroallergens and passive smoke.

Part Nine

Genetic Testing

Chapter 55

What Can the New Gene Tests Tell Us?

A cartoon appearing almost half a century ago in the *New Yorker* featured a young boy facing his father as he reviews his son's report card. "What do you think the trouble with me is, Dad," he asks with artful innocence, "heredity or environment?" In one timeless scene the cartoonist managed to convey our fascination with genetics and the ongoing debate over just how much we can attribute to the genes we inherit from our parents.

Lately we have learned a lot about our genetic legacy. We now know that, in fact, all diseases have a genetic component, whether inherited or resulting from the body's response to environmental stresses like viruses or toxins. The successes of the international Human Genome Project that aims to describe all human DNA have even enabled researchers to pinpoint errors in genes—the smallest units of heredity—that cause or contribute to disease.

The Human Genome Project

The daunting goal of the 13-year Human Genome Project, begun in 1990, is to determine the sequence of the 3 billion building blocks of human DNA—the genome—by 2003. Except for identical twins, everyones' DNA sequence is unique—it's the foundation for all our diversity. Our similarities far outweigh our differences, however: only a tenth of a percent of all our DNA varies from person to person.

Reprinted with permission © 1997, *The Judges' Journal*, Summer 1997, Vol. No. 36, Issue No. 3, revised March 1999.

Scientists in the Human Genome Project are using DNA from a variety of sources to construct a composite reference human genome sequence. All data is freely available over the Internet, and researchers outside the Project are exploring applications in fields as diverse as medicine, agriculture, forensics (DNA identification of individuals) and other areas.

The ultimate goal is to use this information to develop new ways to treat, cure, or even prevent the thousands of diseases that afflict humankind. But the road from gene identification to effective therapies is long and fraught with challenges. In the meantime, companies are racing ahead with commercialization by designing diagnostic tests to detect errant genes in people suspected of having particular diseases or at risk for developing them.

An increasing number of gene tests are becoming available (*See Table 55.1: Some DNA-Based Gene Tests Currently Available*), although the scientific community continues to debate the best way to deliver them to a public and medical community who are unaware of their scientific and social implications. While some of these tests have greatly improved and even saved some lives, scientists themselves remain unsure of how to interpret many of them. Also, patients taking the tests face significant risks of jeopardizing their employment and insurance status. And because genetic information is shared, these risks can extend beyond them to their family members as well.

DNA-Based Gene Tests

Gene tests for the disorders listed below are available from clinical genetics laboratories around the country. Although several hundred gene tests are available, they only detect rare conditions that are usually caused by DNA changes in a single gene. Our most common diseases, such as hypertension, heart disease, diabetes, and many cancers, have more complex genetics that probably involve several genes that interact with environmental conditions to cause disease. There are no gene tests for these conditions yet, but this will undoubtedly change as we learn more about our DNA.

Even so, many more tests are in the works as dozens of new companies vie to spin genetic data into gold. In the United States alone over four hundred laboratory programs aim to develop gene tests for disorders ranging from arthritis to obesity, and the list grows daily. The technology continues to advance rapidly, and future versions will allow simultaneous testing for hundreds of different genetic mistakes. The volume of available personal genetic data is on the brink of exploding, increasing the urgency of addressing ethical, legal, and social issues surrounding the data. This was not unexpected, and Human Genome Project planners have dedicated at least 3% of the budget to grappling with these issues since the project began over 8 years ago.

Beginning with a short introduction to ground the reader in the DNA science underlying the gene tests, this article explains some of the tests, their limitations, and the extraordinary potential of DNA medicine for the twenty first century.

What's a Gene? A Short Primer on DNA Science

A gene is simply a piece of DNA, the chemical that stores coded information on how to reproduce, build, and maintain our bodies. Genes contain instructions that tell the body how, when, and where to make proteins, which are the true workhorses of our trillions of cells. All living organisms are made up largely of proteins, which provide the structural components of all our cells and tissues as well as specialized enzymes for all essential chemical reactions. Through these proteins, our genes determine how well we process foods, detoxify poisons, and respond to infections. Although our cells have the same genes, not all genes are active in all cells. Heart cells synthesize proteins required for that organ's structure and function, liver cells make liver proteins, and so on.

Our DNA is our genome. In humans and other higher organisms, a DNA molecule consists of two ribbon-like strands that wrap around each other, resembling a twisted ladder. The ladder rungs are made up of chemicals called bases, which are abbreviated A, T, C, and G. Each rung consists of a pair of bases, either A and T or C and G. We have 3 billion base pairs (or 6 billion bases) of DNA in most of our cells; this is our genome. With the exception of identical twins, the sequence of the bases—the order of As, Ts, Cs, and Gs—is different for everyone, which is what makes each of us unique. Variation in base sequence, along with environmental factors, accounts for all our diversity, including disease and health.

DNA is coiled into chromosomes. The DNA making up our genome is divided into tightly coiled packets called chromosomes that reside in the nucleus of each cell. Each chromosome is a single long DNA molecule, with the lengths of the different chromosomes ranging from 50 million to 250 million bases. Scientists can distinguish

Table 55.1 Some DNA-Based Gene Tests Currently Available, continued on next page.

Test Name	Symptoms
Alpha-1-antitrypsin deficiency (AAT)	Emphysema and liver disease
Amyotrophic lateral sclerosis (ALS) Lou Gehrig's Disease;	progressive motor function loss leading to paralysis and death
Ataxia telangiectasia (AT)	Progressive brain disorder resulting in loss of muscle control and cancers
Gaucher disease (GD)	Enlarged liver and spleen, bone degeneration
Inherited breast and ovarian cancer (BRCA 1 and 2)	Early onset tumors of breasts and ovaries
Hereditary nonpolyposis colon cancer (CA)	Early onset tumors of colon and sometimes other organs
Charcot-Marie-Tooth (CMT)	Loss of feeling in ends of limbs
Congenital adrenal hyperplasia (CAH)	Hormone deficiency; ambiguous genitalia and male pseudohermaphroditism
Cystic fibrosis (CF)	Disease of lung and pancreas resulting in thick mucous accumulations and chronic infections
Duchenne muscular dystrophy/ Becker muscular dystrophy (DMD)	Severe/mild muscle wasting, deterioration, weakness
Dystonia (DYT)	Muscle rigidity, repetitive twisting movements
Fanconi anemia, group C (FA)	Anemia, leukemia, skeletal deformities
Factor V-Leiden (FVL)	Bleeding disorder
Fragile X syndrome (FRAX)	Leading cause of inherited mental retardation

Table 55.1 Some DNA-Based Gene Tests Currently Available, continued from previous page.

Test Name	Symptoms
Hemophilia A and B (HEMA and HEMB)	Bleeding disorders
Huntington disease (HD)	Usually midlife onset; progressive, lethal, degenerative neurological disease
Myotonic dystrophy (MD)	Progressive muscle weakness; most common form of adult muscular dystrophy
Neurofibromatosis type 1 (NF1)	Multiple benign nervous system tumors that can be disfiguring; cancers
Phenylketonuria (PKU)	Progressive mental retardation due to missing enzyme; correctable by diet
Adult Polycystic Kidney Disease (APKD)	Kidney failure and liver disease
Prader Willi/Angelman syndromes (PW/A)	Decreased motor skills, cognitive impairment, early death
Sickle cell disease (SS)	Blood cell disorder; chronic pain and infections
Spinocerebellar ataxia, type 1 (SCA1)	Involuntary muscle movements, reflex disorders, explosive speech
Spinal muscular atrophy (SMA)	Severe, usually lethal progressive muscle wasting disorder in children
Thalassemias (THAL)	Anemias—reduced red blood cell levels
Tay-Sachs Disease (TS)	Fatal neurological disease of early childhood; seizures, paralysis

the chromosomes by size, distinctive staining patterns, and other characteristics.

Most cells have 46 chromosomes, with one set of 23 from each of our parents. Each set of 23 contains 22 chromosomes that are designated by numbers (1-22) plus either an X or Y sex-determining chromosome. Females receive 22 non-sex-determining chromosomes plus an X chromosome from each parent and males get the 22 chromosomes from each parent plus an X chromosome from one parent and a Y from the other. Sperm and egg cells only have 23 chromosomes (but when they join in fertilization the new cell will then have 46).

Chromosomes are not continuous strings of genes. Genes are interspersed among millions of bases of DNA that do not code for proteins (noncoding DNA) and whose functions are largely unknown. In fact, genes constitute only a tiny fraction of the human genome—a mere 3%. Scientists estimate that we have about 80,000 genes, whose sizes range from fewer than 1 thousand to several million bases. We have two copies of every gene, one from each of our parents. Gene lengths range from 1000 to well over 1 million bases.

From Diversity to Disease

For all our outward variation, we are surprisingly alike at the DNA level. Differences account for only a tenth of a percent of our DNA (about 3 million base pairs). Yet DNA base sequence variations are responsible for all our physical differences and influence many of our other characteristics as well.

Sequence variation can occur in our genes, and the resulting different forms of the same gene are called alleles. People can have two identical or two different alleles for a particular gene, depending on what they inherited from each parent. Variation also occurs outside the genes in the noncoding part of our DNA.

Mutations. While most DNA variation is normal, harmful sequence changes sometimes occur in our DNA that cause or contribute to disease. DNA sequence changes—called mutations—are either passed down from parent to child (in the sperm or egg cells) or acquired during a person's lifetime. The vast majority of diseases are due to acquired changes, known as sporadic mutations. These mutations can arise spontaneously during normal functions, as when a cell divides, or in response to environmental stresses such as toxins, radiation, hormones, and perhaps even diet. Nature provides us with a system of finely tuned repair enzymes that find and fix most DNA errors. But as we age, our repair systems may become less efficient and allow us to accumulate uncorrected mutations. This can result in diseases such as cancer.

Depending on where in our genome they occur, mutations can have devastating effects or none at all. If they are small and fall in the vast sea of noncoding sequences, no one might be the wiser. Changes within genes, however, can result in faulty proteins that function at less-than-normal levels or those that are completely nonfunctional, causing disease.

Some Commonly Inherited Disorders

- Congenital heart defects (encompasses a variety of malformations)
- Cystic fibrosis
- Polycystic kidney disease
- Hemochromatosis
- Neural tube defects
- Hypercholesterolemia
- Diabetes, type 1
- Cleft lip and palate
- Down Syndrome
- Fragile-X mental retardation
- Sickle cell anemia
- Tay Sachs
- Duchenne Muscular Dystrophy
- Hemophilia A
- Marfan Syndrome

Sometimes even a tiny change in DNA sequence in a single gene will lead to a serious disease. The substitution of just a single base, for example, results in sickle cell anemia. Other diseases are caused by deletions or additions of single or multiple bases. Too many repetitions of a particular sequence of three DNA bases can doom a person to Huntington's disease (a fatal neurological disorder), Fragile X syndrome (the most common form of inherited mental retardation), or myotonic dystrophy (a muscle wasting disease). Other diseases can result from large rearrangements of DNA.

Single-gene diseases. Some 4000 diseases are thought to be due to mutations in individual genes (but a different gene for each disease) that is inherited from one or both parents. Most of these disorders are very rare, accounting for only about 3% of all disease. Some occur more frequently in particular ethnic groups. Among the more common inherited disorders for which single, causative genes have been identified are sickle cell anemia (African Americans and Hispanics), cystic fibrosis (Caucasians), and Tay Sachs (Ashkenazi Jews).

Complex diseases. For our most common diseases the causes are much more complex. The common scourges afflicting Western civilization are thought to be due to a variety of gene mutations, perhaps acting together, or to a combination of genes and environmental factors. Heart disease, diabetes, hypertension, cancers, Alzheimer's disease (AD), schizophrenia, and manic depression are all examples of complex diseases.

Except for rare forms of these disorders that are inherited in some families, single mutated genes associated with complex diseases are not considered causative. Rather, they confer a susceptibility or predisposition to their bearers and, given a particular combination of genes and environmental factors, will allow a disease to develop. Untangling the genetic and environmental contributions to complex disease will be one of the greatest challenges for medical researchers in the next century.

Finding disease genes. To find a gene that is a likely candidate for involvement in disease, scientists must search for DNA changes that are present only in people who have the disease. Searching randomly through three billion base pairs of DNA for tiny changes that may be linked with diseases is no easy task. Scientists labored through 10 years of tedious, painstaking work to find the genes associated with Huntington's disease and cystic fibrosis. Thanks to the HGP, researchers now have some guidance from chromosome maps, which have dramatically sped up the discovery of disease-associated genes and have reduced a typical gene search from years (at a cost of several million dollars) to months in some cases.

Once the disease-associated genes themselves or their approximate chromosomal regions are finally identified, academic and commercial laboratories often translate these findings into gene tests that can detect the particular mutations associated with a disease.

Gene Tests

Gene tests (also called DNA-based tests) are the newest and most sophisticated of the techniques used to test for genetic, or inherited, disorders. They involve direct examination of the DNA molecule itself. Other genetic tests include biochemical tests for gene products (proteins, including enzymes), and microscopic examination of stained or fluorescent chromosomes.

Why Use Genetic Tests?

Genetic tests are used mainly for

- carrier screening—identifying unaffected individuals who carry one copy of a gene for a disease that requires two copies for the disease to develop,
- prenatal diagnostic testing,
- newborn screening,
- presymptomatic testing for predicting or estimating a risk of developing adult-onset disorders such as some cancers and Huntington's disease,
- confirmational diagnosis of a symptomatic individual, and
- forensic/identity testing using an individual's DNA.

In gene tests, scientists scan a patient's DNA sample for mutations. A DNA sample can be obtained from any tissue, including blood. (Although mature red blood cells have no chromosomes, white blood cells also present in whole blood have the normal complement of 46 chromosomes.) The cost of testing can range from hundreds to thousands of dollars, depending on the sizes of the genes and the numbers of mutations tested.

Saving lives. Gene testing already has dramatically improved some lives. Some of these tests are used to clarify a diagnosis and direct a physician toward appropriate treatments. Aggressive monitoring for and removal of colon growths, for example, in those inheriting a gene for familial adenomatous polyposis, a rare type of colon cancer, has saved many lives. Other tests identify people at high risk for conditions that may be preventable. Several in vitro fertilization (IVF) clinics offer prospective parents who are at high risk for some genetic diseases (such as Tay Sachs and Huntington's disease) a way to ensure that they will not pass on the defective gene to their children. The clinics also offer them the option of remaining ignorant of their own genetic status, which many choose. After fertilization of the egg outside the mother's body, scientists test resulting embryos for gene mutations associated with a particular disease, and embryos without the mutation are selected preferentially for uterine implantation. Foiling Mother Nature does not come cheap, though. One company estimates that parents can expect to pay about $25,000 for one child conceived this way

On the horizon is a gene test that will provide doctors with a simple diagnostic test for a common iron-storage disease, transforming it from a usually fatal condition to a preventable or treatable disorder. In the summer of 1996, researchers reported finding a gene flaw associated with hemochromatosis, a common hereditary disorder characterized by excess iron storage. Hemochromatosis appears in midlife, when the iron that has accumulated in various organs begins to wreak damage resulting in a range of problems from diabetes and cirrhosis to liver cancer and cardiac dysfunction. A simple and effective treatment has been available for centuries: excess iron is depleted through bloodletting, or phlebotomy. But diagnosis is difficult, and if the condition is left untreated an early death will ensue. Yet when the disease is identified at an early stage, life expectancy can be normal.

Because it is one of the most common inherited diseases, and effectively treated if diagnosed early (or even prevented from ever occurring in the siblings and children of those affected), this disease stands as a model of the great potential of gene-based diagnostics.

Some limitations. Some complexities of current gene tests are outlined below in discussions of tests for Huntington's disease and cystic fibrosis, two disorders caused by single-gene defects, and the tests that may provide some information on predispositions to the more complex Alzheimer's disease, and to a rare, inherited type of breast and ovarian cancer.

Many in the medical establishment feel that uncertainties surrounding test interpretation, current lack of available medical options for most of these diseases, their potential for provoking anxiety, and risks for discrimination and social stigmatization could outweigh the benefits of testing. A task force established by the Human Genome Project to study the scientific and social aspects of genetic testing also emphasizes that genetic testing of children for adult onset diseases should not be undertaken unless direct medical benefit will accrue to the child and this benefit would be lost by waiting until the child has reached adulthood.

A limitation of all medical testing is the possibility for laboratory errors. These might be due to sample misidentification, errors resulting from contamination of the chemicals used for testing, or other sources

Huntington's disease (HD). The test for HD predicts with chilling certainty the future development of this devastating neurological condition that strikes in midlife, causing progressive and unrelenting physical and mental deterioration. HD is inherited in a dominant fashion, which means that people with one mutated HD-associated gene will develop the disease. People who have a parent with HD will themselves have a 1 in 2 chance (50% risk) of suffering the same illness. The majority of these high-risk people choose not to be tested when they understand all the implications: the psychological impact of knowing that they will (or will not) get the disease, the absence of preventive treatments, and the risk of affecting insurance and employment status.

Cystic fibrosis (CF). Although CF is also a disease associated with changes in a single-gene, the issues involved in testing for mutations in this large gene are much more complex than those for HD.

CF is the most common serious inherited disorder in Caucasian populations, affecting about 1 person in 2500 in the United States. In its most severe form, CF causes an accumulation of thick mucous in the lungs, creating an ideal breeding ground for bacteria, and damage to the gastrointestinal and reproductive systems. CF is inherited in a recessive fashion, meaning that one must inherit mutations in the gene from both parents to develop the disorder. If an individual has one mutated and one normal gene they are known as CF carriers and will not develop the disorder. If two carriers have a child, however, the chance is 1 in 4 that they will both pass a mutated gene to their child, who will then have two mutated genes and be affected.

An astounding 700 mutations have been found in the gene associated with CF, and few correlations have been made between specific mutations and disease severity. Interpretation of a positive test can be difficult, therefore, as it cannot predict the severity of the disease in any individual. However, if the mutation is the same as one already present in the family it is possible that some inferences can be made.

Another limitation of current CF gene tests is that they probe for only the most common mutations. Several companies screen for a panel of 70 of the most common mutations, which detects about 90% of CF mutations in Caucasians, and considerably fewer in African Americans, Hispanics, and Asians. A negative test, therefore, could not rule out CF. This limitation poses difficult quandaries for people making reproductive decisions.

Because of these limitations, many in the medical community believe that, while CF genetic testing can be useful, it should only be carried out by health care providers who are familiar with the tests and their interpretation. Doctors in the American College of Medical Genetics support carrier testing and counseling for couples in which 1 or both reproductive partners either has CF or has an affected relative. Because the mutation is so common in Caucasian populations (about 1 person in 25 is a carrier), in the future widespread testing may be recommended, but only when adequate educational support and genetic counseling is available and there is adequate experience with the sensitivity of the test for CF mutations in the ethnic and racial groups tested.

Alzheimer's disease (AD). Information available from the current susceptibility test for AD is even less informative. AD is a progressive brain disorder usually striking in mid to late life and causing devastating memory loss and impaired thinking. There are two forms of AD. A rare, early onset, simply inherited type (35 to 60 years) accounts for about 5% of all cases. The much more common form of AD (sporadic AD), the subject of a controversial gene test, is a complex disease characterized by a later onset (around 70 to 80 years). Scientists believe it is caused by a combination of genes and environmental factors. The most common form of mental impairment of old age, sporadic AD now affects some 4 million people in the U.S., and predictions are for 14 million cases by 2040.

Researchers have found three different forms of a gene called ApoE that appear to modify the risk of developing the common, sporadic type of AD. The gene codes for a protein, called apolipoprotein E, that appears to be involved with transporting cholesterol in the blood. Evidence suggests that African Americans and Hispanics do not exhibit the same gene-related AD risk that whites do.

A gene test was developed in 1995 to identify the presence of the different forms of this gene. The test is not recommended as a predictive test on healthy people, as no definitive information can be gained because AD is known to develop without the high risk form of the gene, some people with this gene form never develop the disease, it can't be used to predict age of onset or severity, and no current treatments or preventive methods are available. People being tested run the usual social risks concerning family and psychological issues, as well as insurance and employment discrimination. For these reasons, use of this test to predict a predisposition to AD has been discouraged by professional genetics groups. The usefulness of the gene test to diagnose the presence of AD in a patient with symptoms of the disease is still under investigation, and one must consider the potential for the same social risks as explained above.

Breast cancer. Predisposition tests for people at high risk for a very rare, inherited form of breast cancer have been marketed to doctors and patients since 1996. However, less than 10% of breast cancer cases are inherited (also called familial). The majority of cases are sporadic and occur in women with no family history of the disease. No gene tests yet exist for diagnosing or determining a susceptibility to sporadic breast cancer, but at least 50 genes have been suggested for involvement in the disease. The remainder of this discussion focuses on the gene tests that attempt to estimate an individual's risk for developing the rare, inherited form of breast cancer.

Mutations in two genes, called BRCA1 and BRCA2 (for BReast CAncer), have been associated with the development of inherited breast cancer in some individuals. Research has suggested that women with a strong family history of the disease who carry these mutations run an increased risk of developing breast cancer, although just how much is the subject of continuing controversy. Some women with the mutations, however, never develop breast cancer.

Women with BRCA1 mutations also face a higher risk of ovarian cancer compared with those in the general population. Men with BRCA1 mutations show no increased risk of breast cancer, but a slightly increased risk of prostate cancer. Men with BRCA2 mutations have a slightly higher risk of breast cancer.

Researchers say interpreting the results of BRCA1 and BRCA2 mutation tests is very difficult, as little is known about the risk associated with each of the hundreds of different mutations found in these genes. Also, no proven preventive or management strategies exist, so doctors are unsure of what kind of follow up to recommend. Increased surveillance, including frequent mammograms, is a possibility, but studies have not shown their usefulness in women under 50. Some women opt to remove healthy breasts (or ovaries) as a preventive measure, although there can be no assurance that all tissue has been removed. A recent study reported that preventive mastectomy reduced the risk of breast cancer by 90% for healthy women at high risk for the disease, but that study did not examine whether the women carried the BRCA1 or BRCA2 mutations.

An important point to remember is that women taking the gene tests run the usual psychological and social risks already mentioned, and these risks will very likely reach their daughters as well. Because of profound uncertainties surrounding the breast cancer tests, their use outside the research laboratory has been discouraged by the American Society for Human Genetics and the National Breast Cancer Coalition, among others.

On the other side are those who call it paternalistic to deny information to high-risk women. A negative test, of course, can provide immense relief to someone whose family has been plagued by breast cancer, although their chances of getting the disease remain the same as those of the general population. Some have used a positive test result to guide them toward preventive surgery or to help them decide whether or not to take estrogen after menopause. (Some studies suggest a connection between breast cancer and taking estrogen.) Those already diagnosed with breast cancer have used the test to help them choose between a radical mastectomy or a lumpectomy and radiation therapy, although the benefits are each are not clear for those with BRCA mutations.

The marketing of breast cancer tests spurred the National Cancer Institute to establish a cancer genetics network across the country to expand opportunities for genetic testing for cancer predisposition and keep it within a research setting. Those participating would have access to counseling and current clinical information and the opportunity to take part in intervention studies.

On a more optimistic note for the future, researchers are now conducting clinical trials using the normal version of the BRCA1 gene itself to treat advanced ovarian cancer patients. While this research is at a very early stage, the hope is that this and other similar trials will pave the way to completely new ways of treating previously intractable diseases and usher in an age of gene-based therapies.

Gene-Based Medicines and Gene Therapy for a New Millennium

Within the next decade, researchers will find most human genes. Explorations into the function of each gene—a major challenge extending far into the next century—will shed light on how faulty genes play a role in disease causation. With this knowledge in hand, commercial efforts will shift away from diagnostics and toward developing a new generation of therapeutics based on genes. Drug design will be revolutionized as researchers create new classes of medicines based on a reasoned approach using gene sequence and protein structure information rather than the traditional trial-and-error method. The drugs, targeted to specific sites in the body, will not have the side effects prevalent in many of today's medicines.

The potential for using genes themselves to treat disease—known as gene therapy—is the most exciting application of DNA science, and has captured the imaginations of the public as well as the biomedical community. This rapidly developing field holds great potential for treating or even curing genetic and acquired diseases, using normal genes to replace or supplement a defective gene or to bolster immunity to disease (e.g., by adding a gene that suppresses tumor growth or one that inhibits the replication of a virus like HIV). Over 350 clinical gene-therapy trials are now in progress worldwide, most for different kinds of cancers. Performed on patients in advanced stages of disease, the goal of most current studies is just establishing the safety of gene therapy rather than determining its effectiveness. The technology itself still faces many obstacles before it can become a practical approach for treating disease.

Using Genes to Treat Disease

Researchers have taken an intriguing step toward developing new treatments for cystic fibrosis, cancers, AIDS, hemophilia and several other diseases, using the genes themselves as medicine. This type of treatment is called gene therapy, and the hope is to treat, cure, and ultimately prevent disease. The science of gene therapy is in its infancy, however, and the goal of and most current gene-therapy clinical trials is only to demonstrate safety of the procedure, not its effectiveness. A partial listing of diseases that presently are the focus of clinical gene therapy trials follow.

- Canavan disease
- Cystic fibrosis
- Familial hypercholesterolemia
- Gaucher's disease
- Hemophilia B
- Various advanced cancers
- HIV infection
- Coronary artery disease
- Rheumatoid arthritis
- Hematological malignancies (leukemias)

The atlas of human biology generated by the Human Genome Project will provide an enormous store of genes for studying, and ultimately preventing, the ills that beset us. As the genetic factors underlying all of these conditions slowly come to light, the challenge will be to use the information responsibly.

For More Information

Promoting Safe and Effective Genetic Testing in the United States: Final Report of the Task Force on Genetic Testing, September 1997.

This task force was created by the National Institutes of Health-Department of Energy Human Genome Project. The report reviews some of the scientific aspects of genetic testing as well as current societal problems that have arisen as a result and those likely to be posed by future developments. (www.nhgri.nih.gov/Elsi/TFGT_final/).

Alliance of Genetic Support Groups

www.medhelp.org/geneticalliance/resources.html
Extensive resource listing of a variety of topics in addition to listing links to support group organizations.

Genetic/Rare Condition Web Page

www.kumc.edu/gec/support/groups.html
An excellent resource list for many genetic diseases, support groups and information.

Genetic Counselors and Clinics

http://www.kumc.edu/gec/prof/genecntr.html

Human Genome Project and Related Genetics Issues

A comprehensive collection of information on the Human Genome Project, explanatory material on genetics, and links to a wealth of related information. Sponsored by the U.S. Department of Energy's Human Genome Program.

Human Genome Management Information System HGMIS
423-574-0597
E-mail: caseydk@ornl.gov
http://www.ornl.gov/hgmis

—Denise K. Casey

Denise K. Casey is a freelance science writer.
E-mail: casey_dk@yahoo.com

Chapter 56

Newborn Screening

There is much public attention surrounding the use of DNA for genetic testing. What the lay public fails to realize is that genetic testing in the form of newborn screening has been in use for two to three decades. While newborn screening is not considered as fancy as the polymerase chain reaction amplification or allelic-specific oligonucleotide hybridization, the testing of protein products of genes or metabolites of metabolic pathways is an indirect genetic test.

Newborn screening has clearly proved quite effective for selected disorders. For example, cretinism from untreated hypothyroidism is now a medical rarity, and patients with late or untreated phenylketonuria no longer populate residential treatment programs. While early identification of patients with hypothyroidism or phenylketonuria has not eliminated all of the problems associated with these disorders, there is no argument that newborn screening is particularly effective for these two disorders and has been implemented in all fifty states. Thus, hypothyroidism and phenylketonuria are good examples of the success of newborn screening as a public health measure.

Reprinted with permission © *The Genetic Drift Newsletter*, Vol. 15. Winter 1998. Published by the Mountain States Regional Genetic Services Network for associates and those interested in Human Genetics. Contributions by C. Holly Nyerges, MSN, CPNP (NM), Benjamin Wilfond, MD (AZ), Peter A. Lane, MD (CO), and Carol Green, MD (CO).

Issues Relating to Early Hospital Discharge and the Impact on Newborn Genetic Screening Programs

For more than three decades, newborn screening has been a successful example of a population-based screening program to detect and treat disorders which cause preventable mental retardation and morbidity. However, some trends in managed care and demand for cost containment are raising concerns for state newborn screening programs across the country. The greatest impact thus far relates to increasing frequency in early hospital discharge (i.e., hospital stays of 24 hours or less) of healthy infants after birth.

When newborn screening started in 1962, hospital stays allowed for the ideal timing of specimen collection between 48 and 96 hours following birth and for the infants to be monitored. Early newborn screening specimen collection (i.e. before 48 hours of age) is primarily a result of early discharge. This practice affects newborn genetic screening programs in two ways: (1) by decreasing the ability to detect infants with inborn errors of metabolism who have not had adequate nutritional intake, and (2) by not being able to minimize the impact on families that is generated by a high number of false positive test results requiring further testing and follow-up to reach a confirmed diagnosis.

The results of a 1994 study of the impact of early discharge on newborn screening in California showed the following:

- Two-thirds of specimens were collected before 24 hours.
- 10% of specimens were collected before 12 hours.
- 50% of low birth weight (LBW) specimens were collected before 24 hours (7% before transfusions).
- Larger hospitals had more early discharges than smaller hospitals.

Issues Related to Specific Screening Tests

Phenylketonuria

Screening tests for phenylketonuria (PKU) are affected by "too early" specimen collection because there is a physiological rise in phenylalanine levels for the first 10 hours following birth gradually falling back to the level one hour post birth at approximately 24 hours of age. At a cutoff level of 4 mg/dl, a significant number of normal results will be falsely positive if collected during the first 24 hours. California found a false positive rate as high as 11/1000 before 24 hours compared to 1.1/1000 between 24-48 hours. Lowering the cut-off level for specimens collected before 24 hours resulted in more false positives without an increase in confirmed cases.

Early discharge can also result in false negative newborn screening results. For example, discharge of an infant with PKU may occur before blood phenylalanine levels have increased to sufficient levels to be detected by the newborn screen. Hence, the early screen would miss an infant with PKU. This scenario is particularly likely for infants with hyperphenylalaninemia, who do not have classical PKU, but still have an error of phenylalanine metabolism.

Hypothyroidism

The detection of primary hypothyroidism presents a similar problem because of a thyroid stimulating hormone (TSH) surge at birth which peaks at around six hours and then gradually declines to reach normal cut-off values by the fifth day of life. Since the majority of screening programs in the US take the lowest 10% of T4 results and run TSH analysis to determine a positive screening result for primary hypothyroidism, specimens collected during the first 24 hours will have a high false positive rate.

Maple Syrup Urine Disease

Screening for maple syrup urine disease (MSUD), by detection of elevation of leucine, is optimal at 24-48 hours of age. This elevation is subject to the same considerations as PKU but the medical issues are more complex in that life-threatening symptoms may become evident before screening results are available.

Homocystinuria

Early specimen collection affects screening for homocystinuria (HCU) by increasing the number of false negative results, since the measured metabolite methionine is often not elevated above normal levels during the first week of life. The optimal time to screen for homocystinuria is actually at 3 to 4 weeks of age.

Congenital Adrenal Hyperplasias

There are four different forms of congenital adrenal hyperplasia (CAH) that can be detected through newborn screening: salt-wasting, simple virilizing, non-classical late onset, and cryptic. The analyte tested is 17-hydroxyprogesterone (17-OHP). At birth, 17-OHP is normally elevated and undergoes a rapid decline to adult normal levels by one to three weeks of age. During the first week of life, the levels of 17-OHP show marked variation. Thus, early specimen collection is expected to result in an unacceptably high number of false positives.

Sickle Cell Disease, Biotinidase Deficiency, and Galactosemia

Other conditions screened for, but not dependent on the time of specimen collection, include tests for sickle cell disease, biotinidase deficiency, and galactosemia. The screening tests for these conditions rely on red cell components. These test results are affected by blood transfusions and specimens must be collected before transfusion for valid results.

Potential Strategies and Solutions

It is evident from the above information that early discharge has the potential to adversely affect the accuracy of newborn screening for the majority of conditions included in the panels of most newborn screening programs. Several strategies are being implemented to remedy this problem. The most important of these may be the legislation signed in the fall of 1997 by President Clinton whereby health insurers must cover 48 hour hospital stays for mothers and babies for a normal delivery and 96 hours for Cesarean sections. This will hopefully decrease the number of specimens collected at less than 24 hours. This legislation went into effect January 1998.

The 1992 AAP and ACOG Guidelines state that all newborns must be screened prior to discharge regardless of age or feeding status of the infant and that the optimal time to collect a sample is at 3 days of age. Most state programs have initiated a routine second screen if the newborn was screened before 24 hours of age. These second screens are collected between 1-2 weeks of age for some programs and 1-4 weeks for others. Some states are narrowing the period of time for the second screen to no later than two weeks of age because of the concern of delayed detection and treatment.

There are seven states that have implemented a routine second screen on the entire screening panel as a safeguard. They include Delaware, Oregon, New Mexico, Nevada, Texas, Colorado, and Utah. All these states consider a routine second screen to be an effective means (both medically and economically) of detecting clinically significant disorders not detected on the original screen.

In the state of Oregon, the routine second screen has resulted in 38 confirmed cases in whom diagnosis would either have been missed or delayed. Since 1991, five PKU cases have been picked up on the second screen. Oregon has also found that the routine second screening enhances practitioners' involvement in the screening process since second screening specimens are collected in their offices. They receive copies of both screening results for all the infants in their care and hopefully discuss these with the parents. Despite this apparent success in Oregon, there is much controversy in the newborn screening community concerning the effectiveness of the routine second screen. The following questions need to be considered in any discussion:

- Is it effective in detecting treatable cases?

- Is the comparative cost/benefit positive? (In comparison to improved testing sensitivity, liability costs, etc.)

- What is the appropriate time of collection for a second screen? (1-2 weeks, 2-4 weeks, etc.)

- What other factors may play a role in whether a second screening test is performed? (Are race and socioeconomic factors significant?)

- Should the second screen be recommended or required? (Is there discrimination if not required?)

Screening for Cystic Fibrosis

While newborn screening for cystic fibrosis (CF) has been feasible since 1979 using the IRT (immunoreactive trypsinogen test), and there have been slowly accumulating observational data regarding the potential benefits of such testing, it is not routinely performed in most states. In part, this is because CF is different from the classic model of PKU newborn screening in which a relatively simple intervention must be initiated within a short time frame (weeks) in order to avoid a significant complication (severe mental retardation). In contrast, cystic fibrosis is a chronic and gradually progressive disease and the potential benefit of newborn screening may be harder to discern.

Issues Regarding Identification of Hemoglobinopathy Carriers by Neonatal Screening

The primary purpose of neonatal screening for hemoglobinopathies is to identify infants with sickle cell disease, for whom early diagnosis, parental education, prophylactic penicillin, and comprehensive medical care markedly reduce morbidity and mortality.

In 1987, an NIH consensus development panel concluded that "the benefits of screening (for sickle cell disease) are so compelling that universal screening should be provided. State law should mandate the availability of these services while permitting parental refusal." During the subsequent 10 years, the number of states that conduct newborn screening for hemoglobinopathies has increased dramatically. Currently, 43 states and the District of Columbia screen newborns for sickle cell disease. In the Mountain States Region, 4 of 6 states (Arizona, Colorado, New Mexico, and Wyoming) screen all newborns for sickle cell disease.

Logistically, the provision of appropriate education and counseling services to families of hemoglobinopathy carriers identified by newborn screening is a formidable and potentially costly task. Approximately 50 infants who are carriers for hemoglobin variants are identified for each individual with sickle cell disease. Thus, thousands of carrier infants are identified each year by neonatal screening programs in the United States.

In many states, the large number of such cases far exceeds the capacity of clinical genetics programs and genetic counselors. Many states have long-standing contracts with community-based sickle cell organizations or with academic sickle cell centers to provide follow-up services. Frequently, but not always, education and counseling are provided by health care professionals (nurses, social workers, etc.) who have extensive knowledge of and experience with hemoglobinopathies. To help ensure the highest quality for the services, many have advocated that a national program be established to set minimum standards of education and training for hemoglobinopathy educators/counselors and to provide for a certification process.

In September 1995, a national symposium was held to address the legal, ethical, technical and logistical issues concerning the follow-up of hemoglobinopathy carriers identified through neonatal screening. Participants included representatives from newborn screening programs and sickle cell organizations, geneticists, ethicists, hematologists, and consumers. There was a clear consensus that families of hemoglobinopathy carriers should be notified of the results and that appropriate education and counseling should be available. As a direct outgrowth of that conference, the CORN Sickle Cell, Thalassemia and Other Hemoglobin Variants Committee (with advice and support from the CORN Newborn Screening Committee) developed guidelines for the follow up of hemoglobinopathy carriers detected by newborn screening.

490

These guidelines (available through the Mountain States Regional Genetic Services Network coordinator) were recently endorsed by the Steering Committee of CORN and are summarized below:

- Ideally, education about newborn screening, which usually includes testing for sickle cell disease, should be provided to families during prenatal care well in advance of the time of delivery. A mechanism should be in place in State Newborn Screening Programs so that all results of sickle cell newborn screening can be made available to parents of all infants who are tested.

- Parents of all infants who are detected to be carriers of hemoglobin variants should be offered appropriate education, counseling and testing.

- Individuals who counsel should have appropriate training and credentials in order to insure the highest quality of services for families of carriers detected by newborn screening.

- Newborn screening programs should have a mechanism for monitoring and assessing the approaches to, responses to, and costs of providing carrier education and counseling services.

Meanwhile, the Sickle Cell Disease Association of America has initiated the lengthy process of developing a national certification program for hemoglobinopathy counselors.

Top Ten Pitfalls in Newborn Screening

Assuming That the Result of the Newborn Screening Test Is Negative (or Normal) Because You Have Not Heard Otherwise.

There are many reasons why the primary care provider may not be notified about an abnormal newborn screening result: difficulty finding and notifying a provider, a test might have never been sent, or an error in delivery of the result to the primary health care provider. The primary care provider of record at the birth of an infant assumes the responsibility to assure that a screen was obtained and that the results are duly recorded in the medical records. In light of the increasing complexity of the health care system, many newborn screening programs are working to facilitate proper dissemination of newborn screening results.

Assuming That a Negative (or Normal) Result of Newborn Screening Definitively Excludes the Conditions Screened For.

"False negative" test results may occur for a wide variety of reasons including human error such as sample transposition and the statistically "built in" false negative tests. For example, approximately 30% of hypothyroidism is missed in babies who were tested before the second week of life. If the primary care provider observes symptoms, which could be the result of one of the disorders on the newborn screening panel in your state, it is appropriate to confirm the results. Any baby with symptoms which might be caused by PKU, hypothyroidism, sickle cell disease, galactosemia, cystic fibrosis or any other disorder for which newborn screening was negative should have specific diagnostic testing performed by an appropriate diagnostic laboratory.

Submitting a Newborn Screening Sample with Incomplete or Illegible Information.

All states design the newborn screening forms to suit the specific panel of tests they perform and each piece of requested information is essential. Nevertheless, all newborn screening programs receive samples with inaccurate or incomplete information. The submitter of the sample cannot, of course, be responsible when families deliberately provide misinformation. The submitter is, however, responsible for providing legible information that is correct so far as she/he is aware. When the screening lab requires multiple copies, all copies must be legible (often a problem with hospital card stamps). When a newborn screening form asks for information about the use of antibiotics, history of transfusion or prematurity, that information is necessary for accurate interpretation of test results. Date of birth is always necessary for proper identification of the newborn, and date of sample for test interpretations. Precise information on age in hours may be necessary for the increasingly complex interpretation of results for early screening.

Ordering a Solubility Test (Sickledex, Sickleprep) as the Follow Up in an Infant with Positive Newborn Screen for Hemoglobinopathy.

Diagnostic follow-up testing is required after a positive newborn screen to exclude a false positive result and to define the specific diagnosis. The false positive rate and the differential diagnosis varies with the disease for which screening is performed and with the nature of the test. Confirmation testing for infants with abnormal hemoglobinopathy screening tests (hemoglobin Barts excepted) should always include hemoglobin electrophoresis. The solubility test (Sickledex, Sickle-prep) should never be performed in this setting because it is often falsely negative in infants with sickle cell disease, does not define the specific hemoglobinopathy present, and fails to differentiate individuals with disease from those with hemoglobin traits.

Similarly, for other conditions on a newborn screen, specific protocols and policies for confirmatory testing have been developed by each newborn screening program. For example, in Colorado, a result of 4 mg/dl on the screen for PKU should be followed by a repeat screen; while a baby with one level of more than 4 mg/dl or two levels of 4 mg/dl each should have diagnostic testing sent to a specific laboratory for phenylalanine and tyrosine levels.

Consultants are available for each disorder and can assist with routine follow-up and with unusual circumstances in which follow-up might need to be tailored to a particular newborn's situation.

Prescribing a PKU Treatment Formula Before Confirming the Diagnosis of PKU.

A significant number of babies with a positive screening test for PKU ultimately prove to be unaffected. After a positive screen, diagnostic test results can be completed in hours to days and treatment begun in a timely fashion, once the diagnosis is confirmed. If treatment is started after the screen only, this may interfere with subsequent diagnostic testing. Also, the PKU diet may be harmful to a child without PKU.

The diet for PKU needs to be carefully calculated by a trained registered dietitian to give a precise amount of essential amino acids by combination of the metabolic formula with human milk or infant formula. In contrast, if a state screens for galactosemia using a test with a low rate of false-positive results, an immediate diet change might be required while diagnostic tests are pending.

Each state has recommendations that take into consideration the specific tests performed in the screening laboratory and the nature of the population served. Guidance regarding any necessary treatment while follow-up screening or diagnostic testing is pursued will be provided.

Not Collecting a Newborn Screening Sample Prior to Blood Transfusion Because the Baby Is "Too Young" or Has Not Yet Been Fed.

Transfusion will alter the results of certain newborn screening tests. If a baby is transfused and then screened using an assay affected by transfusion of red cells, the transfusion will affect the test results. For example, when red cells are transfused prior to screening for hemoglobinopathy, the newborn screening laboratory will be testing donor hemoglobins. One test for galactosemia uses the Beutler Assay to measure in red blood cells the activity of galactose-1-phosphate uridyltransferase, the enzyme deficient in galactosemia. The enzyme is present in red cells and thus the transfused red cells will affect the test results. The appropriate strategy always is to collect a newborn screening sample immediately before transfusion in the very young newborn.

Not Collecting a Newborn Screening Sample Prior to Transfer of the Infant to Another Institution.

Sick and premature babies, some of whom require transfer for more intensive/specialized care, are at no lower risk than healthy newborns for disorders detected by newborn screening. States may have explicit regulations about responsibility for screening when a baby is transferred from or to a nursery. Regardless of specific regulations, it is appropriate for a newborn screen to be sent by the hospital or institution from which the baby is transferred and for the receiving hospital or institution to verify that screen was sent and subsequently to repeat the screen if appropriate.

Not Collecting an Adequate Newborn Screening Sample.

In each state, a variable percentage of healthy babies are never screened. Reasons for failing to screen a healthy baby vary. A sample may have been collected but failed to reach the laboratory, or the newborn screening laboratory may receive a sample that is inadequate for testing because of insufficient sample, unacceptable collection, or sample contamination. Despite the fact that records will show a sample was collected, that baby was never screened. In other cases, no sample is ever collected. This may be a result of human or system error, and is one reason that the primary care provider must ascertain that each baby has been screened.

Home births present special issues, as the lay midwife or delivering family member who would be responsible to collect and send the screening sample may be uninformed about the purpose and process of newborn screening.

Assuming That an Abnormal Newborn Screen Is a False Positive Because the Baby Is Well and/or Because One or More Factors Known To Be Associated with False Positive Results Are Present.

The screening process is successful when affected babies are identified before onset of symptoms. The corollary is that the appearance of good health is not evidence against the presence of the disorder. Even in the presence of special clinical circumstances known to be associated with an increased frequency of physiologic false positive screening tests, a baby who tests positive may be truly affected. For example, the baby who is premature or tested very early, and who has a positive test for thyroid disease, may have real disease and needs prompt confirmation testing.

Referring to the Newborn Screening Test as a "PKU Test".

This is a very common practice among hospital staff and practicing physicians. It is misleading to refer to the newborn screen as "a PKU test", because tests for other diseases are included. Parent confusion about the full scope of testing may impact compliance with follow-up should the newborn screen be abnormal. It is good practice to use the term "newborn screen" and to inform the family of the breadth of the newborn screen.

For Further Information

Carol Clericuzio, MD
Department of Pediatrics
The University of New Mexico
Albuquerque, NM 87131

Part Ten

Pregnancy Tests and Newborn Care

Chapter 57

Pregnancy Tests:

Routine Screening, Maternal Serum Screening (AFP and MMS), and Percutaneous Umbilical Blood Sample (PUBS)

Routine Screening

During your first obstetric appointment, your health-care provider should discuss a plan for future visits and lab tests with you, based on your personal medical situation. The frequency of visits may vary if you have any risk factors, a history of obstetrical difficulties, chronic health problems or, are expecting more than one child. Your clinician generally establishes a regular schedule of prenatal visits so your health and that of your developing baby can be carefully monitored. A normal singleton pregnancy schedule might be as follows:

- Monthly visits until you are 28 weeks pregnant
- Visits every 2 weeks from 28 weeks to 36 weeks
- Weekly visits from 36 weeks until delivery (usually around 40 weeks)

At each routine prenatal visit, the clinician should check your weight and blood pressure; perform urine tests to monitor protein and sugar; and check the position, size and heartbeat of the fetus. You won't necessarily need a pelvic exam or additional lab tests at each appointment, but the doctor should note findings on your chart. It's important to ask any questions you may have and to be

---

Excerpts from "Pregnancy–Tests and Procedures," reprinted with permission © February 1997, The Johns Hopkins University, available on InteliHealth at www.intelihealth.com.

informed of the results of the doctor's examination and the tests that are done.

On the basis of your medical history, the results of your routine exams and tests, and the clinician's customary style of practice, you may require additional tests to further evaluate your baby's health and growth or check for possible birth defects. Such tests can't detect every problem or assure you of a perfect baby, but they often provide valuable medical information. Now is the time to discuss the purpose and possible risks of any test that's suggested, and decide if it's appropriate for you.

Pregnancy Tests

Probably the very first test you'll use during your pregnancy is a home pregnancy test to determine if you are indeed pregnant. These over-the-counter "home" tests are now so sensitive that they can sometimes detect pregnancy before you've even missed a period.

For the most accurate results, it's best to wait until you're at least a few days late. Once your period is a week or more overdue, the reliability of tests like e.p.t.-Plus or First Response is close to 100 percent when done properly. These tests work by measuring the level of human chorionic gonadotropin (hCG), a hormone that's produced by pregnant women and is present in urine. You simply place some fresh urine on the dipstick and watch for a change in color, which indicates a positive (pregnant) result.

If the test is positive, see your doctor to confirm the pregnancy and start prenatal care. If, on the other hand, the test is negative, wait a few days to see if you get your period before checking with your doctor. Even a woman whose period is usually regular may be late on occasion due to disruptions such as travel or stress.

If you suspect you are pregnant, your doctor will perform a blood test, which is more reliable than a home urine test. Blood tests can detect pregnancy as early as 10 days after conception—about 4 days before your period would usually be expected, if you have a regular 28-day cycle. By the time you're even 1 day late, these tests can confirm pregnancy with 100 percent accuracy.

Like home urine tests, blood tests measure hCG but are more accurate. These are referred to as "quantitative tests". There are several types of blood tests for pregnancy, but the newer ones, favored by most OB/GYNs, are called beta hCG tests and measure the concentration of a part of the hCG molecule called the beta-subunit. Only a few drops of blood are required for the test.

Maternal Serum Screening Tests

These are blood tests used to determine whether you have a higher-than-average risk of delivering a baby with certain birth defects. They measure substances in your blood that may change when disorders are present, but are also done to women without risk factors—usually after other tests have produced abnormal results. Maternal serum screening tests include alpha-fetoprotein (AFP) and multiple marker screenings (MMS).

Alpha-fetoprotein (AFP)

AFP is a protein produced by the fetus as it grows, found in both the fetus's blood and the amniotic fluid; small amounts also cross the placenta into your bloodstream. By taking a blood sample from you during weeks 15 through 18, your health-care provider can determine based on the concentration of AFP in your blood whether your unborn baby has a higher-than-normal risk of certain birth defects that include:

- Down syndrome, a chromosome abnormality causing mental retardation and a characteristic physical appearance;

- Neural tube defects such as spina bifida, an exposed spinal cord due to failure of the vertebrae to develop completely;

- Anencephaly, the absence of the brain and top of the skull.

AFP testing poses no risk to the developing fetus and can detect 80 percent of cases of open spinal defects. Abnormal results don't necessarily mean your baby has a medical disorder; a higher-than-normal reading might signal that your baby is older than was previously estimated or that you are carrying twins, triplets or even more babies. But a high reading may indicate a neural tube defect, so your clinician will likely perform further testing. A lower than normal result can mean that your baby is younger than was thought or has Down syndrome. Most abnormal results do not indicate that your baby has a birth defect, so try to stay calm and see what further testing shows. Amniocentesis is the test performed in the presence of abnormal AFP levels. This test is safest when done by an experienced obstetrician—gynecologist. The test is often prescribed for expecting mothers older than age 35, when the father is over 55, or if inherited disorders run in either family.

Multiple Marker Screening (MMS)

These tests measure levels of the hormones estriol and human chorionic gonadotropin (hCG) in the mother's blood, as well as AFP. In most pregnancies, higher-than-normal levels of hCG or lower-than-average of estriol indicate the fetus has Down syndrome. Screening tests can also include sonography and amniocentesis. Multiple marker tests are often recommended for women over age 35, who already have a higher risk of birthing a Down syndrome baby, but can also be performed in younger women who don't have risk factors of a Down syndrome baby. Usually, the same blood sample is used for all the tests and is drawn between the 15th and 18th week of pregnancy.

Percutaneous Umbilical Blood Sample (PUBS Test)

This test is done in a manner similar to amniocentesis, except that the ultrasound-guided needle is inserted into a blood vessel of the unborn infant's umbilical cord to obtain a tiny sample of fetal blood. A PUBS test can be done in weeks 18 through 36. It is used to check abnormal amniocentesis results, diagnose causes of growth late in pregnancy, or determine if the fetus has been exposed in the uterus to a potentially harmful infectious disease, such as German measles or toxoplasmosis, an infection transmitted by eating infected meat or coming in contact with cat feces. Both diseases may cause mild or no symptoms in the mother but, put an unborn baby at risk of devastating birth defects.

Results usually take 3 days. Since this test is quite new, there's no definite research on its reliability, but it's thought to be highly accurate. It poses risks similar to amniocentesis, but is associated with a slight, additional danger of premature delivery or early rupture of the membranes.

HIV Testing

Both the American College of Obstetricians and Gynecologists (ACOG) and the American Academy of Pediatrics (AAP) recommend that all pregnant women receive HIV education and counseling, and if they consent, performance of an HIV test. That's because HIV and AIDS are on the rise among women of child-bearing age.

There are known benefits to determining an expectant mother's HIV status. Treatments exist which can significantly lower her risk of transmitting the virus to her baby before birth or prolong the life of an infected baby, if begun in the first months of life. The ACOG and the AAP strongly urge mothers-to-be to consider an HIV blood test during pregnancy.

Chapter 58

OB/GYN Ultrasound

What Is Ultrasound?

Ultrasound is like ordinary sound except it has a frequency (or pitch) higher than people can hear. Ultrasound is sent into the body from a scanning instrument (transducer) placed on the patient's skin. The sound is reflected off structures inside the body and is analyzed by a computer to make a picture of these structures on a television screen. The moving pictures can be recorded on film or videotape. Diagnostic ultrasound is commonly called sonography or ultrasonography.

Why Do Patients Have an Ultrasound Examination?

The most common reason for having an ultrasound examination is to help you doctor determine when your baby is due, or to make sure your baby is growing as it should. Your doctor may also want an ultrasound examination to determine the baby's position, or to see if you are carrying twins or triplets. With ultrasound, the amount of fluid around your baby can be seen. Ultrasound also may be used to detect some birth defects.

Is There Any Special Preparation for the Examination?

In most cases, no special preparation is needed for the examination. In some cases, you may be asked to drink some water an hour

Reprinted with permission © 1997 *What You Should Know About Your Ultrasound Examination–OB*, American Institute of Ultrasound in Medicine.

before the examination. The reason for this is that sometimes it is easier to see the pregnancy by looking through a full bladder.

Who Will Perform the Examination?

In most cases you will be examined by a specially trained person called a sonographer. The pictures will then be reviewed and read by a doctor. In some cases, you may also be examined by the doctor.

Will It Hurt?

There is no pain from an ultrasound examination. If you have been asked to fill your bladder, this may cause some discomfort. In early pregnancy it may be necessary to put a special transducer (scanner) in your vagina, so the very small baby can be seen. You will be able to empty your bladder before this type of exam is done. It will not hurt, but you may feel some pressure. It does not hurt the baby.

For scanning, a gel-like material is put on your abdomen and the transducer is placed on your skin. The gel makes it possible for the scanner to see through your skin into your body. The gel may feel cold and, even though it wipes off easily, it is a good idea to wear clothes that can be washed. The gel does not usually stain clothing.

Can I See My Baby Move?

The baby's heartbeat and movement of its body, arms, and legs can be seen by ultrasound, depending on the age of the baby. The baby can be seen moving during an ultrasound examination many weeks before the mother can feel movement.

Will I Learn the Sex of My Baby?

Sometimes it is possible to see the sex of the baby and sometimes it is not. If the baby is lying in an inconvenient position, the baby's sex cannot be determined.

Does an Ultrasound Examination Guarantee a Normal Baby?

No. The ability to detect abnormalities depends on many things. For instance, the size and position of you baby may not allow certain abnormalities to be seen. Some types of abnormalities cannot be seen, because they are too small or not visible by ultrasound.

Will I Need More Than One Ultrasound Examination?

In many cases you may have only one examination, but for a variety of reasons your physician may order additional scans during your pregnancy.

Is Ultrasound Safe?

The American Institute of Ultrasound in Medicine, an association of physicians, sonographers, scientists, and engineers, has a Bioeffects Committee that meets regularly to consider safety issues and evaluate reports dealing with bioeffects and safety of ultrasound. The AIUM has adopted the following statement:

> There are no known harmful effects associated with the medical use of sonography. Widespread clinical use of diagnostic ultrasound for many years has not revealed any harmful effects. Studies in humans have revealed no direct link between the use of diagnostic ultrasound and any adverse outcome. Although the possibility exists that biological effects may be identified in the future, current information indicates that the benefits to patients far outweigh the risks, if any.

Chapter 59

Gestational Diabetes

What Is Gestational Diabetes and What Causes It?

Diabetes (actual name is diabetes mellitus) of any kind is a disorder that prevents the body from using food properly. Normally, the body gets its major source of energy from glucose, a simple sugar that comes from foods high in simple carbohydrates (e.g., table sugar or other sweeteners such as honey, molasses, jams and jellies, soft drinks, and cookies), or from the breakdown of complex carbohydrates such as starches (e.g., bread, potatoes, and pasta). After sugars and starches are digested in the stomach, they enter the blood stream in the form of glucose. The glucose in the blood stream becomes a potential source of energy for the entire body, similar to the way in which gasoline in a service station pump is a potential source of energy for your car. But, just as someone must pump the gas into the car, the body requires some assistance to get glucose from the blood stream to the muscles and other tissues of the body. In the body, that assistance comes from a hormone called insulin. Insulin is manufactured by the pancreas, a gland that lies behind the stomach. Without insulin, glucose cannot get into the cells of the body where it is used as fuel. Instead, glucose accumulates in the blood to high levels and is excreted or "spilled" into the urine through the kidneys.

Excerpts from "Understanding Gestational Diabetes," National Institute of Child Health and Human Development (NICHD), NIH Publication updated September 1996.

When the pancreas of a child or young adult produces little or no insulin we call this condition juvenile-onset diabetes or Type I diabetes (insulin-dependent). This is not the type of diabetes you have. Unlike women with Type I diabetes, women with gestational diabetes have plenty of insulin. In fact, they usually have more insulin in their blood than women who are not pregnant. However, the effect of their insulin is partially blocked by a variety of other hormones made in the placenta, a condition often called insulin resistance.

The placenta performs the task of supplying the growing fetus with nutrients and water from the mother's circulation. It also produces a variety of hormones vital to the preservation of the pregnancy. Ironically, several of these hormones such as estrogen, cortisol, and human placental lactogen (HPL) have a blocking effect on insulin, a "contra-insulin" effect. This contra-insulin effect usually begins about midway (20 to 24 weeks) through pregnancy. The larger the placenta grows, the more these hormones are produced, and the greater the insulin resistance becomes. In most women the pancreas is able to make additional insulin to overcome the insulin resistance. When the pancreas makes all the insulin it can and there still isn't enough to

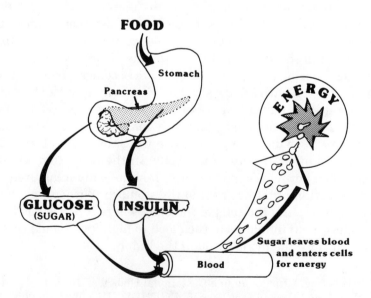

Figure 59.1. *Insulin: The Key to Turning Food into Energy*

overcome the effect of the placenta's hormones, gestational diabetes results. If we could somehow remove all the placenta's hormones from the mother's blood, the condition would be remedied. This, in fact, usually happens following delivery.

How Does Gestational Diabetes Differ from Other Types of Diabetes?

There are several different types of diabetes. Gestational diabetes begins during pregnancy and disappears following delivery. Another type is referred to as juvenile-onset diabetes (in children) or Type I (in young adults). These individuals usually develop their disease before age 20. People with Type I diabetes must take insulin by injection every day. Approximately 10 percent of all people with diabetes have Type I (also called insulin-dependent diabetes).

Type II diabetes or noninsulin-dependent diabetes (formerly called adult-onset diabetes) is also characterized by high blood sugar levels, but these patients are often obese and usually lack the classic symptoms (fatigue, thirst, frequent urination, and sudden weight loss) associated with Type I diabetes. Many of these individuals can control their blood sugar levels by following a careful diet and exercise program, by losing excess weight, or by taking oral medication. Some, but not all, need insulin. People with Type II diabetes account for roughly 90 percent of all diabetics.

Who Is at Risk for Developing Gestational Diabetes and How Is It Detected?

Any woman might develop gestational diabetes during pregnancy. Some of the factors associated with women who have an increased risk are obesity; a family history of diabetes; having given birth previously to a very large infant, a stillbirth, or a child with a birth defect; or having too much amniotic fluid (polyhydramnios). Also, women who are older than 25 are at greater risk than younger individuals. Although a history of sugar in the urine is often included in the list of risk factors, this is not a reliable indicator of who will develop diabetes during pregnancy. Some pregnant women with perfectly normal blood sugar levels will occasionally have sugar detected in their urine.

The Council on Diabetes in Pregnancy of the American Diabetes Association strongly recommends that all pregnant women be screened for gestational diabetes. Several methods of screening exist. The most common is the 50-gram glucose screening test. No special preparation is necessary for this test, and there is no need to fast before the test. The test is performed by giving 50 grams of a glucose drink and then measuring the blood sugar level 1 hour later. A woman with a blood sugar level of less than 140 milligrams per deciliter (mg/dl) at 1 hour is presumed not to have gestational diabetes and requires no further testing. If the blood sugar level is greater than 140 mg/dl the test is considered abnormal or "positive." Not all women with a positive screening test have diabetes. Consequently, a 3-hour glucose tolerance test must be performed to establish the diagnosis of gestational diabetes.

If your physician determines that you should take the complete 3-hour glucose tolerance test, you will be asked to follow some special instructions in preparation for the test. For 3 days before the test, eat a diet that contains at least 150 grams of carbohydrates each day. This can be accomplished by including one cup of pasta, two servings of fruit, four slices of bread, and three glasses of milk every day. For 10 to 14 hours before the test you should not eat and not drink anything but water. The test is usually done in the morning in your physician's office or in a laboratory. First, a blood sample will be drawn to measure your fasting blood sugar level. Then you will be asked to drink a full bottle of a glucose drink (100 grams). This glucose drink is extremely sweet and occasionally makes some people feel nauseated. Finally, blood samples will be drawn every hour for 3 hours after the glucose drink has been consumed.

If two or more of your blood sugar levels are higher than the diagnostic criteria, you have gestational diabetes. This testing is usually performed at the end of the second trimester or the beginning of the third trimester (between the 24th and 28th weeks of pregnancy) when insulin resistance usually begins. If you had gestational diabetes in a previous pregnancy or there is some reason why your physician is unusually concerned about your risk of developing gestational diabetes, you may be asked to take the 50-gram glucose screening test as early as the first trimester (before the 13th week). Remember, merely having sugar in your urine or even having an abnormal blood sugar on the 50-gram glucose screening test does not necessarily mean you have gestational diabetes. The 3-hour glucose tolerance test must be abnormal before the diagnosis is made.

What Can Be Done to Reduce Problems Associated with Gestational Diabetes?

In addition to your obstetrician, there are other health professionals who specialize in the management of diabetes during pregnancy including internists or diabetologists, registered dietitians, qualified nutritionists, and diabetes educators. Your doctor may recommend that you see one or more of these specialists during your pregnancy. In addition, a neonatologist (a doctor who specializes in the care of newborn infants) should also be called in to manage any complications the baby might develop after delivery.

One of the essential components in the care of a woman with gestational diabetes is a diet specifically tailored to provide adequate nutrition to meet the needs of the mother and the growing fetus. At the same time the diet has to be planned in such a way as to keep blood glucose levels in the normal range (60 to 120 mg/dl). Specific details about diet during pregnancy are discussed later.

An obstetrician, diabetes educator, or other health care practitioner can teach you how to measure your own blood glucose levels at home to see if levels remain in an acceptable range on the prescribed diet. The ability of patients to determine their own blood sugar levels with easy-to-use equipment represents a major milestone in the management of diabetes, especially during pregnancy. The technique called "self blood glucose monitoring" (discussed in detail later) allows you to check your blood sugar levels at home or at work without costly and time-consuming visits to your doctor. The values of your blood sugar levels also determine if you need to begin insulin therapy sometime during pregnancy. Short of frequent trips to a laboratory, this is the only way to see if blood glucose levels remain under good control.

What Is Self Blood Glucose Monitoring?

Once you are diagnosed as having gestational diabetes, you and your health care providers will want to know more about your day-to-day blood sugar levels. It is important to know how your exercise habits and eating patterns affect your blood sugars. Also, as your pregnancy progresses, the placenta will release more of the hormones that work against insulin. Testing your blood sugar level at important times during the day will help determine if proper diet and weight gain have kept blood sugar levels normal or if extra insulin is needed to help keep the fetus protected.

Self blood glucose monitoring is done by a special device to obtain a drop of your blood and test it for your blood sugar level. Your doctor or other health care provider will explain the procedure to you. Make sure that you are shown how to do the testing before attempting it on your own. Some items you may use to monitor your blood sugar levels are:

- Lancet—a disposable, sharp needle-like sticker for pricking the finger to obtain a drop of blood.

- Lancet device—a spring-loaded finger sticking device.

- Test strip—a chemically treated strip to which a drop of blood is applied.

- Color chart—a chart used to compare against the color on the test strip for blood sugar level.

- Glucose meter - a device which "reads" the test strip and gives you a digital number value.

Your health care provider can advise you where to obtain the self-monitoring equipment in your area. You may want to inquire if any places rent or loan glucose meters, since it is likely you won't be needing it after your baby is born.

How Often and When Should I Test?

You may need to test your blood several times a day. Generally, these times are fasting (first thing in the morning before you eat) and 2 hours after each meal. Occasionally, you may be asked to test more frequently during the day or at night. As each person is an individual, your health care provider can advise the schedules best for you.

How Should I Record My Test Results?

Most manufacturers of glucose testing products provide a record diary, although some health care providers may have their own version.

You should record any test result immediately because it's easy to forget what the reading was during the course of a busy day. You should always have this diary with you when you visit your doctor or other health care provider or when you contact them by phone. These results are very important in making decisions about your health care.

Are There Any Other Tests I Should Know About?

In addition to blood testing, you may be asked to check your urine for ketones. Ketones are by-products of the breakdown of fat and may be found in the blood and urine as a result of inadequate insulin or from inadequate calories in your diet. Although it is not known whether or not small amounts of ketones can harm the fetus, when

514

large amounts of ketones are present they are accompanied by a blood condition, acidosis, which is known to harm the fetus. To be on the safe side, you should watch for them in your urine and report any positive results to your doctor.

How Do I Test for Ketones?

To test the urine for ketones, you can use a test strip similar to the one used for testing your blood. This test strip has a special chemically treated pad to detect ketones in the urine. Testing is done by passing the test strip through the stream of urine or dripping the strip in and out of urine in a container. As your pregnancy progresses, you might find it easier to use the container method. All test strips are disposable and can be used only once. This applies to blood sugar test strips also. You cannot use your blood sugar test strips for urine testing, and you cannot use your ketone test strips for blood sugar testing.

When Do I Test for Ketones?

Overnight is the longest fasting period, so you should test your urine first thing in the morning every day and any time your blood sugar level goes over 240 mg/dl on the blood glucose test. It is also important to test if you become ill and are eating less food than normal. Your health care provider can advise what's best for you.

Is It Ever Necessary to Take Insulin?

Yes, despite careful attention to diet some women's blood sugars do not stay within an acceptable range. A pregnant woman free of gestational diabetes rarely has a blood glucose level that exceeds 100 mg/dl in the morning before breakfast (fasting) or 2 hours after a meal. The optimum goal for a gestational diabetic is blood sugar levels that are the same as those of a woman without diabetes.

There is no absolute blood sugar level that necessitates beginning insulin injections. However, many physicians begin insulin if the fasting sugar exceeds 105 mg/dl or if the level 2 hours after a meal 120 mg/dl on two separate occasions. Blood sugar levels measured by you at home will help your doctor know when it is necessary to begin insulin. The ability to perform self-blood glucose monitoring has made it possible to begin insulin therapy at the earliest sign of high sugar levels, thereby preventing the fetus from being exposed to high levels of glucose from the mother's blood.

515

Chapter 60

Amniocentesis and Chorionic Villus Sampling (CVS)

Testing for Birth Defects

Many women undergo tests during pregnancy to check for birth defects, genetic disorders, and other problems. A few of the most common tests are ultrasound scans, the alpha-fetoprotein (AFP) test, amniocentesis, and chorionic villi sampling (CVS). Each of these can be helpful in diagnosing problems, but the tests are not necessary for every pregnancy. Check with your doctor about what tests, if any, are appropriate for you.

Amniocentesis

This test examines the cells shed by the fetus into the surrounding amniotic fluid. Performed about 16 weeks into pregnancy, the test involves inserting a long, thin needle through the mother's abdomen to extract fluid from the womb. The cells must be cultured in a laboratory and it may take up to a month for test results to be ready. The test is a reliable indicator of chromosomal abnormalities such as Down syndrome or genetic disorders such as Tay-Sachs disease, Hunter's syndrome, and others. While usually safe, amniocentesis can trigger cramping, leakage of amniotic fluid, and vaginal bleeding, and it may increase the risk of miscarriage by about 0.5 to 1 percent. The test is only done

This chapter contains text from "Healthy Pregnancy, Healthy Baby," by Rebecca D. Williams, *FDA Consumer,* March-April 1999, and Morbidity and Mortality Weekly Report, July 21, 1995.

on women at increased risk of having babies with genetic disorders or to assess the maturity of the baby's lungs in the last trimester.

Chorionic Villi Sampling (CVS)

Performed between 10 and 12 weeks of pregnancy, CVS can detect the same genetic abnormalities as amniocentesis. It involves inserting a catheter or needle into the womb and extracting some of the chorionic villi (cells from the tissue that will become the placenta). The chorionic villi contain the same chromosomes as the fetus. The test is relatively safe but it has a greater risk of miscarriage than amniocentesis. While there has been some concern that the test itself may be associated with limb deformities, many geneticists believe that CVS performed between 10 and 12 weeks of pregnancy does not increase that risk.

Use of CVS and Amniocentesis

In the United States, the current standard of care in obstetrical practice is to offer either CVS or amniocentesis to women who will be older than 35 years of age when they give birth, because these women are at increased risk for giving birth to infants with Down syndrome and certain other types of aneuploidy. Karyotyping of cells obtained by either amniocentesis or CVS is the standard and definitive means of diagnosing aneuploidy in fetuses. The risk that a woman will give birth to an infant with Down syndrome increases with age. For example, for women 35 years of age, the risk is 1 per 385 births (0.3%), whereas for women 45 years of age, the risk is 1 per 30 births (3%). The background risk for major birth defects (with or without chromosomal abnormalities) for women of all ages is approximately 3%.

Before widespread use of amniocentesis, several controlled studies were conducted to evaluate the safety of the procedure. The major finding from these studies was that amniocentesis increases the rate for miscarriage (i.e., spontaneous abortions) by approximately 0.5%. Subsequent to these studies, amniocentesis became an accepted standard of care in the 1970s. In 1990, more than 200,000 amniocentesis procedures were performed in the United States.

In the 1960s and 1970s, exploratory studies were conducted revealing that the placenta (i.e., chorionic villi) could be biopsied through a catheter and that sufficient placental cells could be obtained to permit certain genetic analyses earlier in pregnancy than through amniocentesis. In the United States, this procedure was initially evaluated in a controlled trial designed to determine the miscarriage rate. The difference in fetal-loss rate was estimated to be 0.8% higher after CVS compared with amniocentesis, although this difference was not statistically significant. Because that study was designed to determine miscarriage rates, it had limited statistical power to detect small increases in risks for individual birth defects.

CVS had become widely used worldwide by the early 1980s. The World Health Organization (WHO) sponsors an international Registry of CVS procedures; data in the International Registry probably represent less than half of all procedures performed worldwide. More than 80,000 procedures were reported to the International Registry from 1983-1992; approximately 200,000 procedures were registered from 1983-1995. CVS is performed in hospitals, outpatient clinics, selected obstetricians' offices, and university settings; these facilities are often collectively referred to as prenatal diagnostic centers. Some investigators have reported that the availability of CVS increased the overall utilization of prenatal diagnostic procedures among women over 35 years of age, suggesting that access to first-trimester testing may make prenatal chromosome analysis appealing to a larger number of women. Another group of obstetricians did not see an increase in overall utilization when CVS was introduced. The increase in CVS procedures was offset by a decrease in amniocentesis, suggesting that the effect of CVS availability on the utilization of prenatal diagnostic testing depends on local factors. In the United States, an estimated 40% of pregnant women over 35 years of age underwent either amniocentesis or CVS in 1990.

Indications for Amniocentesis and CVS

Although maternal age-related risk for fetal aneuploidy is the usual indication for CVS or amniocentesis, prospective mothers or fathers of any age might desire fetal testing when they are at risk for passing on certain mendelian (single-gene) conditions. In a randomized trial conducted in the United States, 19% of women who underwent CVS were younger than 35 years of age. DNA-based diagnoses of mendelian conditions, such as cystic fibrosis, hemophilia, muscular dystrophy, and hemoglobinopathies, can be made by direct analysis of uncultured chorionic villus cells (a more efficient method than culturing amniocytes). However, amniocentesis is particularly useful to prospective parents who have a family history of neural tube defects, because alpha-fetoprotein (AFP) testing can be done on amniotic fluid but cannot be done on CVS specimens.

519

When testing for chromosomal abnormalities resulting from advanced maternal age, CVS may be more acceptable than amniocentesis to some women because of the psychological and medical advantages provided by CVS through earlier diagnosis of abnormalities. Fetal movement is usually felt and uterine growth is visible at 17-19 weeks' gestation, the time when abnormalities are detected by amniocentesis; thus, deciding what action to take if an abnormality is detected at this time may be more difficult psychologically. Using CVS to diagnose chromosomal abnormalities during the first trimester allows a prospective parent to make this decision earlier than with amniocentesis.

Amniocentesis is usually performed at 15-18 weeks' gestation, but more amniocentesis procedures are now being performed at 11-14 weeks' gestation. "Early" amniocentesis (defined as earlier 15 weeks' gestation) remains investigational, because the safety of the procedure is currently being evaluated with controlled trials.

Limb Deficiencies Among Infants Whose Mothers Underwent CVS

Certain congenital defects of the extremities, known as limb deficiencies or limb reduction defects, have been reported among infants whose mothers underwent CVS.

Reports of clusters of infants born with limb deficiencies after CVS were first published in 1991. Three studies illustrate the spectrum of CVS-associated defects. Data from these studies suggest that the severity of the outcome is associated with the specific time of CVS exposure. Exposure at >70 days' gestation has been associated with more limited defects, isolated to the distal extremities, whereas earlier exposures have been associated with more proximal limb deficiencies and orofacial defects. For example, in a study involving 14 infants exposed to CVS at 63-79 days' gestation and examined by a single pediatrician, 13 had isolated transverse digital deficiencies. In another study in Oxford of five infants exposed to CVS at 56-66 days' gestation, four had transverse deficiencies with oromandibular hypogenesis. In a review of published worldwide data, associated defects of the tongue or lower jaw were reported for 19 of 75 cases of CVS-associated limb deficiencies. Of those 19 infants with oromandibular-limb hypogenesis, 17 were exposed to CVS before 68 days' gestation. In this review, 74% of infants exposed to CVS at 270 days' gestation had digital deficiencies without proximal involvement.

Recommendations

An analysis of all aspects of CVS and amniocentesis indicates that the occasional occurrence of CVS-related limb defects is only one of several factors that must be considered in counseling prospective parents about prenatal testing. Factors that can influence prospective parents' choices about prenatal testing include their risk for transmitting genetic abnormalities to the fetus and their perception of potential complications and benefits of both CVS and amniocentesis. Prospective parents who are considering the use of either procedure should be provided with current data for informed decision making. Individualized counseling should address the following:

Indications for Procedures and Limitations of Prenatal Testing

- Counselors should discuss the prospective parents' degree of risk for transmitting genetic abnormalities based on factors such as maternal age, race, and family history.

- Prospective parents should be made aware of both the limitations and usefulness of either CVS or amniocentesis in detecting abnormalities.

Potential Serious Complications from CVS and Amniocentesis

- Counselors should discuss the risk for miscarriage attributable to both procedures: the risk from amniocentesis at 15-18 weeks' gestation is approximately 0.25%-0.50% (1/400-1/200), and the miscarriage risk from CVS is approximately 0.5%-1.0% (1/200-1/100).

- Current data indicate that the overall risk for transverse limb deficiency from CVS is 0.03%-0.10% (1/3,000-1/1,000). Current data indicate no increase in risk for limb deficiency after amniocentesis at 15-18 weeks' gestation.

- The risk and severity of limb deficiency appear to be associated with the timing of CVS: the risk earlier than 10 weeks' gestation (0.20%) is higher than the risk from CVS done earlier than 10 weeks' gestation (0.07%). Most defects associated with CVS at 210 weeks' gestation have been limited to the digits.

Timing of Procedures

- The timing of obtaining results from either CVS or amniocentesis is relevant because of the increased risks for maternal morbidity and mortality associated with terminating pregnancy during the second trimester compared with the first trimester.

- Many amniocentesis procedures are now done at 11-14 weeks' gestation; however, further controlled studies are necessary to fully assess the safety of early amniocentesis.

Chapter 61

Electronic Fetal Monitoring

The unborn baby's heart rate is an important indicator of how things are going. The heartbeat can be monitored by a care-giver with a special stethoscope called a fetoscope or by an electronic fetal monitor.

Electronic fetal monitors, which are FDA-approved medical devices, measure the baby's heart rate continuously in one of two ways: externally or internally. With external monitors, two belts are placed around the mother's abdomen. One belt uses ultrasound to monitor the baby's heartbeat while the other measures the length of contractions. Internal monitors measure the baby's heart rate through an electrode attached to the baby's scalp.

Both types of monitors usually require the mother to stay in bed so the belts or electrodes stay in place.

Although measuring and recording every heartbeat sounds ideal, not everyone thinks the technology is an advantage.

"When I started delivering babies in 1971," says FDA's Phill Price, M.D., "physicians really believed that electronic fetal monitoring would be a tool that would tell us if a baby was going to be in trouble. But the last 8 to 10 years have told us that electronic fetal monitoring has not done a lot to actually improve the overall care of mothers or babies."

The theory behind the continuous monitoring is that the care-giver could note a change in the baby's heart rate immediately and take

This chapter contains text from *FDA Consumer*, December 1992 by Dori Stehlin and Online Publication of the U.S. Preventative Services Task Force, Feb. 1997 by Carolyn DiGuiseppi.

immediate action to prevent any harm to the baby. That action, almost always, is a Caesarean section.

The harm doctors are most concerned about is oxygen starvation, which can lead to conditions such as cerebral palsy.

However, in the last 25 years the incidence of cerebral palsy has remained the same—3 per 1,000 whether the patient was monitored or not, says Price.

Some babies are going to have problems, and in all likelihood those problems occurred during the nine months of pregnancy, he explains. "To think that because I waited 5 or 10 or 15 minutes before doing a C-section the baby will come up with cerebral palsy is ludicrous," he says. "If you have a nurse who listens every 15 minutes in the first stage of labor and every five minutes in the second stage, you can get the same outcome."

"If I'm physically present, I can be pretty sure if things are fine or if things are starting to go wrong," says Barbara Good, a certified nurse-midwife in Takoma Park, Md.

But Wayne Cohen, M.D., of the Albert Einstein College of Medicine in New York City, says he has serious doubts about replacing electronic monitors with "old-fashioned" intermittent listening to the heart rate, because a monitor can pick up very uncommon patterns that might be missed by the intermittent method. While he agrees with Price that some of those uncommon patterns may indicate brain damage that occurred before labor even began, "I don't think our knowledge is sophisticated enough yet to be able to be say when we see a very abnormal pattern that no benefit can be accrued by delivering as quickly as possible."

Accuracy of Fetal Monitoring

The principal screening technique for fetal distress and hypoxia during labor is the measurement of fetal heart rate. Abnormal decelerations in fetal heart rate and decreased beat-to-beat variability during uterine contractions are considered to be suggestive of fetal distress. The detection of these patterns during monitoring by auscultation or during electronic monitoring (cardiotocography) increases the likelihood that the fetus is in distress, but the patterns are not diagnostic. In addition, normal or equivocal heart rate patterns do not exclude the diagnosis of fetal distress. Precise information on the frequency of false-negative and false-positive results is lacking, however, due in large part to the absence of an accepted definition of fetal distress. For many years, acidosis and hypoxemia as determined by fetal scalp blood pH were used for this purpose in research and clinical practice, but it is now clear that neither finding is diagnostic of fetal distress.

Electronic fetal heart rate monitoring can detect at least some cases of fetal distress, and it is often used for routine monitoring of women in labor. In 1991, the reported rate of electronic fetal monitoring in the U.S. was 755/1,000 live births. The published performance characteristics of this technology, derived largely from research at major academic centers, may overestimate the accuracy that can be expected when this test is performed for routine screening in typical community settings. Two factors in particular that may limit the accuracy and reliability achievable in actual practice are the method used to measure fetal heart activity and the variability associated with cardiotocogram interpretations.

Measurement of Fetal Heart Rate

The measurement of fetal heart activity is performed most accurately by attaching an electrode directly to the fetal scalp, an invasive procedure requiring amniotomy and associated with occasional complications. This has been the technique used in most clinical trials of electronic fetal monitoring.

Other noninvasive techniques of monitoring fetal heart rate, which include external Doppler ultrasound and periodic auscultation of heart sounds by clinicians, are more appropriate for widespread screening but provide less precise data than the direct electrocardiogram using a fetal scalp electrode. In studies comparing external ultrasound with the direct electrocardiogram, about 20-25% of tracings differed by at least 5 beats per minute.

A second factor influencing the reliability of widespread fetal heart rate monitoring is inconsistency in interpreting results. Several studies have documented significant intra- and interobserver variation in assessing cardiotocograms even when tracings are read by experts in electronic fetal monitoring. It would be expected that routine performance of electronic monitoring in the community setting with interpretations by less experienced clinicians would generate a higher proportion of inaccurate results and potentially unnecessary interventions than has been observed in the published work of major research centers.

Recommendations of Other Groups

The American College of Obstetricians and Gynecologists states that all patients in labor need some form of fetal monitoring, with more intensified monitoring indicated in high-risk pregnancies; the choice of technique (electronic fetal monitoring or intermittent auscultation) is based on various factors, including the resources available. The Canadian Task Force on the Periodic Health Examination advises against routine electronic fetal monitoring in normal pregnancies but found poor evidence regarding the inclusion or exclusion of its routine use in high-risk pregnancies.

Discussion

Electronic fetal monitoring has become an accepted standard of care in many settings in the U.S. for the management of labor. Birth certificate data suggest that this technology was used in about three fourths of all live births in 1991; in certain academic centers the rate may be as high as 86-100%. As discussed above, there are important questions regarding the definition of fetal distress, as well as about the accuracy and reliability of electronic fetal monitoring in discriminating accurately between pregnancies with and without this disorder. It is also unclear whether the use of this technology results in significantly improved outcome for the baby when compared to active clinical monitoring. Adequately conducted trials generalizable to obstetric care in the U.S. have not reported a reduction in perinatal mortality, although sample sizes are not adequate to exclude a benefit.

Evidence does support a reduced risk of neonatal seizures, but the benefit was mainly seen in women with complicated labors (i.e., induced, augmented with oxytocin, or prolonged), and it is not clear that there are long-term adverse effects associated with the types of seizures prevented. Follow-up of study subjects at 9 months to 4 years of age has not revealed any long-term neurologic benefits from electronic monitoring. If anything, effect estimates suggest an increased risk of cerebral palsy and low developmental scores in electronically monitored infants, possibly due to false reassurance and consequent delayed intervention.

In addition to the maternal risks associated with electronic fetal monitoring, including increased rates of cesarean or operative vaginal (e.g., forceps) delivery, general anesthesia and maternal infection, and the possible increased risk of adverse neonatal neurologic outcome, increased use of this technology is associated with increased costs of labor care. The widespread use of electronic fetal monitoring in low-risk pregnancies in the face of uncertain benefits, and certain maternal risks and costs, has been attributed to concerns about litigation.

It has been estimated that nearly 40% of all obstetric malpractice losses are due to fetal monitoring problems, and this may be a major motivating factor behind the widespread use of electronic fetal monitoring during labor.

Clinical Intervention

Routine electronic fetal monitoring is not recommended for low-risk women in labor when adequate clinical monitoring including intermittent auscultation by trained staff is available. There is insufficient evidence to recommend for or against electronic fetal monitoring over intermittent auscultation for high-risk pregnancies.

For pregnant women with complicated labor (i.e., induced, prolonged, or oxytocin augmented), recommendations for electronic monitoring plus scalp blood sampling may be made on the basis of evidence for a reduced risk of neonatal seizures, although the long-term neurologic benefit to the neonate is unclear and must be weighed against the increased risk to the mother and neonate of operative delivery, general anesthesia, and maternal infection, and a possible increased risk of adverse neurologic outcome in the infant. There is currently no evidence available to evaluate electronic fetal monitoring in comparison to no monitoring.

Chapter 62

Medical Care and Your Newborn

By the time you hold your new baby in your arms for the first time, chances are you have already chosen one of the most important people in his early life—his pediatrician. You and your baby will probably visit the pediatrician more often during the first year than at any other time.

You may have had a prenatal visit with your baby's doctor-to-be to discuss some specifics, such as when he or she will see your newborn for the first time, office hours and on-call hours, who fills in for your doctor when he or she is out of the office, and how the office handles after-hours emergencies. You may have also learned your pediatrician's views on certain issues. In this way, you've begun to forge a relationship with your baby's doctor that should last through the bumps, bruises, and midnight fevers to come.

What Will Happen Right after Birth?

Depending on your desires and the rules of the hospital or birth center where your baby is delivered, his first exam will either take place in the nursery or at your side. His weight, length, and head circumference will be measured. His temperature will be taken, and his breathing and heart rate will be measured. The doctor or nurse will monitor the color of his skin and his activity. He'll receive special eye drops to ward off infection and a shot of vitamin K to prevent excessive bleeding. He'll eventually be given his first bath, and his umbilical cord stump will be cleaned.

Most hospitals and birthing centers provide personal instructions (and sometimes videos) to new parents that cover feeding, bathing, and other important aspects of newborn care.

When Will We See the Doctor?

The hospital or birth center where you deliver your baby will notify your pediatrician of his birth. If you have had any medical problems during pregnancy, or if any medical problems for your baby are suspected, the doctor may be alerted about the birth ahead of time and be standing by.

The doctor you have chosen for your newborn will probably give your baby a full physical examination within 24 hours of birth. You and your doctor will have the chance to talk about your new baby and the many aspects of parenting. This is also a good opportunity to ask any questions you have about your new baby's care. Find out when the pediatrician would like to see your newborn again. Most healthy newborns are routinely examined at the doctor's office when they are about two to four weeks old.

What Happens at the First Office Visit?

During the first office visit, your doctor will assess your baby in a variety of ways to see how he is doing. The first office visit will differ from doctor to doctor, but you can probably expect:

- Measurement of your baby's weight, length, and head circumference to assess how he's been doing since birth

- Testing of your newborn's vision, hearing, and reflexes

- A total physical examination to check for any abnormalities of the body or organ function

- Questions about how you are doing with the new baby and how your baby is eating and sleeping

- Advice on what you can expect in the coming month

- A discussion of your home environment and how it might affect your baby's health. For example, smoking in the house can negatively affect your baby's health in a number of ways.

Also, if the results of screening tests performed on your newborn after birth are available, they may be discussed with you. Bring to your doctor any questions or concerns you have at this time. Make sure to write down any specific instructions he or she gives you regarding special baby care. Keep a permanent medical record for your baby that includes information about his growth, immunizations, medications, and any problems or illnesses.

What Immunizations Will My Baby Receive?

A baby receives some natural immunity against many infectious diseases from his mother. A mother's infection-preventing antibodies are passed to her baby through the umbilical cord before the baby is born. This immunity is only temporary, but your baby will develop his own immunity against many infectious diseases. Breast-fed babies receive antibodies and enzymes in breast milk that help protect them from some infections and even some allergic conditions.

Most infants will receive their first artificial immunization, a hepatitis B vaccine (HBV), at birth or shortly after. This immunization is given in three doses. Although no other immunizations will be needed at this time, it's not too early to familiarize yourself with the standard immunization schedule.

When Should I Call the Doctor?

Since small problems can indicate big problems for newborns, don't hesitate to call your pediatrician if you have concerns. There are some difficulties that you should be aware of during this first month:

- Excessive drowsiness can be hard to spot in a newborn since most sleep so much. But if you suspect your infant is sleepier than normal, call your doctor. Sometimes this could mean there is an infection present in a baby's system.

- Eye problems can be caused by blockage of one or both tear ducts. Normally the ducts open on their own before too long, but sometimes they remain clogged, which can cause mucus-like tearing of the eyes. The white discharge can crust up on a baby's eyes and make it difficult for him to open his eyes, and the blockage can lead to infection. If you suspect a serious infection, such as pink-eye (conjunctivitis), call your pediatrician immediately. If your baby has an infection, your doctor will need to examine him and may prescribe special drops and a special method of cleaning your baby's eyes with sterile water.

• Fever in a newborn (rectal temperature above 100.4 degrees F) should be reported to your doctor right away.

• Extreme floppiness or jitters in a baby could be a sign of underlying problems. Report them to your doctor immediately.

• A runny nose can make it difficult for a baby to breathe, especially when he's feeding. You can help ease your baby's discomfort by using a rubber bulb aspirator to gently suction mucus from his nose. Be sure to call your doctor—even a common cold can be dangerous for a newborn.

• While breast-fed newborns generally have loose, mustard-colored stools, very loose and watery stools could indicate illness. The danger here for a baby is dehydration, which can show up as a dry mouth and a noticeable reduction in urine output (fewer than six wet diapers in 24 hours). Call your doctor if your newborn's stools seem watery or loose or if they often occur at other times besides after feeding.

Part Eleven

Sexually Transmitted Disease (STD) Tests

Chapter 63

Introduction to Sexually Transmitted Diseases

Sexually transmitted diseases (STDs), once called venereal diseases, are among the most common infectious diseases in the United States today. More than 20 STDs have now been identified, and they affect more than 13 million men and women in this country each year. The annual comprehensive cost of STDs in the United States is estimated to be well in excess of $10 billion.

Understanding the basic facts about STDs—the ways in which they are spread, their common symptoms, and how they can be treated— is the first step toward prevention. The National Institute of Allergy and Infectious Diseases (NIAID), a part of the National Institutes of Health provides this important information. Research investigators supported by NIAID are looking for better methods of diagnosis and more effective treatments, as well as for vaccines and topical microbicides to prevent STDs. It is important to understand at least five key points about all STDs in the U.S. today:

1. STDs affect men and women of all backgrounds and economic levels. They are most prevalent among teenagers and young adults. Nearly two-thirds of all STDs occur in people younger than 25 years of age.

2. The incidence of STDs is rising, in part because in the last few decades, young people have become sexually active earlier yet

National Institute of Allergy and Infectious Diseases (NIAID), NIH, June 1998.

are marrying later. In addition, divorce is more common. The net result is that sexually active people today are more likely to have multiple sex partners during their lives and are potentially at risk for developing STDs.

3. Most of the time, STDs cause no symptoms, particularly in women. When and if symptoms develop, they may be confused with those of other diseases not transmitted through sexual contact. Even when an STD causes no symptoms, however, a person who is infected may be able to pass the disease on to a sex partner. That is why many doctors recommend periodic testing or screening for people who have more than one sex partner.

4. Health problems caused by STDs tend to be more severe and more frequent for women than for men, in part because the frequency of asymptomatic infection means that many women do not seek care until serious problems have developed.

    *   Some STDs can spread into the uterus (womb) and fallopian tubes to cause pelvic inflammatory disease (PID), which in turn is a major cause of both infertility and ectopic (tubal) pregnancy. The latter can be fatal.

    *   STDs in women also may be associated with cervical cancer. One STD, human papillomavirus infection (HPV) causes genital warts and cervical and other genital cancers.

    *   STDs can be passed from a mother to her baby before, during, or immediately after birth; some of these infections of the newborn can be cured easily, but others may cause a baby to be permanently disabled or even die.

5. When diagnosed and treated early, many STDs can be treated effectively. Some infections have become resistant to the drugs used to treat them and now require newer types of antibiotics. Experts believe that having STDs other than AIDS increases one's risk for becoming infected with the AIDS virus.

Chapter 64

Testing for HIV

Should You Have the HIV Test?

This chapter talks about testing for HIV, the virus that causes AIDS. To find out if you should take the test to know if you have HIV, (sometimes called the AIDS test), answer these questions.

Have you—

- had sex without knowing for sure if the person or persons you had sex with do not have HIV?

- had sex with someone you know has HIV or AIDS?

- had a disease passed on by sex, like genital herpes or syphilis? (Having these diseases makes it easier to get HIV.)

- had sex with many men or women or had sex with someone who has had sex with many men or women?

- had sex with someone who has used needles to take drugs?

- shared needles or equipment to take drugs?

This chapter includes text from "Taking the HIV (AIDS) Test, How to Help Yourself," National Institute of Allergy and Infectious Diseases (NIAID), Fact Sheet, available at: www.niaid.nih.gov/publications/help/test.htm, NIH Publication No. 95-3322; "New Ways to Prevent and Treat AIDS" by Mike Kubic, *FDA Consumer* January-February 1997, revised May 1997 and January 1998, *Publication No. (FDA) 98-1268;* and "FDA Talk Paper" by Lenore Gelb, August 6, 1996.

If you have answered "yes" to any of these questions, you should think about having the HIV test.

How HIV Testing Can Help You

If tests show you don't have HIV, you can learn how to stay HIV-free. (Someone who does not have HIV is called HIV-negative.)

If tests show you do have HIV, you can get medical care right away to help you:

- Stay healthy longer
- Avoid getting some illnesses caused by HIV
- Get early treatment for illnesses that do occur

Testing is the only way to know if you have HIV, and testing is the first step to getting medical care, counseling, and support if you need it.

Before You Take the Test

Taking the HIV test can help you, but it is a big step. You should think about how having HIV could affect your life. These steps can help you prepare to take the test.

1. Consider telling someone you trust that you are having the HIV test. Support of a family member or friend can mean a lot.

2. Find out how private your test results will be. Ask the clinic if anyone but you can learn your test results.

3. Set a time to get your results. Don't put it off. The test can only help you when you find out what it shows.

How the HIV Test Works

The HIV test shows if you have signs in your blood of the virus that causes AIDS. HIV testing has four steps.

1. You go to the clinic or doctor's office. A nurse or counselor tells you about the test. You can ask questions and talk about your fears and concerns.

2. You decide to have the test. A nurse or aide takes some blood from your arm using a needle.

3. Your blood is tested for signs of HIV. If the first test (called ELISA) is positive (shows signs of HIV), the blood will be tested again. If the second test is positive, another kind of test (called a Western blot) will be done to confirm the result.

4. Test results come back to the clinic. A nurse or counselor tells you when to come in, what the results mean, and how to help yourself.

New Ways to Prevent and Treat AIDS

Preventing and treating AIDS is one of the Food and Drug Administration's top priorities. A new class of drugs, a home blood test collection kit, an oral diagnostic test, an HIV antigen test, an HIV-1 antigen test for blood supply, and an HIV viral load test are among the most recent in a long line of products FDA has approved to prevent, diagnose and treat infection with HIV, the virus that causes AIDS.

HIV Tests

The 1992 National Health Interview Survey by the Centers for Disease Control and Prevention found that only 20 percent of people at increased risk for HIV infection—such as intravenous drug users, male homosexuals, and prostitutes—agreed to be tested for HIV. More than twice that many people in the same risk group said they might use a home testing and counseling service if one were available. At the time, however, testing could be done only by a professional.

The situation changed, in May 1996, when FDA approved the first HIV test system with a home-use blood collection kit. The only one on the market, as of December 1997, is the Home Access Express HIV-1 Test System. It is hoped that home testing will make diagnosis easier and more accessible, especially in populations among whom the recent rise in cases of HIV is greatest, such as women, African Americans, and Hispanics. The tests are highly reliable and are designed to protect the user's anonymity.

FDA's approval on June 3, 1996, of OraSure Western blot, a laboratory test that does not require a blood sample, is also expected to increase participation in testing for HIV. Instead of pricking a finger—a procedure shunned by many individuals—OraSure uses a treated cotton pad to collect an oral specimen from between the gum and cheek.

The sample is tested for antibodies to HIV by a procedure that has been shown to be highly accurate. An earlier version of OraSure used a less reliable method to screen for HIV antibodies, and people who tested positive had to undergo a standard blood test to confirm the presence of the virus.

In March 1996, FDA approved the Coulter HIV-1 p24 Antigen Assay, the first blood screening test to detect antigens rather than antibodies. In screening routinely carried out since the mid-1980s, technicians check donated blood for HIV-1 antibodies by using enzyme-linked immunosorbent assay (ELISA) test kits. Since a small number of ELISA test results are nonspecific or falsely positive, the standard procedure uses a second, more specific test—the Western blot test—to validate the positive results from ELISA testing.

The Coulter test, which is used in addition to ELISA, screens blood for antigens—proteins found on the surface of the virus—that are detectable about one week earlier than HIV antibodies. The new test reduces the so-called "window" period, typically up to three months long, during which standard blood tests show no HIV antibodies, even though the donor may be infected.

The Amplicor HIV-1 Monitor Test, another new blood test approved last year, enables physicians to predict the risk of HIV disease progression by precisely measuring virus levels in blood. The test, which amplifies copies of genetic material from the virus by using polymerase chain reaction technology, is based on clinical studies showing that higher virus levels can be correlated with increased risk that the disease will progress to AIDS, and AIDS-related infection or death.

FDA Approves First Urine–Based HIV Test

The Food and Drug Administration has approved the first HIV test that uses urine samples. All previously approved HIV tests use either blood or oral fluid samples. The new urine-based test detects the presence of antibodies to HIV-1, the virus that causes the vast majority of U.S. AIDS cases, using an enzyme-linked immunosorbent assay (ELISA) method.

The test is approved to screen for HIV-1 infection and may be useful for medical purposes when the collection of blood samples is impractical. The test is manufactured by the Calypte Biomedical Corporation of Berkeley, Calif., and will be marketed as the Calypte HI-1 Urine EIA. It will also be marketed by Seradyn Inc. of Indianapolis, Indiana as the Seradyn Sentinel HIV-1 Urine EIA.

The test can be ordered only by a physician. Samples will be analyzed in certified medical laboratories. Any initially reactive sample will be retested twice. If even one of the second tests is reactive, the screening test will be considered positive, although this positive result does not always indicate HIV infection. For confirming a positive screening test, anyone testing positive with the Calypte test must be retested with a more accurate test using a blood sample.

A patient information sheet provided with the new test will outline the limitations of urine HIV-1 testing in addition to the usual information on HIV and AIDS provided to people before HIV testing. After reading the information sheet, the person being tested will initial the statement confirming the receipt of the pre-test counseling, peel off the sample label and apply it to the urine collection cup.

FDA's approval was based on clinical studies demonstrating that the test is sufficiently accurate for screening in medical and public health settings. The urine-based ELISA test is not approved to screen blood donors. For that purpose, more accurate ELISA tests using blood samples are required. In the clinical studies, urine and blood samples were taken from 298 patients diagnosed with AIDS and tested with both the Calypte HIV-1 Urine EIA and a licensed ELISA test using a blood specimen. The urine test was positive as an initial screening test 99.3% of the time in persons known to have AIDS. In asymptomatic HIV-1 infected patients, the test would be expected to miss 1 or 2 people in every 100. Other studies showed that the urine-based test would give a falsely positive result in one or two people out of 100 without HIV-1 antibodies in their blood, compared to one in 1000 with a blood-based ELISA test.

To Find Out More

To learn more about HIV and where to get the test in your city or town, call:

- 1-800-342-AIDS (1-800-342-2437)
- Your local health department

People at these numbers can answer your questions about HIV. They can also send you booklets that have more information.

Remember: If the HIV test is positive, it will mean that you have the HIV virus that causes AIDS. It will mean you can get medical care and support services to help you if you need them.

More information about AIDS and HIV is also available from FDA's Office of AIDS and Special Health Issues on the World Wide Web at www.fda.gov/.

Chapter 65

Pelvic Inflammatory Disease

Aside from AIDS, the most common and serious complication of sexually transmitted diseases (STDs) among women is pelvic inflammatory disease (PID), an infection of the upper genital tract. PID can affect the uterus, ovaries, fallopian tubes, or other related structures. Untreated, PID causes scarring and can lead to infertility, tubal pregnancy, chronic pelvic pain, and other serious consequences.

Each year in the United States, more than 1 million women experience an episode of acute PID, with the rate of infection highest among teenagers. More than 100,000 women become infertile each year as a result of PID, and a large proportion of the 70,000 ectopic (tubal) pregnancies occurring every year are due to the consequences of PID. In 1997 alone, an estimated $7 billion was spent on PID and its complications.

Symptoms

The major symptoms of PID are lower abdominal pain and abnormal vaginal discharge. Other symptoms such as fever, pain in the right upper abdomen, painful intercourse, and irregular menstrual bleeding can occur as well. PID, particularly when caused by chlamydial infection, may produce only minor symptoms or no symptoms at all, even though it can seriously damage the reproductive organs.

National Institute of Allergy and Infectious Diseases, NIH, June 1998.

Risk Factors for PID

- Women with STDs—especially gonorrhea and chlamydial infection—are at greater risk of developing PID; a prior episode of PID increases the risk of another episode because the body's defenses are often damaged during the initial bout of upper genital tract infection.

- Sexually active teenagers are more likely to develop PID than are older women.

- The more sexual partners a woman has, the greater her risk of developing PID.

Recent data indicate that women who douche once or twice a month may be more likely to have PID than those who douche less than once a month. Douching may push bacteria into the upper genital tract. Douching also may ease discharge caused by an infection, so the woman delays seeking health care.

Diagnosis

PID can be difficult to diagnose. If symptoms such as lower abdominal pain are present, the doctor will perform a physical exam to determine the nature and location of the pain. The doctor also should check the patient for fever, abnormal vaginal or cervical discharge, and evidence of cervical chlamydial infection or gonorrhea. If the findings of this exam suggest that PID is likely, current guidelines advise doctors to begin treatment.

If more information is necessary, the doctor may order other tests, such as a sonogram, endometrial biopsy, or laparoscopy to distinguish between PID and other serious problems that may mimic PID. Laparoscopy is a surgical procedure in which a tiny, flexible tube with a lighted end is inserted through a small incision just below the navel. This procedure allows the doctor to view the internal abdominal and pelvic organs, as well as take specimens for cultures or microscopic studies, if necessary.

Treatment

Because culture of specimens from the upper genital tract are difficult to obtain and because multiple organisms may be responsible for an episode of PID, especially if it is not the first one, the doctor will prescribe at least two antibiotics that are effective against a wide range of infectious agents. The symptoms may go away before the infection is cured. Even if symptoms do go away, patients should finish taking all of the medicine. Patients should be re-evaluated by their physicians two to three days after treatment is begun to be sure the antibiotics are working to cure the infection.

About one-fourth of women with suspected PID must be hospitalized. The doctor may recommend this if the patient is severely ill; if she cannot take oral medication and needs intravenous antibiotics; if she is pregnant or is an adolescent; if the diagnosis is uncertain and may include an abdominal emergency such as appendicitis; or if she is infected with HIV (human immunodeficiency virus, the virus that causes AIDS).

Many women with PID have sex partners who have no symptoms, although their sex partners may be infected with organisms that can cause PID. Because of the risk of re-infection, however, sex partners should be treated even if they do not have symptoms.

Consequences of PID

Women with recurrent episodes of PID are more likely than women with a single episode to suffer scarring of the tubes that leads to infertility, tubal pregnancy, or chronic pelvic pain. Infertility occurs in approximately 20 percent of women who have had PID.

Most women with tubal infertility, however, never have had symptoms of PID. Organisms such as *C. trachomatis* can silently invade the fallopian tubes and cause scarring, which blocks the normal passage of eggs into the uterus.

A women who has had PID has a six-to-tenfold increased risk of tubal pregnancy, in which the egg can become fertilized but cannot pass into the uterus to grow. Instead, the egg usually attaches in the fallopian tube, which connects the ovary to the uterus. The fertilized egg cannot grow normally in the fallopian tube. This type of pregnancy is life threatening to the mother, and almost always fatal to her fetus. It is the leading cause of pregnancy-related death in African-American women.

In addition, untreated PID can cause chronic pelvic pain and scarring in about 20 percent of patients. These conditions are difficult to treat but are sometimes improved with surgery.

Another complication of PID is the risk of repeated attacks of PID. As many as one-third of women who have had PID will have the disease at least one more time. With each episode of re-infection, the risk of infertility is increased.

Prevention

Women can play an active role in protecting themselves from PID by taking the following steps:

- Signs of discharge with odor or bleeding between cycles could mean infection. Early treatment may prevent the development of PID.

- If used correctly and consistently, male latex condoms will prevent transmission of gonorrhea and partially protect against chlamydial infection.

Chapter 66

Chlamydial Infection

Chlamydial ("kla-mid-ee-uhl") infection is the most common bacterial sexually transmitted disease (STD) in the United States today. The U.S. Centers for Disease Control and Prevention estimates that more than 4 million new cases occur each year. The highest rates of chlamydial infection are in 15–19 year old adolescents regardless of demographics or location. Pelvic inflammatory disease (PID), a serious complication of chlamydial infection, has emerged as a major cause of infertility among women of childbearing age. Chlamydial infection is caused by a bacterium, *Chlamydia trachomatis*, and can be transmitted during vaginal, oral, or anal sexual contact with an infected partner. A pregnant woman may pass the infection to her newborn during delivery, with subsequent neonatal eye infection or pneumonia. The annual cost of chlamydial infection is estimated to exceed $2 billion.

Symptoms

Most chlamydial infections are silent, causing no symptoms. However, men and women with *C. trachomatis* may experience abnormal genital discharge or pain during urination. These early symptoms may be mild. If symptoms occur, they usually appear within one to three weeks after exposure. Two of every three infected women and one or two of every four infected men have no symptoms whatsoever. As a

National Institute of Allergy and Infectious Diseases, NIH, June 1998.

result, often the disease may not be diagnosed and treated until complications develop.

Diagnosis

Chlamydial infection can be confused with gonorrhea because the symptoms of both diseases are similar; in some populations they occur together. The most reliable way to diagnose chlamydial infection is for a clinician to send a sample of secretions from the patient's genital area to a laboratory that will look for the organism using one of a wide variety of quick and inexpensive laboratory tests. Although attempting to grow the organism in specialized tissue culture in the laboratory is one of the most definitive tests, it is expensive and technically difficult to do, and test results are not available for three or more days.

Scientists have developed several rapid tests for diagnosing chlamydial infection that use sophisticated techniques and a dye to detect bacterial proteins. Although these tests are slightly less accurate, they are less expensive, more rapid, and can be performed during a routine checkup. These tests use a process called DNA amplification to detect the genes of the organisms in genital secretions. Recently, the U.S. Food and Drug Administration approved this process for detection of *C. trachomatis* in urine. This is a major step in diagnosing chlamydial infection because it does not require an invasive sample; it can be used in settings where performing a pelvic examination is not convenient or not feasible, e.g., in college health units and at health fairs. Results from the urine test are available within 24 hours.

Treatment

Doctors usually prescribe antibiotics such as a one-day course of azithromycin or a seven-day course of doxycycline to treat chlamydial infection. Other antibiotics such as erythromycin or ofloxacin also are effective. Penicillin, which is often used for treating some other STDs, is not effective against chlamydial infections.

Pelvic Inflammatory Disease

Each year up to 1 million women in the United States develop PID, a serious infection of the reproductive organs. As many as half of all cases of PID may be due to chlamydial infection, and many of these occur without symptoms.

Prevention

Because chlamydial infection often occurs without symptoms, people who are infected may unknowingly infect their sex partners. Many doctors recommend that all persons who have more than one sex partner, especially women under 25 years of age, be tested for chlamydial infection regularly, even in the absence of symptoms. Using condoms or diaphragms during sexual intercourse may help reduce the transmission of chlamydia.

Chapter 67

Genital Herpes

Genital herpes is a contagious viral infection that affects an estimated one out of four (or 45 million) Americans. Doctors estimate that as many as 500,000 new cases may occur each year. The infection is caused by the herpes simplex virus (HSV). There are two types of HSV, and both can cause genital herpes. HSV type 1 most commonly causes sores on the lips (known as fever blisters or cold sores), but it can cause genital infections as well. HSV type 2 most often causes genital sores, but it also can infect the mouth.

Symptoms

Eighty percent of people with genital herpes are unaware of their disease because they never develop any symptoms or do not recognize them. When symptoms do occur, they vary widely from person to person. Symptoms of a first episode of genital herpes usually appear within two to 10 days of infection, and first episodes last an average of two to three weeks. Early symptoms can include an itching or burning sensation; pain in the legs, buttocks, or genital area; vaginal discharge; or a feeling of pressure in the abdominal region.

Within a few days, sores (also called lesions) appear at the site of infection. Lesions also can occur inside the vagina and on the cervix in women, or in the urinary passage of women and men. Small red

National Institute of Allergy and Infectious Diseases (NIAID), NIH, June 1998.

bumps appear first, develop into blisters, and then become painful open sores. Over a period of days, the sores become crusted and then heal without scarring. Other symptoms that may accompany the first or primary episode of genital herpes can include fever, headache, muscle aches, painful or difficult urination, vaginal discharge, and swollen glands in the groin area.

Recurrences

In genital herpes, after invading the skin or mucous membranes, the virus travels to the sensory nerves at the end of the spinal cord. Even after the skin lesions have disappeared, the virus remains inside the nerve cells in an inactive, latent state. In most people, the virus will reactivate monthly. It travels along the nerves to the skin, where it multiplies on the surface at or near the site of the original herpes sores, causing new sores to erupt. It also can reactivate without causing any visible sores. At these times, small amounts of the virus may be shed at or near sites of the original infection, in genital secretions, or from barely noticeable lesions. This shedding occurs without any pain or discomfort, it may last only a day, but it is possible to infect a sex partner during this time.

The symptoms of recurrent episodes usually are milder than those of the first episode and typically last about a week. The frequency and severity of the recurrent episodes vary greatly. While some people recognize only one or two recurrences in a lifetime, others may experience several outbreaks a year.

Diagnosis

The sores of genital herpes in its active stage may be visible to the naked eye. Several laboratory tests may be needed, however, to distinguish herpes sores from other infections. The most accurate method of diagnosis is by viral culture, in which a new sore is swabbed or scraped and the sample is added to a laboratory culture containing healthy cells. When examined under a microscope after one to two days, the cells show changes that indicate growth of the herpes virus.

A newer, more rapid, but somewhat less accurate way of diagnosing herpes involves detection of viral protein components in lesion swabs. These tests should be done when the sores first appear to ensure the most reliable results. Other laboratory tests also are available to physicians. It is important to recognize that the virus is hard to find and that although clinicians commonly fail to detect the virus in an active sore, this does not mean that a person does not have genital herpes.

A blood test cannot determine whether a person has an active genital herpes infection. A blood test, however, can detect antibodies to the virus, which indicate that the person has been infected with HSV at some time and has produced antibodies to it. (Antibodies are proteins made by a person's immune system to fight infections.) Unlike antibodies to some other viruses, however, antibodies to HSV only partially protect an individual against another infection with a different strain or a different type of herpes virus, and they do not prevent a reactivation of the latent virus. The standard blood tests only reliably indicate whether a patient has had a herpes infection, but it cannot tell if it is oral or genital.

New blood tests have been developed that can distinguish whether a person has had prior type 1 or type 2 infection, or both. These tests, however, are available mainly in research hospitals and are not currently available in the doctor's office.

Treatment

During an active herpes episode, whether primary or recurrent, it is important to follow a few simple steps to speed healing and to avoid spreading the infection to other sites of the body or to other people:

- Keep the infected area clean and dry to prevent secondary infections from developing.

- Try to avoid touching the sores; wash hands after contact with the sores.

- Avoid sexual contact from the time symptoms are first recognized until the sores are completely healed, i.e., the scab has fallen off and new skin has formed over the site of the lesion.

Researchers have shown that the oral form of acyclovir (Zovirax®) is a superior and safe treatment that helps patients with first or recurrent episodes of genital herpes.

The U.S. Food and Drug Administration recently approved two new drugs, famciclovir (Famvir®) and valacyclovir (Valtrex®), to treat recurrent episodes of genital herpes. Famciclovir also has been approved for use in suppressing viral activity and preventing recurrences.

Complications

Usually, genital herpes infections do not cause permanent disability or long-term damage in healthy adults. In people who have suppressed immune systems, however, HSV episodes can be long-lasting and unusually severe. A pregnant woman who develops a first episode of genital herpes can pass the virus to her fetus and may be at higher risk for premature delivery. Half of the babies infected with herpes either die or suffer neurologic damage. A baby born with herpes can develop encephalitis (inflammation of the brain), severe rashes, and eye problems.

HSV and AIDS

Genital herpes, like other genital ulcer diseases, increases the risk of acquiring HIV, the virus that causes AIDS, by providing an accessible point of entry for HIV. Also, prior to effective therapy for AIDS, persons with HIV had severe herpes outbreaks, and this may help transmit both herpes and HIV infections to others.

Prevention

People with early signs of a herpes outbreak or with visible sores should not have sexual intercourse until the sores have healed completely. Between outbreaks, using condoms during sexual intercourse may offer partial protection. Use of chronic suppressive acyclovir therapy offers promise for reducing transmission.

Chapter 68

Vaginitis

Vaginitis Due to Vaginal Infections

Vaginitis is an inflammation of the vagina characterized by discharge, odor, irritation, and/or itching. The cause of vaginitis may not always be determined adequately solely on the basis of symptoms or a physical examination. For a correct diagnosis, a doctor should perform laboratory tests including microscopic evaluation of vaginal fluid. A variety of effective drugs are available for treating vaginitis.

Vaginitis often is caused by infections, which cause distress and discomfort. Some infections are associated with more serious diseases. The most common vaginal infections are bacterial vaginosis, trichomoniasis, and vaginal yeast infection or candidiasis. Some vaginal infections are transmitted through sexual contact, but others such as yeast infections probably are not, depending on the cause.

Bacterial Vaginosis

Bacterial vaginosis (BV) is the most common cause of vaginitis symptoms among women of childbearing age. Previously called nonspecific vaginitis or *Gardnerella*-associated vaginitis, BV is associated with sexual activity. BV reflects a change in the vaginal ecosystem. This imbalance, including pH changes, occurs when different types of bacteria outnumber the normal ones. Instead of *Lactobacillus* bacteria

The National Institute of Allergy and Infectious Diseases (NIAID), NIH, June 1998.

being the most numerous, increased numbers of organisms such as *Gardnerella vaginalis, Bacteroides, Mobiluncus,* and *Mycoplasma hominis* are found in the vaginas of women with BV. Investigators are studying the role that each of these microbes may play in causing BV, but they do not yet understand the role of sexual activity in developing BV. A change in sexual partners and douching may increase the risk of acquiring bacterial vaginosis.

Symptoms. The primary symptom of BV is an abnormal, odorous vaginal discharge. The fish-like odor is noticeable especially after intercourse. Nearly half of the women with clinical signs of BV, however, report no symptoms. A physician may observe these signs during a physical examination and may confirm the diagnosis by doing tests of vaginal fluid.

Diagnosis. A healthcare worker can examine a sample of vaginal fluid under a microscope, either stained or in special lighting, to detect the presence of the organisms associated with BV. They can make a diagnosis based on the absence of lactobacilli, the presence of numerous "clue cells" (cells from the vaginal lining that are coated with BV organisms), a fishy odor, and decreased acidity or change in pH of vaginal fluid.

Treatment. All women with BV should be informed of their diagnoses, including the possibility of sexual transmission, and offered treatment. They can be treated with antibiotics such as metronidazole or clindamycin. Generally, male sex partners are not treated. Many women with symptoms of BV do not seek medical treatment, and many asymptomatic women decline treatment.

Complications. Researchers have shown an association between BV and pelvic inflammatory disease (PID), which can cause infertility and tubal (ectopic) pregnancy. BV also can cause adverse outcomes of pregnancy such as premature delivery and low-birth-weight infants.

Trichomoniasis

Trichomoniasis, sometimes referred to as "trich", is a common STD that affects 2 to 3 million Americans yearly. It is caused by a single-celled protozoan parasite called *Trichomonas vaginalis*. Trichomoniasis is primarily an infection of the urogenital tract; the urethra is the most common site of infection in man, and the vagina is the most common site of infection in women.

Symptoms. Trichomoniasis, like many other STDs, often occurs without any symptoms. Men almost never have symptoms. When women have symptoms, they usually appear within four to 20 days of exposure. The symptoms in women include a heavy, yellow-green or gray vaginal discharge, discomfort during intercourse, vaginal odor, and painful urination. Irritation and itching of the female genital area, and on rare occasions, lower abdominal pain also can be present. The symptoms in men, if present, include a thin, whitish discharge from the penis and painful or difficult urination.

Treatment. Because men can transmit the disease to their sex partners even when symptoms are not present, it is preferable to treat both partners to eliminate the parasite. Metronidazole is the drug used to treat people with trichomoniasis. It usually is administered in a single dose. People taking this drug should not drink alcohol because mixing the two substances occasionally can cause severe nausea and vomiting.

Complications. Research has shown a link between trichomoniasis and two serious sequelae. Data suggest that trichomoniasis is associated with increased risk of transmission of HIV and may cause a woman to deliver a low-birth-weight or premature infant. Additional research is needed to fully explore these relationships.

Prevention. Use of male condoms may help prevent the spread of trichomoniasis, although careful studies have never been done that focus on how to prevent this infection.

Vaginal Yeast Infection

Vaginal yeast infection or vulvovaginal candidiasis is a common cause of vaginal irritation. Doctors estimate that approximately 75 percent of all women will experience at least one symptomatic yeast infection during their lifetimes.

Symptoms. The most frequent symptoms of yeast infection in women are itching, burning, and irritation of the vagina. Painful urination and/or intercourse are common. Vaginal discharge is not always present and may be minimal. The thick, whitish-gray discharge is typically described as cottage-cheese-like in nature, although it can vary from watery to thick in consistency. Most male partners of women with yeast infection do not experience any symptoms of the infection.

A transient rash and burning sensation of the penis, however, have been reported after intercourse if condoms were not used. These symptoms are usually self-limiting.

Diagnosis. Because few specific signs and symptoms are usually present, this condition cannot be diagnosed by the patient's history and physical examination. The doctor usually diagnoses yeast infection through microscopic examination of vaginal secretions for evidence of yeast forms.

Scientists funded by the National Institute of Allergy and Infectious Diseases (NIAID) have developed a rapid simple test for yeast infection, which will soon be available for use in doctors' offices. If such a test were available for home screening, it would help them to appropriately use yeast medication.

Treatment. Various antifungal vaginal medications are available to treat yeast infection. Women can buy some antifungal creams, tablets, or suppositories (butoconazole, miconazole, clotrimazole, and tioconazole) over the counter for use in the vagina. But because BV, trichomoniasis, and yeast infection are difficult to distinguish on the basis of symptoms alone, a woman with vaginal symptoms should see her physician for an accurate diagnosis before using these products.

Other Causes of Vaginitis

Although most vaginal infections in women are due to bacterial vaginosis, trichomoniasis, or yeast, there may be other causes as well. These causes may include allergic and irritative factors or other STDs.

Chapter 69

Syphilis

Syphilis, once a cause of devastating epidemics, can be effectively diagnosed and treated with antibiotic therapy. In 1996, 11,387 cases of primary and secondary syphilis in the United States were reported to the U.S. Centers for Disease Control and Prevention. Although treatment is available, the early symptoms of syphilis can be very mild, and many people do not seek treatment when they first become infected. Of increasing concern is the fact that syphilis increases the risk of transmitting and acquiring the human immunodeficiency virus (HIV) that causes AIDS.

Symptoms

The first symptom of *primary syphilis* is an ulcer called a chancre ("shan-ker"). The chancre can appear within 10 days to three months after exposure, but it generally appears within two to six weeks. Because the chancre may be painless and may occur inside the body, it may go unnoticed. It usually is found on the part of the body exposed to the partner's ulcer, such as the penis, the vulva, or the vagina. A chancre also can develop on the cervix, tongue, lips, or other parts of the body. The chancre disappears within a few weeks whether or not a person is treated. If not treated during the primary stage, about one-third of people will progress to chronic stages.

National Institute of Allergy and Infectious Diseases (NIAID), NIH, July 1998.

Secondary syphilis is often marked by a skin rash that is characterized by brown sores about the size of a penny. The rash appears anywhere from three to six weeks after the chancre appears. While the rash may cover the whole body or appear only in a few areas, the palms of the hands and soles of the feet are almost always involved. Because active bacteria are present in these sores, any physical contact—sexual or nonsexual—with the broken skin of an infected person may spread the infection at this stage. The rash usually heals within several weeks or months. Other symptoms also may occur, such as mild fever, fatigue, headache, sore throat, as well as patchy hair loss, and swollen lymph glands throughout the body. These symptoms may be very mild and, like the chancre of primary syphilis, will disappear without treatment. The signs of secondary syphilis may come and go over the next one to two years.

If untreated, syphilis may lapse into a *latent* stage during which the disease is no longer contagious and no symptoms are present. Many people who are not treated will suffer no further consequences of the disease. Approximately one-third of those who have secondary syphilis, however, go on to develop the complications of late, or *tertiary*, syphilis, in which the bacteria damage the heart, eyes, brain, nervous system, bones, joints, or almost any other part of the body. This stage can last for years, or even for decades. Late syphilis, the final stage, can result in mental illness, blindness, other neurologic problems, heart disease, and death.

Neurosyphilis: Syphilis bacteria frequently invade the nervous system during the early stages of infection, and approximately 3 to 7 percent of persons with untreated syphilis develop neurosyphilis. Some persons with neurosyphilis never develop any symptoms. Others may have headache, stiff neck, and fever that result from an inflammation of the lining of the brain. Some patients develop seizures. Patients whose blood vessels are affected may develop symptoms of stroke with resulting numbness, weakness, or visual complaints. In some instances, the time from infection to developing neurosyphilis may be up to 20 years. Neurosyphilis may be more difficult to treat and its course may be different in people with HIV infection.

Diagnosis

Syphilis has sometimes been called "the great imitator" because its early symptoms are similar to those of many other diseases. Sexually active people should consult a doctor about any suspicious rash or sore in the genital area. Those who have been treated for another

STD, such as gonorrhea, should be tested to be sure they have not also acquired syphilis.

There are three ways to diagnose syphilis: a doctor's recognition of its signs and symptoms; microscopic identification of syphilis bacteria; and blood tests. The doctor usually uses these approaches together to detect syphilis and decide upon the stage of infection.

To diagnose syphilis by identifying the bacteria, the doctor takes a scraping from the surface of the ulcer or chancre, and examines it under a special "darkfield" microscope to detect the organism itself. Blood tests also provide evidence of infection, although they may give false- negative results (not show signs of infection despite its presence) for up to three months after infection. False-positive tests also can occur; therefore, two blood tests are usually used. Interpretation of blood tests for syphilis can be difficult, and repeated tests are sometimes necessary to confirm the diagnosis.

The blood-screening tests most often used to detect evidence of syphilis are the VDRL (Venereal Disease Research Laboratory) test and the RPR (rapid plasma reagin) test. The false-positive results (showing signs of infection when it is not present) occur in people with autoimmune disorders, certain viral infections, and other conditions.

Therefore, a doctor will administer a confirmatory blood test when the initial test is positive. These tests include the fluorescent treponemal antibody-absorption (FTA-ABS) test that can accurately detect 70 to 90 percent of cases. Another specific test is the *T. pallidum* hemagglutination assay (TPHA). These tests detect syphilis antibodies (proteins made by a person's immune system to fight infection). They are not useful for diagnosing a new case of syphilis in patients who have had the disease previously because once antibodies are formed, they remain in the body for many years. These antibodies, however, do not protect against a new syphilis infection. In some patients with syphilis (especially in the latent or late stages), a lumbar puncture (spinal tap) must be done to check for infection of the nervous system.

Treatment

Syphilis usually is treated with penicillin, administered by injection. Other antibiotics can be used for patients allergic to penicillin. A person usually can no longer transmit syphilis 24 hours after beginning therapy. Some people, however, do not respond to the usual doses of penicillin. Therefore, it is important that people being treated for syphilis have periodic blood tests to check that the infectious agent has been completely destroyed. Persons with neurosyphilis may need to be retested for up to two years after treatment. In all stages of syphilis, proper treatment will cure the disease, but in late syphilis, damage already done to body organs cannot be reversed.

Effects of Syphilis in Pregnant Women

It is likely that an untreated pregnant woman with active syphilis will pass the infection to her unborn child. About 25 percent of these pregnancies result in stillbirth or neonatal death. Between 40 to 70 percent of such pregnancies will yield a syphilis-infected infant.

Prevention

The open sores of syphilis may be visible and infectious during the active stages of infection. Any contact with these infectious sores and other infected tissues and body fluids must be avoided to prevent spread of the disease. As with many other STDs, methods of prevention include using condoms during sexual intercourse. Screening and treatment of infected individuals, or secondary prevention, is one of the few options for preventing the advance stages of the disease. Testing and treatment early in pregnancy is the best way to prevent syphilis in infants and should be a routine part of prenatal care.

Chapter 70

Gonorrhea

In 1995, 392,848 cases of gonorrhea in the United States were reported to the U.S. Centers for Disease Control and Prevention (CDC). The Institute of Medicine, however, estimates that 800,000 cases of gonorrhea occur annually in the United States. The annual cost of gonorrhea and its complications is estimated at close to $1.1 billion.

Gonorrhea is caused by a bacterium, *Neisseria gonorrhoeae*, that grows and multiplies quickly in moist, warm areas of the body including the reproductive tract, the oral cavity, and the rectum. Although in women the cervix usually is the initial site of infection, the disease can spread to and infect the uterus (womb) and fallopian tubes, resulting in pelvic inflammatory disease (PID). This can cause infertility and ectopic (tubal) pregnancy.

The disease is most commonly spread during sexual intercourse—vaginal, oral, and anal. Gonorrhea of the rectum can occur in people who practice anal intercourse and also may occur in women due to spread of the infection from the vaginal area.

Gonorrhea can be passed from an infected woman to her newborn infant during delivery, causing eye infections in the baby. When the infection occurs in the genital tract, mouth, or rectum of a child, it is due most commonly to sexual abuse.

National Institute of Allergy and Infectious Diseases (NIAID), NIH, June 1998.

Symptoms

The early symptoms of gonorrhea often are mild, and many women who are infected have no symptoms of the disease. If symptoms of gonorrhea develop, they usually appear within two to ten days after sexual contact with an infected partner, although a small percentage of patients may be infected for several months without showing symptoms. The initial symptoms in women include a painful or burning sensation when urinating and/or vaginal discharge that is yellow or bloody. More advanced symptoms, which indicate progression to PID, include abdominal pain, bleeding between menstrual periods, vomiting, or fever. Men are more often symptomatic than women. They usually have a discharge from the penis and a burning sensation during urination that may be severe. Symptoms of rectal infection include discharge, anal itching, and sometimes painful bowel movements.

Diagnosis

Three techniques, gram stain, detection of bacterial genes or nucleic acid (DNA), and culture, are generally used to diagnose gonorrhea. Many doctors prefer to use more than one test to increase the chance of an accurate diagnosis. The gram stain is quite accurate for men but is not very sensitive for women. Only one in two women with gonorrhea have a positive gram stain. The test involves placing a smear of the discharge from the penis or the cervix (the opening to the uterus) on a slide and staining the smear with a dye. The slide is examined under a microscope for the presence of the bacteria. A doctor usually can give test results to the patient at the time of an office or clinic visit. More often, urine or cervical swabs are used for a new test that detects the genes of the bacteria. These tests are as accurate as culture and are used widely.

The culture test involves placing a sample of the discharge onto a culture plate and incubating it up to two days to allow the bacteria to multiply. The sensitivity of this test depends on the site from which the sample is taken. Cervical samples detect infection approximately 90 percent of the time. The doctor also can take a throat culture to detect pharyngeal gonorrhea.

Treatment

Because penicillin-resistant cases of gonorrhea are common, other antibiotics are used to treat most patients with gonococcal infections.

One of the most effective medicines to treat patients is ceftriaxone, which the doctor can inject in a single dose. Other effective antibiotics that a patient can take by mouth include a single dose of cefixime, ciprofloxacin, or ofloxacin. Pregnant women and patients younger than 18 years old should not take ciprofloxacin or ofloxacin.

Gonorrhea can occur together with chlamydial infection, another common sexually transmitted disease (STD). Therefore, doctors usually prescribe a combination of antibiotics, such as ceftriaxone and doxycycline or azithromycin. Single-dose oral therapy is available. All sexual partners of a person with gonorrhea should be tested and treated if infected whether or not they have symptoms of infection.

Complications

The most common consequence of untreated gonorrhea is PID, a serious infection of the female reproductive organs that occurs in an estimated 1 million American women each year. Gonococcal PID often appears immediately after the menstrual period. PID can scar or damage cells lining the fallopian tubes, resulting in infertility in as many as 10 percent of women affected. If the tube is only partially scarred, proper passage of the fertilized egg into the uterus is prevented. If this happens, the egg may implant in the tube; this is called ectopic or tubal pregnancy and is life threatening if not detected early. Rarely, untreated gonorrhea can spread to the blood or the joints.

An infected pregnant woman may give the infection to her infant as the baby passes through the birth canal during delivery. A doctor can prevent infection of the eye, called ophthalmia neonatorum, by applying silver nitrate or other medications to the baby's eyes immediately after birth. Because of the risks from gonococcal infection to both mother and child, doctors recommend that a pregnant woman have at least one test for gonorrhea.

Gonorrhea also increases the risk of HIV infection (HIV, human immunodeficiency virus, causes AIDS), so prevention and early treatment of gonorrhea is critically important.

Prevention

By using male condoms correctly and consistently during sexual activity, sexually active people can reduce their risk of gonorrhea and its complications.

Part Twelve

Payment of Medical Tests

Chapter 71

Guide to Health Insurance

If you have ever been sick or injured, you know how important it is to have health coverage. But if you're confused about what kind is best for you, you're not alone.

What types of health coverage are available? If your employer offers you a choice of health plans, what should you know before making a decision? In addition to coverage for medical expenses, do you need some other kind of insurance? What if you are too ill to work? Or, if you are over 65, will Medicare pay for all your medical expenses?

These are questions that today's consumers are asking; and these questions aren't necessarily easy to answer.

This chapter should help. It discusses the basic forms of health coverage and includes a checklist to help you compare plans. It answers some commonly asked questions and also includes thumbnail descriptions of other forms of health insurance, including hospital-surgical policies, specified disease policies, catastrophic coverage, hospital indemnity insurance, and disability, long-term care, and Medicare supplement insurance.

Making Sense of Health Insurance

The term **health insurance** refers to a wide variety of insurance policies. These range from policies that cover the costs of doctors and hospitals to those that meet a specific need, such as paying for

Excerpts from *Guide to Health Insurance* © April 1997, reprinted with permission of the Health Insurance Association of America.

long-term care. Even disability insurance–which replaces lost income if you can't work because of illness or accident–is considered health insurance, even though it's not specifically for medical expenses.

But when people talk about health insurance, they usually mean the kind of insurance offered by employers to employees, the kind that covers medical bills, surgery, and hospital expenses. You may have heard this kind of health insurance referred to as **comprehensive** or **major medical** policies, alluding to the broad protection they offer. But the fact is, neither of these terms is particularly helpful to the consumer.

Today, when people talk about broad health care coverage, instead of using the term major medical, they are more likely to refer to **fee-for-service** or **managed care**. These terms apply to different kinds of coverage or health plans. Moreover, you'll also hear about specific kinds of managed care plans: **health maintenance organizations** or **HMOs, preferred provider organizations** or **PPOs**, and **point-of-service (POS)** plans.

Fee-For-Service

This type of coverage generally assumes that the medical provider (usually a doctor or hospital) will be paid a fee for each service rendered to the patient–you or a family member covered under your policy. With fee-for-service insurance, you go to the doctor of your choice; and you or your doctor or hospital submits a claim to your insurance company for reimbursement. You will only receive reimbursement for covered medical expenses, the ones listed in your benefits summary.

When a service is covered under your policy, you can expect to be reimbursed for some but generally not all of the cost. How much you will receive depends on the provisions of the policy on **co-insurance** and **deductibles**.

Managed Care

The three major types of managed care plans are **health maintenance organizations (HMOs), preferred provider organizations (PPOs)**, and **point-of-service (POS)** plans.

Managed care plans generally provide comprehensive health services to their members, and offer financial incentives for patients to use the providers who belong to the plan. In managed care plans, instead of paying for each service that you receive separately, your coverage is paid in advance. This is called prepaid care.

One of the interesting things about health maintenance organizations is that they deliver care directly to patients. Patients sometimes go to a medical facility to see the nurses and doctors or to a specific doctor's office. Another common model is a network of individual practitioners. In these individual practice associations (IPAs), you will get your care in a physician's office. (More than half the people enrolled in HMOs are in IPAs.)

Preferred provider organizations and point-of-service plans are categorized as managed care plans. (Indeed, many people call POS plans an HMO with a point-of-service option.) From the consumer's point of view, these plans combine features of fee-for-service and HMOs. They offer more flexibility than HMOs, but premiums are likely to be somewhat higher.

Always look carefully at the description of the plans you are considering for the conditions of payment. Check with your employer, your benefits manager, or your state department of insurance to find out about laws that may regulate who is responsible for payment.

Self-Insured Plans

Your employer may have set up a financial arrangement that helps cover employees' health care expenses. Sometimes employers do this and have the health plan administered by an insurance company; but sometimes there is no outside administrator. With self-insured health plans, certain federal laws may apply; thus, if you have problems with a plan that isn't state regulated, it's probably a good idea to talk to an attorney who specializes in health law.

How Do I Get Health Coverage?

Health insurance is generally available through groups and to individuals. Premiums–the regular fee that you pay for health insurance coverage–are generally lower for group coverage. When you receive group insurance at work, the premium usually is paid through your employer.

Group insurance is typically offered through employers, although unions, professional associations, and other organizations also offer group insurance. As an employee benefit, group health insurance has many advantages. Much–although not all–of the cost may be borne by the employer. Premium costs are frequently lower because economies of scale in large groups make administration less expensive With group insurance, if you enroll when you first become eligible for coverage, you generally will not be asked for evidence that you are insurable. (Enrollment usually occurs when you first take a job, and/or during a specified period each year, which is called open enrollment.) Some employers offer employees a choice of fee-for-service and managed care plans. In addition, some group plans offer dental insurance as well as medical.

Individual insurance is a good option if you work for a small company that does not offer health insurance or if you are self-employed. Buying individual insurance allows you to tailor a plan to fit your needs from the insurance company of your choice. It requires careful shopping, because coverage and costs vary from company to company. In evaluating policies, consider what medical services are covered, what benefits are paid, and how much you must pay in deductibles and co-insurance. You may keep premiums down by accepting a higher deductible.

Pre-existing Conditions: Federal Law

Many people worry about coverage for pre-existing conditions, especially when they change jobs. Changes in federal law help assure continued health insurance coverage for employees and their dependents. Effective July 1, 1997, insurers may impose only one 12-month waiting period for any pre-existing condition treated or diagnosed in the previous six months. Your prior health insurance coverage will be credited toward the pre-existing condition exclusion period as long as you have maintained continuous coverage without a break of more than 62 days. Pregnancy is not considered a pre-existing condition, and newborns and adopted children who are covered within 30 days are not subject to the 12-month waiting period.

If you have had group health coverage for two years, and you switch jobs and go to another plan, that new health plan cannot impose another pre-existing condition exclusion period. If, for example, you have had prior coverage of only eight months, you may be subject to a four month pre-existing exclusion period when you switch jobs. If you've never been covered by an employer's group plan, and you get a job that offers such coverage, you may be subject to a 12-month pre-existing condition waiting period.

Federal law also makes it easier for you to get individual insurance under certain situations, including if you have left a job where you had group health insurance, or had another plan for more than 18 months without a break of more than 62 days.

If you have not been covered under a group plan and have found it difficult to get insurance on your own, check with your state insurance department to see if your state has a risk pool. Similar to risk pools for automobile insurance, these can provide health insurance for people who cannot get it elsewhere.

What Happens to My Insurance if I Lose My Job?

If you have had health coverage as an employee benefit and you leave your job, voluntarily or otherwise, one of your first concerns will be maintaining protection against the costs of health care. You can do this in one of several ways:

- First, you should know that under a federal law (the Consolidated Omnibus Budget Reconciliation Act of 1985, commonly know as COBRA), group health plans sponsored by employers with 20 or more employees are required to offer continued coverage for you and your dependents for 18 months after you leave your job. (Under the same law, following an employee's death or divorce, the worker's family has the right to continue coverage for up to three years.) If you wish to continue your group coverage under this option, you must notify your employer within 60 days. You must also pay the entire premium, up to 102 percent of the cost of the coverage.

- If COBRA does not apply in your case—perhaps because you work for an employer with fewer than 20 employees—you may be able to convert your group policy to individual coverage. The advantage of that option is that you may not have to pass a medical exam, although an exclusion based on a pre-existing condition may apply, depending on your medical history and your insurance history.

- If COBRA doesn't apply and converting your group coverage is not for you, then, if you are healthy, not yet eligible for Medicare, and expect to take another job, you might consider an interim or short-term policy. These policies are designed to provide medical insurance for people with a short-term need, such as those temporarily between jobs or those making the transition between college and a job. These policies, typically written for two to six months and renewable once, cover hospitalization, intensive care, and surgical and doctors' care provided in the hospital, as well as expenses for related services performed outside the hospital, such as x-rays or laboratory tests.

• Another possibility is obtaining coverage through an association. Many trade and professional associations offer their members health coverage—often HMOs—as well as basic hospital-surgical policies, and disability and long-term care insurance. If you are self-employed, you may find association membership an attractive route.

What To Do When a Medical Bill Is Turned Down

Ask the insurance company why the claim was rejected. If the answer is that the service isn't covered under your policy, and you're sure that it is, check to see that the provider entered the correct diagnosis or procedure code on the insurance claim form. Also check that your deductible was correctly calculated. Make sure that you didn't skip an essential step under your plan, such as pre-admission certification. If everything is in order, ask the insurer to review the claim.

Other Forms of Health Insurance

In addition to broad coverage for medical, surgical, and hospital expenses, there are many other kinds of health insurance.

Hospital-Surgical Policies

Hospital-surgical policies, sometimes called **basic** health insurance, provide benefits when you have a covered condition that requires hospitalization. These benefits typically include room and board and other hospital services, surgery, physicians' nonsurgical services that are performed in a hospital, expenses for diagnostic x-rays and laboratory tests, and room and board in an extended care facility.

Keep in mind that hospital-surgical policies usually do not cover lengthy hospitalizations and costly medical care. In the event that you need these types of services, you may incur large expenses that are difficult to meet unless you have other insurance.

Catastrophic Coverage

Catastrophic coverage pays hospital and medical expenses above a certain deductible; this can provide additional protection if you hold either a hospital-surgical policy or a major medical policy with a lower-than-adequate lifetime limit. These policies typically contain a very high deductible ($15,000 or more), and a maximum lifetime limit high enough to cover the costs of catastrophic illness.

Specified or Dread Disease

Specified or dread disease policies provide benefits only if you get the specific disease or group of diseases named in the policy. For example, a policy might cover only medical care associated with cancer. Because benefits are limited in amount, these policies are not a substitute for broad medical coverage. Nor are specified disease policies available in every state.

Hospital Indemnity Insurance

Hospital indemnity insurance pays you a specified amount of cash benefits for each day that you are hospitalized, generally up to a designated number of days. These cash benefits are paid directly to you, can be used for any purpose, and may be useful in meeting out-of-pocket expenses not covered by other insurance.

Medicare Supplement

Medicare supplement insurance, sometimes called **Medigap** or **MedSupp**, is private insurance that helps cover some of the gaps in Medicare coverage.

Medicare is the federal program of hospital and medical insurance primarily for people age 65 and over who are not covered by an employer's plan; but Medicare doesn't cover all medical expenses. That's where Medsupp comes in.

All Medicare supplement policies must cover certain expenses, such as the daily co-insurance amount for hospitalization and 90 percent of the hospital charges that otherwise would have been paid by Medicare, after Medicare is exhausted. Some policies may offer additional benefits, such as coverage for preventive medical care, prescription drugs, or at-home recovery.

There are 10 standard Medicare supplement policies, designated by the letters A through J. With these standardized policies, it is much easier to compare the costs of policies issued by different insurers. While all 10 standard policies may not be available to you, Plan A must be made available to Medicare recipients everywhere.

Insurers are not permitted to sell policies that duplicate benefits you already receive under Medicare or other policies. If you decide to replace an existing Medicare supplement policy–and you should do so only after careful evaluation–you must sign a statement that you intend to replace your current policy and that you will not keep both policies in force.

People who are 65 or older can buy Medicare supplement insurance without having to worry about being rejected for existing medical problems, so long as they apply within six months after enrolling in Medicare.

Long-term Care

Long-term care policies cover the medical care, nursing care, and other assistance you might need if you ever have a chronic illness or disability that leaves you unable to care for yourself for an extended period of time. These services generally are not covered by other health insurance. You may receive long-term care in a nursing home or in your own home.

Disability Insurance

Disability insurance provides you with an income if illness or injury prevents you from being able to work for an extended period of time. It is an important but often overlooked form of insurance.

There are other possible sources of income if you are disabled. Social Security provides protection, but only to those who are severely disabled and unable to work at all; workers' compensation provides benefits if the illness or injury is work-related; civil service disability covers federal or state government workers; and automobile insurance may pay benefits if the disability results from an automobile accident. But these sources are limited.

Some employers offer short and long-term disability coverage; and if you are self-employed, you can buy individual disability income insurance policies. Generally:

- Monthly benefits are usually 60 percent of your income at the time of purchase, although cost-of-living adjustments may be available.

- If you pay the premiums for an individual disability policy, payments you receive under the policy are not subject to income tax. If your employer has paid some or all of the premiums under a group disability policy, some or all of the benefits may be taxable.

Whether you are an employer shopping for a group disability policy or someone thinking of purchasing disability income insurance, you will need to evaluate different policies. Here are some things to look for:

- Some policies pay benefits only if someone is unable to perform the duties of their customary occupation, while others pay only if the person can engage in no gainful employment at all. Make sure that you know the insurer's definition of disability.

- Some policies pay only for accidents, but it's important to be insured for illness too. Be sure, as you evaluate policies, that both accident and illness are covered.

- Benefits may begin anywhere from one month to six months or more after the onset of disability. A later starting date can keep your premiums down. But remember, if your policy only starts to pay (for example) three months after the disability begins, you may lose a considerable amount of income.

- Benefits may be payable for a period ranging anywhere from one year to a lifetime. Since disability benefits replace income, most people do not need benefits beyond their working years. But it's generally wise to insure at least until age 65 since a lengthy disability threatens financial security much more than a short disability.

A Final Word

If you get health care coverage at work, or through a trade or professional association, or a union, you are almost certainly enrolled under a group contract. Generally, the contract is between the group and the insurer, and your employer has done comparison shopping before offering the plan to the employees. Nevertheless, while some employers only offer one plan, some offer more than one. Compare plans carefully!

If you are buying individual insurance, or any form of insurance that you purchase directly, read and compare the policies you are considering before you buy one, and make sure you understand all of the provisions. Marketing or sales literature is no substitute for the actual policy. Read the policy itself before you buy.

Ask for a summary of each policy's benefits or an outline of coverage. Good agents and good insurance companies want you to know what you are buying. Don't be afraid to ask your benefits manager or insurance agent to explain anything that is unclear.

It is also a good idea to ask for the insurance company's rating. The A.M. Best Company, Standard & Poor's Corporation, and Moody's all rate insurance companies after analyzing their financial records. These publications that list ratings usually can be found in the business section of libraries.

And bear in mind: In some cases, even after you buy a policy, if you find that it doesn't meet your needs, you may have 30 days to return the policy and get your money back. This is called the free look.

Chapter 72

Medicare

Contents

Section 72.1

Medicare Overview

Excerpts from *Medicare & You*, Health Care Financing Administration, 7500 Security Blvd., Baltimore, MD 21244-1850.

Medicare is a health insurance program for:

- People 65 years of age and older
- Certain younger people with disabilities
- People with End-Stage Renal Disease (people with permanent kidney failure who need dialysis or a transplant).

What Is the Original Medicare Plan?

The Original Medicare Plan is the traditional pay-per-visit arrangement. You can go to any doctor, hospital, or other health care provider who accepts Medicare. You must pay the deductible. Then Medicare pays its share, and you pay your share (coinsurance). The Original Medicare Plan has two parts: Part A (Hospital Insurance) and Part B (Medical Insurance). If you are in the Original Medicare Plan now, the way you receive your health care will not change unless you enroll in another Medicare health plan.

What Is Part A (Hospital Insurance)?

Part A (Hospital Insurance) helps pay for care in hospitals and skilled nursing facilities, and for home health and hospice care. If you are eligible, Part A is premium free—that is, you don't pay a premium because you or your spouse paid Medicare taxes while you were working.

Your Fiscal Intermediary can answer your questions on what Part A services Medicare will pay for and how much will be paid.

You are eligible for premium-free Medicare Part A (Hospital Insurance) if:

- You are 65 or older. You are receiving or eligible for retirement benefits from Social Security or the Railroad Retirement Board, or

- You are under 65. You have received Social Security disability benefits for 24 months, or

- You are under 65. You have received Railroad Retirement disability benefits for the prescribed time and you meet the Social Security Act disability requirements, or

- You or your spouse had Medicare-covered government employment, or

- You are under 65 and have End-Stage Renal Disease.

If you don't qualify for premium-free Part A, and you are 65 or older, you may be able to buy it. Contact the Social Security Administration.

What Is Part B (Medical Insurance)?

Part B (Medical Insurance) helps pay for doctors, outpatient hospital care and some other medical services that Part A doesn't cover, such as the services of physical and occupational therapists. Part B covers all doctor services that are medically necessary. Beneficiaries may receive these services anywhere (a doctor's office, clinic, nursing home, hospital, or at home). Your Medicare carrier can answer questions about Part B services and coverage.

You are automatically eligible for Part B if you are eligible for premium-free Part A. You are also eligible if you are a United States citizen or permanent resident age 65 or older. Part B cost $43.80 per month in 1998.*

Part B is voluntary. If you choose to have Part B, the monthly premium is deducted from your Social Security, Railroad Retirement, or Civil Service Retirement payment. Beneficiaries who do not receive any of the above payments are billed by Medicare every 3 months.

If you didn't take Part B when you were first eligible, you can sign-up during 2 enrollment periods:

- **General Enrollment Period:** If you didn't take Part B, you can only sign up during the general enrollment period, January 1 through March 31 of each year. Your Part B coverage is effective July 1. Your monthly Part B premium may be higher. The Part B premium increases 10% for each 12-month period that you could have had Part B but did not take it.

- **Special Enrollment Period:** If you didn't take Part B because you or your spouse currently work and have group health plan coverage through your current employer or union, you can sign up for Part B during the special enrollment period. Under the special enrollment period, you can sign up at any time you are covered under the group plan. In addition, if the employment or group health coverage ends, you have 8 months to sign up. The 8-month period starts the month after the employment ends or the group health coverage ends, whichever comes first. Generally, your monthly Part B premium is not increased when you sign up for Part B during the special enrollment period. Contact the Social Security Administration, or the Railroad Retirement Board to sign up for Part B.

What Are Your "Out-of-Pocket" Costs?

The Original Medicare Plan pays for much of your health care, but not all of it. Your "out-of-pocket"costs for health care will include your monthly Part B premium. In addition, when you get health care services, you will also have to pay deductibles and coinsurance or copayments. Generally, you will pay for your outpatient prescription drugs. You also pay for routine physicals, custodial care, most dental care, dentures, routine foot care, or hearing aids. Physical therapy and occupational therapy services, except for those you get in hospital outpatient departments, are subject to annual limits. The Original Medicare Plan does pay for some preventive care, but not all of it.

Your Out-of-Pocket Costs

Out-of-pocket costs may depend on:

- Whether your doctor accepts assignment.
- How often you need health care.
- What type of health care you need.

If you choose another Medicare health plan or purchase a supplemental policy, out-of-pocket costs may also depend on:

- Which Medicare health plan you choose.
- What extra benefits are covered by the plan.
- What your supplemental health insurance covers.

Help for Low-Income Medicare Beneficiaries

For certain older, low-income or disabled individuals entitled to Medicare Part A, your State Medicaid program will pay some or all of Medicare's premiums, and may also pay Medicare's deductibles and coinsurance if you have Part A, and your bank accounts, stocks, bonds, or other resources do not exceed $4,000 for an individual, or $6,000 for a couple, you may qualify for assistance. If you think you may qualify, contact your State, county, or local medical assistance office.

Section 72.2

Medicare Covered Services

Excerpts from *Medicare & You*, Health Care Financing Administration, 7500 Security Blvd., Baltimore, MD 21244-1850.

Medicare Part A (Hospital Insurance) Covered Services

Hospital Stays

Semiprivate room, meals, general nursing and other hospital services and supplies (but not private duty nursing, a television or telephone in your room, or a private room unless medically necessary). For each benefit period you pay:

- A total of $764 for a hospital stay of 1-60 days.
- $191 per day for days 61-90 of a hospital stay.
- $382 per day for days 91-150 of a hospital stay.**
- All costs for each day beyond 150 days

Skilled Nursing Facility (SNF) Care

Semiprivate room, meals, skilled nursing and rehabilitative services, and other services and supplies. For each benefit period you pay:

- Nothing for the first 20 days.
- Up to $95.50 per day for days 21-100.
- All costs beyond the 100th day in the benefit period.

Contact your Fiscal Intermediary with questions about Skilled Nursing Facility Care and conditions of coverage.

Home Health Care

Intermittent skilled nursing care, physical therapy, speech language pathology services, home health aide services, durable medical equipment (such as wheelchairs, hospital beds, oxygen, and walkers) and supplies, and other services. You pay:

- Nothing for Home Health Care services.
- 20% of approved amount for durable medical equipment (such as wheelchairs, hospital beds, oxygen, and walkers).

Call your Regional Home Health Intermediary with questions about Home Health Care and conditions of coverage.

Hospice Care:***

Pain and symptom relief, and supportive services for the management of a terminal illness. Home care is provided. Also covers necessary inpatient care and a variety of services otherwise not covered by Medicare. You pay:

- Limited costs for outpatient drugs and inpatient respite care (care given to a hospice patient so that the usual care giver can rest).

Call your Regional Home Health Intermediary about Hospice Care and conditions of coverage.

Blood

From a hospital or skilled nursing facility during a covered stay. You pay:

- For the first 3 pints.

*1999 Part A & B premium, coinsurance, and deductible amounts will be available before January 1, 1999.

**You have 60 reserve days that may only be used once. For each reserve day, Medicare pays all covered costs except for a daily coinsurance ($382 in 1998).

***You must meet certain conditions in order for Medicare to cover these services.

Benefit Period:

Starts the day you are admitted to a hospital or Skilled Nursing Facility and ends when you haven't received hospital inpatient or Skilled Nursing Facility care for 60 consecutive days.

Call your Fiscal Intermediary for general questions about your Medicare Part A coverage.

Medicare Part B (Medical Insurance) Covered Services

Medical Expenses:

Doctors' services, inpatient and outpatient medical and surgical services and supplies, physical, occupational and speech therapy, diagnostic tests, and durable medical equipment (DME). You pay:

- $100 deductible (pay once per year).

- 20% of approved amount after the deductible, except in the outpatient setting.

- 50% for most outpatient mental health.

- 20% of first $1,500 for all physical therapy services and 20% of first $1,500 for all occupational therapy services, and all charges thereafter. (Hospital outpatient therapy services do not count towards limit.)

Clinical Laboratory Service:

Blood tests, urinalysis, and more. You pay:

- Nothing for services.

Home Health Care: (If You Don't Have Part A.)

Intermittent skilled care, home health aide services, DME and supplies, and other services. You pay:

- Nothing for services.

- 20% of approved amount for DME.

Outpatient Hospital Services:

Services for the diagnosis or treatment of an illness or injury. You pay:

- No less than 20% of the Medicare payment amount (after the deductible).

Blood:

As an outpatient, or as part of a Part B covered service. You pay:

- For the first 3 pints plus 20% of approved amount for additional pints (after the deductible).

*1999 Part A & B premium, coinsurance, and deductible amounts will be available before January 1, 1999.

Note: Actual amounts you must pay for coinsurance are higher if the doctor does not accept assignment.

Call your Medicare Carrier if you have general questions about your Medicare Part B coverage.

Part B Also Helps Pay For:

- X-rays
- Speech language pathology services
- Artificial limbs and eyes
- Arm, leg, back, and neck braces
- Kidney dialysis and kidney transplants
- Under limited circumstances, heart, lung, and liver transplants in a Medicare-approved facility
- Preventive services
- Very limited outpatient drugs
- Emergency care
- Limited chiropractic services
- Medical supplies: items such as ostomy bags, surgical dressings, splints, and casts
- Breast prostheses following a mastectomy
- Ambulance services (limited coverage)
- The services of practitioners such as clinical psychologists, clinical social workers, and nurse practitioners
- One pair of eyeglasses after cataract surgery with an intraocular lens

Medicare Preventive Services—Added Benefits to Help You Stay Healthy

Screening Mammogram

Once per year for all female Medicare beneficiaries age 40 and older. You pay 20% of the Medicare approved amount with no Part B deductible.

Pap Smear and Pelvic Examination (Includes Clinical Breast Exam)

Once every three years for all female Medicare beneficiaries. Once per year if you are at high risk for cervical or vaginal cancer, or if you are of child bearing age and have had an abnormal Pap Smear in the preceding three years.

You do not pay coinsurance or Part B deductible for the Pap smear (clinical laboratory charge). For doctor services and all other exams, you pay 20% of the Medicare approved amount with no Part B deductible.

Colorectal Cancer Screening

All Medicare beneficiaries age 50 and older are covered with no age limit for having a colonoscopy.

- **Fecal Occult Blood Test**, once every year.

- **Flexible Sigmoidoscopy**, once every four years.

- **Colonoscopy,** once every two years if you are high risk for cancer of the colon.

- **Barium Enema**, can be substituted by the doctor for sigmoidscopy or colonoscopy.

You do not pay coinsurance or Part B deductible for the fecal occult blood test. For all other tests, you pay 20% of the Medicare approved amount after the annual Part B deductible.

Diabetes Monitoring

Includes coverage for glucose monitors, test strips, lancets, and self-management training for all Medicare beneficiaries with diabetes both insulin users and non-users.

You pay 20% of the Medicare approved amount after the annual Part B deductible.

Bone Mass Measurements:

This is available to certain Medicare beneficiaries at risk for losing bone mass, coverage varies with your health status.

You pay 20% of the Medicare approved amount after the annual Part B deductible.

Vacinations

- **Flu Shot:** Once per year for all Medicare beneficiaries.

- **Pneumococcal Vaccination:** One may be all you ever need, ask your doctor. It is available for all Medicare beneficiaries.

- **Hepatitis B Vaccination:** Available to those at high or intermediate risk for hepatitis.

You do not pay coinsurance or Part B deductible for flu or pneumococcal vaccinations. For Hepatitis B vaccination, you pay 20% of the Medicare approved amount after the part B deductible.

More Medicare Health Plan Choices

Starting in 1999, Medicare offers more health plan choices. One of the new health plan choices might be right for you. The choice is yours. No matter what you decide, you are still in the Medicare program. All Medicare health plans must provide all Medicare covered services described above.

To Be Eligible for the Other Medicare Health Plan Choices

- You must have Part A (Hospital Insurance) and Part B (Medical Insurance).

- You must not have End-Stage Renal Disease. (ESRD is permanent kidney failure that requires dialysis or a transplant.) However, ESRD beneficiaries currently in a health plan will be able to remain in the plan they are in.

- You must live in the service area of a health plan. The service area is the geographic area where the plan accepts enrollees.

For plans that require you to use their doctors and hospitals, it is also the area where services are provided. The plan may disenroll you if you move out of the plan's service area. If you are disenrolled, you are automatically covered under the Original Medicare Plan. You can also choose to join a Medicare health plan in your new area.

Your Out-of-Pocket Costs May Depend On

- Which Medicare health plan you choose.
- How often you need health care.
- What type of health care you need.
- Which extra benefits are covered by the plan.
- What your supplemental health insurance covers.
- Whether your doctor accepts assignment (Original Medicare Plan only).

Section 72.3.

1999 Medicare Deductible, Coinsurance, and Premium Amounts

The *Federal Register*, Volume 63, No. 203, pages 56199-56201 and 56212-56214, October 21, 1998, Updated November 19, 1998; and Social Security Act, Title 18, Section 1833(b), Office of the Actuary/HCFA.

Hospital Insurance (Part A)

- **Deductible**—$768 per each Benefit Period.

- **Coinsurance**

  - $192 a day for the 61st through the 90th day, per Benefit Period;

  - $384 a day for each "nonrenewable, lifetime reserve day".

- **Skilled Nursing Facility coinsurance**—$96 a day for the 21st through the 100th day per Benefit Period;

* **Hospital Insurance Premium**—$309 (See NOTE 1)

* **Reduced Hospital Insurance Premium**—$170 (See NOTE 1)

Deductible—$100 per year
Monthly Premium—$45.50 (see NOTE 2)

NOTE:

1. Most people age 65 or older are eligible for premium-free Hospital Insurance (Part A). However, there are some people age 65 or older who do not meet the requirements for premium-free Hospital Insurance. Also, certain disabled individuals who were entitled to premium-free Hospital Insurance lose their entitlement upon having earnings exceeding certain amounts. If you are in either of these categories, you can get Part A by paying a monthly premium. The full Part A premium in calendar year 1999 will be $309 per month. However, if you or your spouse have 30 to 39 quarters of Social Security coverage, your Part A premium, in calendar year 1999, will be $170 per month. For both the full and reduced premiums, a surcharge of 10% is accessed for late enrollment; this surcharge is applied only for a period twice as long as enrollment was delayed.

2. A surcharge of 10% is assessed for each full 12 months (in the same continuous period of eligibility) in which a beneficiary could have been enrolled but was not.

Section 72.4

Assistance for Low-Income Beneficiaries

Medicare Savings for Qualified Beneficiaries, Health Care Financing
Administration (HCFA), 1998.

Medicare Savings for You

The Health Care Financing Administration (HCFA), a Federal
government agency that administers Medicare and Medicaid, and
your State have developed programs that can help pay your Medicare
out-of-pocket expenses. These programs help people who have limited
resources and income to pay for some Medicare expenses. This could
save you hundreds of dollars each year.

If you qualify, you may not have to pay for your:

• Medicare premiums, and in some cases, deductibles, and coinsurance.

Several Programs Offer Help

There are four programs that offer different levels of help. They
are:

• Qualified Medicare Beneficiary (QMB)
• Specified Low-income Medicare Beneficiary (SLMB)
• Qualifying Individual-1 (QI-1)
• Qualifying Individual-2 (QI-2)

You may qualify for one of these programs if:

1. You are entitled to Medicare Part A. If you do not have Part A
   or you are not sure, check your Medicare card or call the Social Security office on 1-800-772-1213 to find out how to get it.

2. Your financial resources, such as bank accounts, stocks, and
   bonds, are not more than $4,000 for one person or $6,000 for a

591

couple. Some things—like the home you live in, one automobile, burial plots, home furnishings, personal jewelry, and life insurance—usually do not count as resources. (If the combined face value of the life insurance policy is less than $1,500, it is not counted.)

3. Your monthly income is at or below a certain level. Income includes Social Security benefits, pensions, and wages as well as interest payments and dividends on stocks and bonds you may own. The amount of help you can get depends upon your monthly income. The monthly income limits for different levels of help are shown below. If your monthly income changes you may move to a different level of help.

To qualify for any of the programs listed below, you must meet requirements (1) and (2) listed above.

Qualified Medicare Beneficiary (QMB)

This program pays your Medicare premiums, deductibles, and coinsurance. You may qualify for it if your monthly income in 1998 was at or below:

- **All states except Alaska and Hawaii:** $691 (individual) $925 (couple).
- **Alaska:** $860 (individual) $1,151 (couple).
- **Hawaii:** $792 (individual) $1,060 (couple).

Specified Low-income Medicare Beneficiary (SLMB).

This program pays your Medicare Part B premium. You may qualify for it if your monthly income in 1998 was at or below:

- **All states except Alaska and Hawaii:** $825 (individual) $1,105 (couple).
- **Alaska:** $1,027 (individual) $1,377 (couple).
- **Hawaii:** $946 (individual) $1,268 (couple).

Qualifying Individual-1 (QI-1)

This program pays your Medicare Part B premium.

- **All states except Alaska and Hawaii:** $926 (individual) $1,241 (couple).

- **Alaska:** $1153 (individual) $1, 547 (couple).

- **Hawaii:** $1,062 (individual) $1,424 (couple).

Qualifying Individual-2 (QI-2)

This program pays for a small part of your Medicare Part B premium.

- **All states except Alaska and Hawaii:** $1194 (individual) 1,603 (couple).

- **Alaska:** $1,489 (individual) $1,999 (couple).

- **Hawaii:** $1,371 (individual) $1,840 (couple).

How Do I Apply for These Programs?

If you think you qualify, you should do the following:

- Contact your State, county, or local medical assistance office. In some States, it could be your local social services office or your local Agency on Aging.

- When you call, ask for information on programs that help pay your Medicare Part B premium or ask how you can get help paying for some of your Medicare expenses.

- Ask for an application.

- Ask what documents you will need.

- Ask if you must apply in person or if you can do it by phone or mail.

- Complete and return the application with necessary documents.

What Documents Do I Need to Apply?

You may often need the following documents when you apply, but it is best to call your State to find out exactly what you will need. Gather these documents **BEFORE your first meeting or visit** with your state, county, or local medical assistance office and take them with you to avoid making more than one visit.

- Proof that you have Medicare Part A
- Recent bank statements
- Property deeds
- Insurance policies
- Financial statements from any stocks or bonds you may own
- Proof of any funeral or burial policies you may have
- Proof of identity
- Proof of residence
- Proof of any income pension check, social security payment, etc.

Where Do I Get More Information about These Programs?

For more information about these programs, call your state, county, or local medical assistance office. Check your phone directory for the office nearest you. You can find these offices listed under Medicaid, Social Services, Medical Assistance, Public Assistance, Human Services or Community Services or call 1-800-638-6833 to speak to a representative from HCFA that will help you in finding the phone number in your State.

Section 72.5

Telemedicine Reimbursement

Telehealth Update, Office for the Advancement of Telehealth, HRSA, December 1998.

Few payers reimburse telemedicine services, but on January 1, 1999, Medicare began paying for teleconsultations in rural health professional shortage areas. This provision, enacted in the Balanced Budget Act of 1997, represents Medicare's first national reimbursement policy for telemedicine services. These new payment regulations are fairly restrictive but provide a significant first step toward covering telehealth services while also raising some important issues about how best to pay for these services.

On January 1, 1999, Medicare joined approximately 11 state Medicaid programs and a handful of private health insurers in paying for telemedicine services. Medicare's move into the telemedicine reimbursement arena represents a step into new and unfamiliar territory for the Health Care Financing Administration. As the largest payer of medical claims in the country, Medicare often sets the standard for how other payers will handle new or innovative services.

First Steps Toward Telemedicine Reimbursement

The Health Care Financing Administration's (HCFA) telemedicine reimbursement rule is a notable change for the Medicare program. The program raises some critical questions for policy makers, practitioners and telemedicine networks on how best to pay for telemedicine services. As policy makers, practitioners and telemedicine service providers sift through the new regulations, several key issues have emerged about which services will be covered, which health care practitioners can take part in a consultation and what kind of telecommunications technology can be used.

Background

While telemedicine technology has made it easy to deliver health care services over a distance, few payers are covering these services. Currently, at least 11 state Medicaid programs and several Blue Cross/ Blue Shield plans and some other private insurers pay for telemedicine services. Several other states have also recently passed laws requiring all insurers to pay for telemedicine services. Medicare, however, has been more cautious. Prior to enactment of the Balanced Budget Act (BBA) of 1997, Medicare did not have an explicit policy to pay for telemedicine services. Nevertheless, telemedicine services that did not traditionally require face-to-face contact between a patient and practitioner, such as EKG or EEG interpretation, teleradiology, and telepathology were covered under Medicare in most areas of the nation, in accordance with individual Medicare carrier policies.

The passage of the BBA required Medicare to pay for telemedicine consultation services using interactive video (i.e., teleconsultation) in rural "Health Professional Shortage Areas" (HPSAs) by Jan. 1, 1999. This signaled a major change in policy. The legislation limits eligibility for coverage to rural HPSAs and prohibits payment for line charges or for facility fees. In addition, Medicare payment is set at the consultant's fee schedule and requires referring and consulting practitioners to share the payment. The final regulation, which was published in the *Federal Register* on Nov. 2, 1998, explains how Medicare initially will pay for these services and which services will be covered.

Site of Coverage

Under the BBA, there is only one type of shortage area applicable to the Medicare teleconsultation regulation: a "geographic" rural HPSA (Health Professional Shortage Area). Although some geographic rural HPSAs encompass an entire county, while others are only located in a portion of a county, HCFA decided to include all rural geographic HPSAs as eligible regardless of whether the entire county is a HPSA or not. The final rule stipulates the use of the site of presentation (patient location) as a proxy, or substitution, for beneficiary residence. However, if the beneficiary can show that he or she lives in a rural HPSA, Medicare will make payment regardless of where the teleconsultation occurred.

Eligible Presenting Practitioners

One of the more contentious issues in the formation of this regulation was deciding which health care practitioners should be paid for consultation. Telemedicine practitioners have used a variety of settings and practitioners for presenting patients to specialists and other consultants. For instance, some health care practitioners will refer a patient for a telemedicine consultation and then let a nurse at the telemedicine site present the patient to the specialist. Other primary care practitioners may present the patient themselves. Under this rule, however, Medicare has strictly defined which practitioners can be paid for participating in a teleconsultation at both ends, based on the parameters specified in the BBA.

Consultants

The BBA's language only allows certain practitioners to be a teleconsultant, and specifies that the referring medical professional is either a physician or a practitioner as defined in the Social Security Act. This act very specifically defines which medical professionals are considered "practitioners" under the Medicare program. As a result, there are some practitioners who are eligible only to act as consulting practitioners and others who are eligible only to act as referring practitioners. For example, clinical nurse specialists, physician assistants, nurse practitioners, and certified nurse-midwifes can act as both referring and consulting practitioners for this provision. However, clinical social workers and clinical psychologists can only act as referring practitioners under this rule. Registered nurses, licensed practical nurses and other types of similar health care professionals cannot present patients for consultations because they are not considered practitioners under the Medicare program as defined by the Social Security Act.

Scope of Coverage

According to HCFA, the BBA limits the scope of coverage to a consultation for which payment may be made under the Medicare program. These services include initial, follow-up, or confirmatory consultations in hospitals, outpatient facilities, or medical offices. Eligible Current Procedural Terminology (CPT) codes are:

- 99241-99245;
- 99251-99355;
- 99261-99263;
- 99271-99275.

The Medicare final rule on teleconsultation specifies that these codes can be used for a number of medical specialties, such as cardiology, dermatology, gastrology, neurology, pulmonary, and psychiatry. According to HCFA, it will cover additional consultations for the same or a new problem if the attending physician or practitioner requests the consultation, and if it is documented in the medical records of the beneficiary.

Sharing of Fees

The BBA mandates that consulting and referring practitioners share payments. HCFA requires that 75 percent of the fee go to the consultant and the remaining 25 percent go to the referring practitioner. HCFA came up with this split based on the relative work for practitioners at both ends. There was also an inherent recognition that different consultations call for different levels of effort. As a result, the fee split reflects the projected level of new work done by each practitioner over the course of various teleconsultations.

Types of Technology Covered

HCFA's payment policy was developed to replicate a standard consultation as closely as possible. Under Medicare, a separate payment for a consultation requires a face to face examination of the patient. This requirement is consistent with the American Medical Association's description of a consultation. To that end, Medicare's teleconsultation rule requires a certain level of interaction between the patient and consulting practitioner because it offers the best substitute for a "face-to-face" consultation.

Regardless of the technology, the patient must be present during the consultation. That is because Medicare does not currently make separate payment for the review and interpretation of a previous examination or dermatology photos. Thus, this policy may preclude the use of standard store-and-forward technologies. In most store-and-forward applications, a practitioner at the remote site will typically examine the patient and send a video clip or a photographic scan, along with the patient's medical record to a distant consulting practitioner. The consulting practitioner will then review the file and make a diagnosis. Medicare will not cover this type of telemedicine application because it does not allow for live interaction between the consulting practitioner and the patient and the referring practitioner at the rural site. Medicare will cover some uses of store-and-forward technology as a consultation if the patient is present and there is real-time video and audio interaction level of video or audio interaction between the consulting practitioner and the patient.

Next Steps

Medicare's telemedicine reimbursement rule represents a significant departure in policy for Medicare and how it pays for telemedicine services. Consequently, this new rule may undergo some changes in the years to come. The Secretary of Health and Human Services has asked HCFA to reexamine some key points, including what services are covered, which medical professionals are eligible to present the patient, and uses of store-and-forward technology. The Department will develop recommendations for Congress within the next year on potential modifications to the reimbursement rule. HCFA will be working with the Agency for Health Care Policy and Research (AHCPR) and Health Resources and Services Administration (HRSA)'s Office for the Advancement of Telehealth in the development of these recommendations.

Chapter 73

Medicaid

Note: The following is a very brief summary of a complex subject. It should be used only as an overview and general guide to the Medicaid program. This summary does not render any legal, accounting or other professional advice; nor is it intended to fully explain all of the provisions or exclusions of the relevant laws, regulations and rulings of the Medicaid program.

Overview of Medicaid

Title XIX of the Social Security Act is a Federal-State matching entitlement program that pays for medical assistance for certain vulnerable and needy individuals and families with low incomes and resources. This program, known as Medicaid, became law in 1965 as a jointly funded cooperative venture between the Federal and State governments ("State" used herein includes the Territories and the District of Columbia) to assist States furnishing medical assistance to eligible needy persons. Medicaid is the largest source of funding for medical and health-related services for America's poorest people. In 1996, it provided health care assistance to more than 36 million persons, at a cost of $160 billion dollars.

This chapter contains text from the following Health Care Financing Administration (HCFA) publications; "Brief Summaries of Medicare & Medicaid, Title XVIII and Title XIX of The Social Security Act" prepared by Mary Onnis Waid, Office of the Actuary, June 25, 1998, and "State Medical Assistance Offices," *Medicare & You*.

Within broad national guidelines established by Federal statutes, regulations and policies, each State: (1) establishes its own eligibility standards; (2) determines the type, amount, duration, and scope of services; (3) sets the rate of payment for services; and (4) administers its own program. Medicaid policies for eligibility, services, and payment are complex, and vary considerably even among similar-sized and/or adjacent States. Thus, a person who is eligible for Medicaid in one State might not be eligible in another State; and the services provided by one State may differ considerably in amount, duration, or scope from services provided in a similar or neighboring State. In addition, Medicaid eligibility and/or services within a State can change during the year.

Basis of Eligibility and Maintenance Assistance Status

Medicaid does not provide medical assistance for all poor persons. Even under the broadest provisions of the Federal statute, Medicaid does *not* provide health care services even for very poor persons *unless* they are in one of the groups designated below. And low income is only one test for Medicaid eligibility for those within these groups; their resources also are tested against threshold levels (as determined by each State within Federal guidelines).

States generally have broad discretion in determining which groups their Medicaid programs will cover and the financial criteria for Medicaid eligibility. To be eligible for Federal funds, however, States are *required* to provide Medicaid coverage for certain individuals who receive Federally assisted income-maintenance payments, as well as for related groups not receiving cash payments. In addition to the Medicaid program, most States have additional "State-only" programs to provide medical assistance for specified poor persons who do not qualify for Medicaid. Federal funds are *not* provided for State-only programs. The following displays the mandatory Medicaid "categorically needy" eligibility groups for which Federal matching funds are provided:

- Individuals are generally eligible for Medicaid if they meet the requirements for the AFDC program that were in effect in their State on July 16, 1996, or— at State option—more liberal criteria;

- Children under age six whose family income is at or below 133% of the Federal poverty level (FPL);

- Pregnant women whose family income is below 133% of the FPL (services to women are limited to: those related to pregnancy, complications of pregnancy, delivery and postpartum care);

- SSI recipients in most States (some States use more restrictive Medicaid eligibility requirements that pre-date SSI);

- Recipients of adoption or foster care assistance under Title IV of the Social Security Act;

- Special protected groups (typically individuals who lose their cash assistance due to earnings from work or from increased Social Security benefits, but who may keep Medicaid for a period of time);

- All children born after September 30, 1983 who are under age 19, in families with incomes at or below the FPL. (This phases in coverage, so that by the year 2002, all such poor children under age 19 will be covered); and

- Certain Medicare beneficiaries

States also have the *option* of providing Medicaid coverage for other "categorically related" groups. These optional groups share the characteristics of the mandatory groups (that is, they fall within defined categories), but the eligibility criteria are somewhat more liberally defined. The broadest optional groups for which States will receive Federal matching funds for coverage under the Medicaid program include:

- Infants up to age one and pregnant women not covered under the mandatory whose family income is no more than 185% of the FPL (the percentage amount is set by each State);

- Children under age 21 who meet what were the AFDC income and resources requirements in effect in their State on July 16, 1996, (even though they do not meet the mandatory eligibility requirements);

- Institutionalized individuals eligible under a "special income level" (the level is set by each State—up to 300% of the SSI Federal benefits rate);

- Individuals who would be eligible if institutionalized, but who are receiving care under home and community-based services waivers;

- Certain aged, blind or disabled adults who have incomes above those requiring mandatory coverage, but below the FPL;

- Recipients of State supplementary income payments;

- Certain working and disabled persons with family income less than 250% of FPL who would qualify for SSI if they did not work;

- TB-infected persons who would be financially eligible for Medicaid at the SSI income level if they were within a Medicaid-covered category (however, coverage is limited to TB-related ambulatory services and TB drugs);

- "Optional targeted low-income children" included within the Children's Health Insurance Program (CHIP) established by the Balanced Budget Act of 1997 (BBA); and

- "Medically needy" persons (described below).

The Medically Needy (MN) program allows States the option to extend Medicaid eligibility to additional qualified persons. These persons would be eligible for Medicaid under one of the mandatory or optional groups, except that their income and/or resources are above the eligibility level set by their State. Persons may qualify immediately, or may "spend-down" by incurring medical expenses that reduce their income to or below their State's MN income level.

The *medically needy* Medicaid program does not have to be as extensive as the *categorically needy* program, and may be quite restrictive in rules as to who is covered and/or as to what services are offered. Federal matching funds are available for MN programs. However, if a State elects to have *any* MN program, there are Federal requirements that certain *groups* and certain *services* must be included. Children under age 19 and pregnant women who are medically needy must be covered; and prenatal and delivery care for pregnant women, and ambulatory care for children must be provided. A State may elect to provide MN eligibility to certain additional groups, and may elect to provide certain additional services within its MN program. In 1996, forty-two States elected to have a MN program, and provided at least some MN services for at least some MN recipients. All remaining States utilize the "special income level" option (above) to extend Medicaid to the "near poor" in medical institutional settings.

The Personal Responsibility and Work Opportunity Reconciliation Act of 1996 (Public Law 104-193)—known as the "welfare reform" bill—made restrictive changes regarding eligibility for Supplemental Security Income (SSI) coverage that will have an impact on the Medicaid program. The new law may be significant for certain aliens' Medicaid coverage. For most legal resident aliens and other qualified aliens who entered the United States on or after August 22, 1996, Medicaid is barred for five years. Medicaid for most aliens entering before that date is a State option, as is coverage after the five year ban, except for emergency services. For aliens who lose SSI benefits because of new restrictions regarding SSI coverage, Medicaid can continue, except for emergency care, only if these persons can be covered for Medicaid under some other eligibility status. Although a number of disabled children lost SSI as a result of changes to the P.L. 104-193, their continued eligibility for Medicaid was assured by Public Law 105-33: the Balanced Budget Act of 1997 (the BBA).

In addition, welfare reform repealed the open-ended Federal entitlement program known as Aid to Families with Dependent Children (AFDC), and replaced it with Temporary Assistance for Needy Families (TANF), which will provide grants to States to be spent on time-limited cash assistance. TANF limits a family's lifetime cash welfare benefits to a maximum of five years, and permits States to impose a wide range of other restrictions as well—in particular, requirements related to employment. However, the impact on Medicaid eligibility is not expected to be significant. Under welfare reform, persons who would have been eligible for AFDC under the AFDC requirements in effect on July 16, 1996, generally will still be eligible for Medicaid. Although most persons covered by TANF will receive Medicaid, the law does not so require.

Title XXI of the Social Security Act, known as the Children's Health Insurance Program (CHIP), is a new program initiated by the BBA. In addition to allowing States to craft or expand an existing State insurance program, CHIP will provide more Federal funds for States to expand Medicaid eligibility to include more children who are currently uninsured. With certain exceptions, these are low-income children who would not qualify for Medicaid based on the plan that was in effect on April 15, 1997. Funds from the CHIP also may be used for providing medical assistance to children during a presumptive eligibility period for Medicaid. This is one of several options for States to select for providing health care coverage for more children, as prescribed within the BBA's Title XXI program.

Medicaid coverage may begin as early as the third month prior to application—*if* the person would have been eligible for Medicaid had he applied during that time. Medicaid coverage generally stops at the end of the month in which a person no longer meets the criteria of any Medicaid eligibility group. The BBA allows States to provide 12 months of continuous Medicaid coverage (without reevaluation) for eligible children under the age of 19.

Scope of Medicaid Services

Title XIX of the Social Security Act (the Medicaid program) allows considerable flexibility within the States' Medicaid plans. However, some Federal requirements are mandatory if Federal matching funds are to be received. A State's Medicaid program *must* offer medical assistance for certain *basic* services to most categorically needy populations. These services generally include:

- inpatient hospital services;

- outpatient hospital services;

- prenatal care;

- vaccines for children;

- physician services;

- nursing facility services for persons aged 21 or older;

- family planning services and supplies;

- rural health clinic services;

- home health care for persons eligible for skilled-nursing services;

- laboratory and x-ray services;

- pediatric and family nurse practitioner services;

- nurse-midwife services;

- Federally-qualified health-center (FQHC) services, and ambulatory services of an FQHC that would be available in other settings; and

- early and periodic screening, diagnostic, and treatment (EPSDT) services for children under age 21.

States also may receive Federal matching funds for providing certain *optional* services. The most common of the 34 currently-approved optional Medicaid services include:

- diagnostic services;
- clinic services;
- intermediate care facilities for the mentally retarded (ICFs/MR);
- prescribed drugs and prosthetic devices;
- optometrist services and eyeglasses;
- nursing facility services for children under age 21;
- transportation services;
- rehabilitation and physical therapy services; and
- home and community-based care to certain persons with chronic impairments.

The Balanced Budget Act included another provision for eligible persons as a State option known as PACE (Programs of All-inclusive Care for the Elderly). PACE provides an *alternative* to institutional care for persons aged 55 and over who require a *nursing facility level* of care. The PACE team offers and manages *all* health, medical and social services, and mobilizes other services as needed to provide preventative, rehabilitative, curative and supportive services. This care is provided in day health centers, homes, hospitals and nursing homes—while helping the person maintain independence, dignity and quality of life. PACE functions within the Medicare program as well as under Medicaid. Regardless of source of payment, PACE providers receive payment only through the PACE agreement, and must make available all items and services covered under both Titles XVIII and XIX without amount, duration or scope limitations, and without application of any deductibles, copayments or other cost sharing. The individuals enrolled in PACE receive benefits solely through the PACE program.

Amount and Duration of Medicaid Services

Within broad Federal guidelines and certain limitations, States determine the amount and duration of services offered under their Medicaid programs. States may limit, for example, the number of days of hospital care or the number of physician visits covered. Two restrictions apply: (1) limits must result in a sufficient level of services to reasonably achieve the purpose of the benefits; and (2) limits on benefits may not discriminate among beneficiaries based on medical diagnosis or condition.

In general, States are required to provide Medicaid coverage for comparable amounts, duration and scope of services to all categorically-needy and categorically-related eligible persons. There are two important exceptions: 1) Medically necessary health care services identified under the EPSDT program for eligible children which are within the scope of mandatory or optional services under Federal law, must be covered even if those services are not included as part of the covered services in that State's Plan (i.e., only these specific children might receive that specific service); and 2) States may request "waivers" to pay for otherwise-uncovered home and community-based services (HCBS) for Medicaid-eligible persons who might otherwise be institutionalized (i.e., only persons so designated might receive HCBS). States have few limitations on the services which may be covered under such waivers as long as the services are cost effective (except that, other than as a part of respite care, they may not provide room and board for such recipients). With certain exceptions, a State's Medicaid Plan must allow recipients to have some informed choices among participating providers of health care, and to receive quality care that is appropriate and timely.

Low Income Assistance, Qualifying for Medicaid, and Filing Medicaid Claims.

Call your state Medical Assistance Office for answers to questions about low income assistance, qualifying for Medicaid, or filing Medicaid claims.

Table73.1. State Medical Assistance Offices; continued on next page.

State Name	Phone Number(s)
Alabama	800-362-1504
Alaska	800-770-5650
American Samoa	011-684-633-4590
Arizona	602-417-4680
Arkansas	501-682-8487
California	800-952-5253
Colorado	303-866-2993
Connecticut	860-424-5008
Delaware	302-577-4901
District of Columbia	202-727-0735; 202-724-5506
Florida	850-488-3560
Georgia	800-282-4536
Guam	1-0-671-734-7264
Hawaii	808-586-5391
Idaho	208-334-5747

Table73.1. State Medical Assistance Offices; continued from previous page.

State Name | Phone Number(s)

Illinois 800-252-8635
Indiana 317-232-4966
Iowa 515-281-8621
Kansas 785-296-3349
Kentucky 502-564-6885
Louisana 504-342-3855; 504-342-5716
Maine 207-624-5277
Maryland 410-767-1432
Massachusetts 800-841-2900
Michigan 800-642-3195
Minnesota 800-657-3739
Mississippi 601-359-6056
Missouri 573-751-3425
Montana 406-444-5900
Nebraska 402-471-9147
Nevada 702-687-4775
New Hampshire 603-271-4344
New Jersey 609-588-2600
New Mexico 505-827-3100
New York 518-486-4803
North Carolina 800-662-7030
North Dakota 800-755-2604
Northern Mariana Islands ....: 011-670-234-8950 ext. 2905
Ohio 800-324-8680
Oklahoma 405-530-3439
Oregon 503-945-5811
Pennsylvania 717-787-1870
Puerto Rico 787-765-1230
Rhode Island 401-464-2121
South Carolina 803-253-6100
South Dakota 605-773-3495
Tennessee 615-741-0213
Texas 512-438-3219
Utah 801-538-6155
Vermont 802-241-2880
Virginia 804-786-7933
Virgin Islands 809-774-4624
Washington 800-562-3022
West Virginia 800-642-3607
Wisconsin 608-266-2522
Wyoming 307-777-5500

Chapter 74

The Hill-Burton Free Care Program

What's Hill-Burton Free Health Care About?

In 1946, Congress passed a law which gave hospitals and other health facilities money for construction and modernization. In return, the facilities that received these Hill-Burton funds agreed to (1) provide a reasonable volume of services to persons unable to pay, and (2) make their services available to all persons residing in the facility's area. The Department of Health and Human Services (DHHS) is responsible for the administration of this program.

The following is a simplified explanation of the Hill-Burton program at most health facilities. Some Hill-Burton facilities may use different eligibility standards and procedures.

What's Available?

Free or low cost health care. Many health facilities must give health care to some people who cannot afford to pay. Hill-Burton facilities must post a sign that says "NOTICE-Medical Care for Those Who Cannot Afford to Pay" in the health facility's Admissions Office, Business Office and Emergency Room.

This chapter contains text from the following U.S. Department of Health & Human Services (DHHS) publications: *Free Hospital Care, Nursing Home Care, and Care Provided in Other Types of Health Facilities Under the Hill-Burton Program*, and *Frequently Asked Questions by Consumers about Receiving Hill-Burton Free or Reduced Cost Care*, 1999.

Who Can Get It?

You may qualify if your income falls within the Poverty Guidelines, published annually by the Department of Health and Human Services. You may also qualify at some facilities if your income is up to double the Poverty Guidelines (or triple the Guidelines for nursing homes).

Where Can You Get It?

At Hill-Burton assisted facilities including hospitals, nursing homes, clinics, etc. Apply at the Admissions Office or Business Office.

When Can You Apply?

At any time—before or after you receive care; even after a bill has been sent to a collection agency.

How Can You Receive It?

Ask for Hill-Burton assistance.

Services Available

- Each Hill-Burton facility can choose which types of services to provide at no charge or reduced charge. They do this in an ALLOCATION PLAN published in the newspaper.

- The facility must give you a written INDIVIDUAL NOTICE which will tell you what types of Hill-Burton free or reduced charge services it provides.

- Only facility costs are covered, not your private doctor's bills. Hill-Burton facilities must provide a specific amount of free or reduced charge care each year, but can stop once they have given that amount.

- To obtain a list of Hill-Burton facilities in your area, write your Department of Health and Human Services' field office at the address listed at the end of the chapter or call the HOT LINE telephone number.

Eligibility

- If your income is less than the current Poverty Guidelines, facility services may be free.

- If your income is greater than, but not more than double the Poverty Guidelines (or triple the Guidelines for nursing homes), Hill-Burton facilities may provide services at full charge, reduced charge, or free. The INDIVIDUAL NOTICE will tell you what income levels qualify for free care.

- The facility may ask you to provide information to verify eligibility, such as proof of income.

- Hill-Burton facilities must make a determination of your eligibility within a set time frame. Time frames depend on when a request is made and on whether the facility is a hospital, nursing home, or other type of facility. See the facility's INDIVIDUAL NOTICE for the time frame in place at the facility.

- The facility must provide you with a written statement which says either when you can get free or reduced charge services or why you have been denied.

Follow These Steps:

1. Ask facility personnel for a copy of the INDIVIDUAL NOTICE. (This notice will tell you exactly where in the facility to apply.)

2. Ask how to apply for Hill-Burton free care. The facility may request that you fill out an application.

3. If you are asked to furnish proof of income eligibility, give this information to the facility (a pay stub may be requested).

4. If you are asked to apply for Medicaid, Medicare, or some other financial assistance program, you must do so.

5. When you return the completed application, ask for a DETERMINATION OF ELIGIBILITY.

Reasons for Denial

The facility may deny your request—

- If your income is more than the current Poverty Guidelines, (or more than twice the Guidelines (or triple the Guidelines for nursing homes) if the facility provides Hill-Burton services to persons with income up to these amounts).

- If the facility has given out its required amount of free care as specified in its ALLOCATION PLAN.

- If the services you requested or received are not covered in the facility's ALLOCATION PLAN.

- If the services you requested or received are to be paid by Medicare/Medicaid, insurance or other financial assistance program.

- If the facility asks you to first apply for Medicaid/Medicare or a financial assistance program, and you do not cooperate.

- If you do not give the facility proof of your income, such as a pay stub.

Complaints

You may file a complaint with your Department of Health and Human Services' field office if you have reason to believe you have been unfairly denied Hill-Burton free care.

- A complaint must be in writing. It can be a letter that simply states the facts and dates concerning the complaint.

- You may call the HOT LINE for help in filing a complaint.

- You may call your local legal aid services for help in filing a complaint.

Frequently Asked Questions

What Services Are Covered Under the Hill-Burton Program?

Each facility chooses which services it will provide at no or reduced cost. The covered services are specified in a notice which is published by the facility and also in a notice provided to all persons seeking services in the facility. Services fully covered by a third-party insurance or a government program (e.g., Medicare and Medicaid) are not eligible for Hill-Burton coverage. However, Hill-Burton may cover services not covered by the government programs.

Private pharmacy and private physician fees are not covered by this program. However, services provided by physicians hired by the facility may be covered under the Hill-Burton program if included in the published notice (Allocation Plan).

Can I Receive Hill-Burton Assistance to Cover My Medicare Deductible and Coinsurance Amounts or Medicaid Co-pay and Spenddown Amounts?

Medicare deductible and coinsurance amounts are not eligible under the program. However, Medicaid co-payment amounts are eligible, except in a long-term care facility. In addition, Medicaid spenddown amounts (the liability a patient must incur before being eligible for Medicaid) are eligible in all Hill-Burton facilities.

Where Can I Get Hill-Burton Free or Reduced Cost Care?

At a Hill-Burton facility. Check the Directory listing available on the internet at http://www.hrsa.dhhs.gov/ or with your HRSA Field Office. The facilities included are hospitals, nursing homes, clinics, etc. Apply at the Admissions, Business or Patient Accounts Office.

Who Can Receive Free Care?

Eligibility is based on a person's family size and income. Income is calculated based on your actual income for the last 12 months or your last 3 month's income times 4, whichever is less. You may qualify if your income falls within the poverty guidelines, as published in the Federal Register every year. You may also qualify for free or reduced cost care at some facilities if your income is up to double (or triple for nursing home services) the poverty guidelines.

What Does Income Include?

Gross income (before taxes), interest/dividends earned, and child support payments **are examples of income.** Assets, food stamps, gifts, loans or one-time insurance payments are examples of items **not included as income** when considering eligibility. For self-employed people, income is determined after deductions for business expenses. For more specific information, see the poverty guidelines.

When Can I Apply for Hill-Burton Assistance?

You may apply for Hill-Burton assistance at any time, before or after you receive care. You may even apply after a bill has been sent to a collection agency. If a hospital obtains a court judgment before you applied for Hill-Burton assistance, the solution must be worked out within the judicial system. However, if you applied for Hill-Burton before a judgment was rendered and are found eligible, you will receive Hill-Burton even if a judgment was rendered while you were waiting for a response to your application.

Is United States Citizenship Required for Hill-Burton Eligibility?

No. However, in order for a person to have a Hill-Burton eligibility determination made, he must have lived in the U. S. for at least 3 months.

Can I Apply for Hill-Burton Assistance on Behalf of an Uninsured Relative or Friend?

Yes. You can apply for Hill-Burton assistance on behalf of any patient for whom you can provide the information required to establish eligibility, i.e., you must be able to provide information regarding the patient's family size and income.

Do I Have to Wait until I Am Sick before I Can Apply for Hill-Burton Assistance?

Hill-Burton is not health insurance. In order to apply for Hill-Burton assistance you must have already received services or know that you will require a specific service in the near future.

What Can I Do if I Have a Complaint Against a Hill-Burton Facility?

If you feel you were unfairly denied free care or reduced cost care, a complaint must be filed in writing to the HRSA Field Office responsible for the particular State involved. You must include: 1) the name and address of the person making the complaint; 2) the name and location of the facility; and 3) a statement of the actions that the complainant considers to violate the requirements of the Hill-Burton program.

What Other Service Obligation Does a Hill-Burton Facility Have?

Under the community service assurance, Hill-Burton facilities are responsible for providing emergency treatment and for treating all persons residing in the service area, regardless of race, color, national origin, creed or Medicare or Medicaid status. This assurance is in effect for the life of the facility. If you feel you were unfairly denied services or discriminated against you should contact the Office for Civil Rights (OCR) at:

U.S. Department of Education
Office for Civil Rights
Customer Service Team
Mary E. Switzer Building
330 C Street, SW
Washington, DC 20202
800-421-3481
202-205-5413
202-260-0471 TDD
202-205-9862 Fax
E-mail: OCR@ED.Gov
Website: http://www.ed.gov/offices/OCR

How Do I Apply for Free Care?

You should contact the Admissions, Business or Patient Accounts Office at a Hill-Burton obligated facility to find out if you qualify for assistance and whether or not a facility provides the specific services needed.

HRSA Field Office Clusters

Northeast Cluster Division of Health Resources

Philadelphia Branch: Delaware, Maryland, Pennsylvania, Virginia, West Virginia, District of Columbia.

Public Ledger Building, Suite 1172
150 S. Independence Mall West
Philadelphia, Pennsylvania 19106-3499
215-861-4401
215-861-4338 Fax

Boston Branch: Connecticut, Main, Massachusetts, New Hampshire, Rhode Island, Vermont.

John F. Kennedy Federal Building
Government Center, Room 1826
Boston, Massachusetts 02203
617-565-1433
617-565-4027 Fax

New York Branch: New York, New Jersey, Puerto Rico, Virgin Islands.

Federal Building, Room 3337
26 Federal Plaza
New York, New York 10278
212-269-2571
212-264-2673 Fax

Southeast FO Division of Health Resources

Alabama, Florida, Georgia, Kentucky, Mississippi, North Carolina, South Carolina, Tennessee.

61 Forsyth St., SW, Suite 3m60
Atlanta, Georgia 30303-8909

Midwest Cluster Division of Health Resources

Chicago Branch: Illinois, Indiana, Michigan, Minnesota, Ohio, Wisconsin.

105 West Adams Street, 17th Floor
Chicago, Illinois 60603
312-353-8121
312-886-3770 Fax

Kansas City Branch: Iowa, Kansas, Missouri, Nebraska.

601 East 12th Street, Room 501
Kansas City, Missouri 64106
816-426-5291
816-426-3633 Fax

West Central Cluster Division of Health Resources

Dallas Branch: Arkansas, Louisiana, New Mexico, Oklahoma, Texas, Colorado, Montana, North Dakota, South Dakota, Utah, Wyoming.

10 Floor, HRSA 4
1301 Young Street
Dallas, Texas 75202
214-767-3921
214-762-3030 Fax

Pacific West Cluster Division of Health Resources

San Francisco Branch: Arizona, California, Hawaii, Nevada, Guam, American Samoa, Republic of Palau, Commonwealth of the Northern Mariana Islands, Republic of the Marshall Islands, Federated States of Micronesia.

Federal Office Building, Room 317
50 United Nations Plaza
San Francisco, California 94102
415-437-8121
415-437-8105 Fax

Seattle Branch: Alaska, Idaho, Oregon, Washington.

2201 Sixth Avenue
Mail Stop RX-27
Seattle, Washington 98121
206-615-2046
206-615-2466 Fax

For Additional Information

Please write to your Department of Health and Human Services field office or call the HOT LINE. The HOT LINE Toll Free number is:

1-800-638-0742
or for Maryland Residents
1-800-492-0359

The HRSA website at http://158.72.83.3/osp/dfcr/obtain/ HBSTATES.HTM continually updates the list of obligated facilities and provides other information about the Hill-Burton program.

Hill-Burton facilities must provide services without discrimination on the basis of race, color, national origin, or creed. They also may not discriminate against Medicare or Medicaid patients. For more information about the Community Service Assurance, you may call the Office for Civil Rights.

1-800-368-1019

Part Thirteen

Additional Help and Information

Chapter 75

Glossary of Important Terms

Auditory Brain Stem Response (ABR) is a special hearing test that can be used to track the nerve signals arising in the inner ear as they travel through the hearing nerve (called the auditory nerve) to the region of the brain responsible for hearing.

Accuracy is the ability of a test to give consistent results.

Allergens are substances that cause an allergic reaction.

Allergy is a specific immunologic reaction to a normally harmless substance.

Angiography is an invasive diagnostic procedure that allows direct visualization of blood vessels in the body. It is performed by the injection of radiographic contrast material (dye) into the blood vessels via a catheter that is placed directly into the artery or vein.

Anterior chamber a space in the front of the eye where a clear fluid flows continuously in and out nourishing nearby tissues. In many people, increased pressure inside the anterior chamber causes glaucoma.

Arteriography is a more specific term for the study that visualizes the arteries.

Atherosclerosis, occurs when a buildup of fat, cholesterol and other substances on the inner walls of the coronary arteries blocks the flow of oxygen-rich blood.

Arrhythmias are problems with the heart's electrical signals which lead to abnormal heart rhythms, rate, or both.

Arthroscopy is one method used by doctors to diagnose knee problems. The doctor manipulates a small, lighted optic tube (arthroscope) that has been inserted into the joint through a small incision in the knee. Images of the inside of the knee joint are projected onto a television screen.

Asymptomatic is a lack or absence of symptoms.

Audiogram is a basic hearing test of one's ability to hear pure tones in each ear.

Biopsy is a procedure in which tissue is removed by a surgeon or other specialist and examined under a microscope by a pathologist. Tissue samples for biopsy can be obtained by either surgery or needle.

Blood test is a laboratory test that is done on the blood that your doctor draws from your arm.

Cardiac catheterization is a diagnostic procedure, a test that can measure blood pressure and blood flow in the heart's chambers, examine the arteries of the heart (coronary arteries), and provide information about the pumping ability of the heart muscle.

Central vision is the area where light is focused onto your macula, cells change the light into nerve signals and tell the brain what you are seeing.

Colonoscopy (koh-luh-NAH-skuh-pee) lets the physician look inside your entire large intestine, from the lowest part, the rectum all the way up through the colon to the lower end of the small intestine.

Computed Tomography provides a single slice image for each revolution of the x-ray tube around the patient. It demonstrates the tissue that was traversed by the x-ray beam during that exposure.

Core needle biopsy uses a somewhat larger needle than used with fine needle aspiration with a special cutting edge. The needle is inserted, under local anesthesia, through a small incision in the skin, and a small core of tissue is removed.

Cystoscope is an instrument made of a hollow tube about the diameter of a drinking straw with several lenses and a light used to see inside the bladder and urethra.

Diabetes (actual name is diabetes mellitus) of any kind is a disorder that prevents the body from using food properly.

Diastolic pressure is the last sound heard as air is released from a blood pressure cuff. It represents the lowest pressure that remains within the artery when the heart is at rest.

Doppler ultrasound is a special form of ultrasound. That can see the structures inside the body and evaluate blood flow at the same time.

Drusen are tiny yellow deposits in the retina.

Ear canals are the tubular openings that carry sounds from the outside of the body to the ear drum.

Ear drum is a thin, transparent membrane located deep within the outer ear canal that vibrates in response to sound waves.

Electrocardiogram records the electrical activity of your heart and is indispensable for evaluating many forms of heart disease.

EEG (electroencephalogram) displays the electrical activity of the brain.

Electronic fetal monitors measure an unborn baby's heart rate continuously in one of two ways: externally or internally.

Electrophysiology Study (EPS) is a diagnostic test used to evaluate and record the electrical activity of your heart providing information about your heart rhythm (the speed and pattern of your heartbeat). It is not a surgical procedure.

Endoscopic retrograde cholangiopancreatography (en-doh-SKAH-pik REH-troh-grayd koh-LAN-jee-oh-PANG-kree-uh-TAH-gruh-fee) (ERCP) is a scope test which enables the physician to diagnose problems in the liver, gallbladder, bile ducts, and pancreas.

Electronystagmogram (ENG) is a special test of the balance mechanism of the inner ear.

Eustachian tube is a tiny passageway that connects the middle ear to the nose. It normally serves to ventilate and equalize pressure to the middle ear.

False positive is a test result indicating someone has a condition that in fact the person does not.

False negative is a test result that does not identify a condition that is in fact present.

Fine needle aspiration uses a very thin needle and syringe to remove either fluid from a cyst or clusters of cells from a solid mass.

Holter monitor test is a daylong continuous recording of your heart's electrical activity

Insomnia is the perception or complaint of inadequate or poor-quality sleep.

Laparoscope is a tube with a light in it.

Lower gastrointestinal (GI) series uses x-rays to diagnose problems in the large intestine, which includes the colon and rectum. The lower GI series may show problems like abnormal growths, ulcers, polyps, and diverticuli.

Lumbar puncture (LP) is done when physicians need to examine the spinal fluid that bathes the brain and spinal cord.

Macula is the light-sensitive layer of tissue at the back of the eye in the center of the retina.

Macrocalcifications are coarse calcium deposits.

Mammogram is an x-ray of the breast.

Microcalcifications are tiny flecks of calcium found in an area of rapidly dividing cells.

Middle ear is a small, air-containing cavity that sits behind the eardrum. When the eardrum vibrates, tiny bones within the middle ear transmit the sound signals to the inner ear. Here nerves are stimulated to relay the sound signals to the brain.

Multiple Sleep Latency Test (MSLT) measures the speed of falling asleep.

Pap test (sometimes called a Pap smear) is a way to examine cells collected from the cervix and vagina. This test can show the presence of infection, inflammation, abnormal cells, or cancer.

Pathologist is a doctor who specializes in identifying tissue changes that are characteristic of disease, including cancer.

Polysomnography is a test that records a variety of body functions during sleep, such as the electrical activity of the brain, eye movement, muscle activity, heart rate, respiratory effort, air flow, and blood oxygen levels.

Positrons are subatomic particles that resemble electrons but carry a positive instead of a negative charge.

Radionuclides are radioactive isotopes which emit ionizing radiation.

Sigmoidoscopy (SIG-moy-DAH-skuh-pee) enables the physician to look at the inside of the large intestine from the rectum through the last part of the colon, called the sigmoid colon.

Signs are an indication of illness, injury, or that something is not right in the body. Signs are observations made by a physician, nurse or other health care professional. Fever, rapid breathing rate, abnormal breathing sounds heard through a stethoscope are signs that may indicate pneumonia.

Sleep apnea is a serious, potentially life-threatening condition. It is a breathing disorder characterized by repeated collapse of the upper airway during sleep, with consequent cessation of breathing.

Spirometry is useful for assessing lung function as well as general health. It is the simplest and most common of the lung function tests.

Symptoms are an indication of disease, illness, injury, or that something is not right in the body. Symptoms are felt or noticed by a patient, but not easily observed by anyone else. For example chills, weakness, achiness, shortness of breath, and a cough are symptoms that might indicate pneumonia.

Systolic blood pressure is the first sound heard and registered on the gauge or mercury column. It represents the maximum pressure in the artery produced as the heart contracts and the blood begins to flow. Blood pressure is at it greatest when the heart contracts and is pumping the blood.

Telemedicine involves the use of computers and telecommunications equipment to provide health care over long distances.

Tumor markers are substances that can often be detected in higher-than-normal amounts in the blood, urine, or body tissues of some patients with certain types of cancer.

Tympanogram is a test that measures how easily the eardrum vibrates back and forth and at what pressure the vibration is the easiest.

Ultrasound is a frequency (or pitch) higher than humans can hear which when sent into the body from a transducer (probe) resting on the patient's skin can reflect off internal structures. The returning echoes are received by the transducer and converted by an electronic instrument into an image on a monitor. These continually changing images can be recorded on videotape or film. Diagnostic ultrasound imaging is commonly called sonography or ultrasonography.

Upper endoscopy enables the physician to look inside the esophagus, stomach, and duodenum (first part of the small intestine). The procedure might be used to discover the reason for swallowing difficulties, nausea, vomiting, reflux, bleeding, indigestion, abdominal pain, or chest pain.

Upper gastrointestinal (GI) series uses x-rays to diagnose problems in the esophagus, stomach, and duodenum (first part of the small intestine). It may also be used to examine the small intestine. The upper GI series can show a blockage, abnormal growth, ulcer, or a problem with the way an organ is working.

Venography is a study of the veins using radiographic contrast, is another type of angiogram.

X-rays are actually electromagnetic waves. When they are passed through a patient's body to a photographic film on the other side, they create a picture of internal body structures called a radiograph.

Chapter 76

Computer Diagnosis and Telemedicine

In Hays, Kan., an infant is born with a heart murmur. Because there is a slight chance of severe cardiac problems when this happens, Robert Cox, M.D., a pediatrician and medical director of rural development and telemedicine at Hays Medical Center, seeks the advice of a cardiologist in Kansas City, which is 270 miles away. Yet the infant and Cox never leave the small town of Hays.

Instead, using interactive videoconferencing, the cardiologist in Kansas City examines the infant and listens to the heartbeat as a technician in Hays holds an instrument similar to a stethoscope against the baby's body. The cardiologist also can view the baby's chest x-ray and electrocardiogram. Because of this technology, Cox says, "Today, we refer only 1 percent of infants with heart murmurs to an out-of-town hospital, instead of 100 percent."

An elderly man who has trouble walking is referred to a small hospital in rural West Virginia. "Even after doing a complete physical exam, no one was sure what the problem was," recalls James Brick, M.D., a rheumatologist and medical director of the telemedicine program at the West Virginia University School of Medicine in Morgantown.

So a medical student at the rural hospital used videoconferencing to present the patient's case to the chairman of the university's neurology department. The neurologist examined the patient, put him through various tests, and made a diagnosis of amyotrophic lateral sclerosis, commonly known as Lou Gehrig's disease.

"Lights, Camera, Telemedicine," *FDA Consumer*, May/June1997.

These doctors are practicing telemedicine, which involves the use of computers and telecommunications equipment to provide health care over long distances. It is actually an extension of one of the oldest, simplest, and most popular forms of electronic medical consultation: a telephone conversation between doctor and patient or a medical generalist and a specialist. But, unlike the telephone, some aspects of telemedicine are regulated by the Food and Drug Administration.

Telemedicine Technology

Teleradiology is the oldest form of telemedicine referenced in the medical literature and one FDA has been involved in since 1977, according to Melvyn Greberman, M.D., of FDA's Center for Devices and Radiological Health. As now practiced, this technology involves creating and transmitting medical images, such as x-rays or computed tomography scans, electronically in the form of a digital signal from one location to another. An expert at a distant site receives the images, evaluates them, helps make a diagnosis, and suggests additional care as needed. The process is much like sending an x-ray by mail or courier—but with telemedicine, the transmission is almost instantaneous.

FDA and the medical community share responsibility for ensuring the safety and effectiveness of the medical devices used in the telemedicine process. For example, photographs of a suspicious skin lesion can be sent electronically as digital images. The images are then reconstructed for display on a monitor and read by the doctor who receives them.

"The question that the doctor should ask is, 'Is the resulting image adequate for the purposes intended?'" FDA's Greberman says. "If an image will be used for diagnosis, then the clinician must be certain that it has sufficient detail to permit accurate interpretation."

For example, he says, the digitized image, which may be compressed to reduce transmission time and storage requirements, should not have degraded significantly in quality when it is viewed as a reconstructed image. "FDA requires a manufacturer to indicate on-screen when compression that results in the loss of some data is used, but the doctor must determine the impact of this compression on the clinical adequacy of the image," he adds.

Another form of telemedicine is interactive videoconferencing, also known as interactive television and interactive teleconferencing. This technique permits two doctors and a patient to confer simultaneously, even though they are at different sites. For example, a camera in an examining room would enable one doctor to present the patient to the other. The other doctor, usually a consultant, also in front of a video camera, would offer an opinion.

Nurses and other health professionals also can use interactive television to monitor patients at home. For example, in Hays, an older woman receives regular visits from a home health nurse via cable television.

The woman's television emits a beep two minutes before the nurse is scheduled to check on her. The patient switches on the television, which also is equipped with a small videocamera. She can see the nurse, and the nurse can see her. The nurse assesses the patient's overall appearance; reviews her temperature, blood pressure, and other vital signs; and reminds her to take her medication.

"With this technology, we found that one home health nurse could visit nine patients in one morning during a blizzard, simply by working from her base station," Kansas doctor Cox says.

The same technology also is used for educational purposes. For example, the Georgia Telemedicine Network, which is based at the Medical College of Georgia in Augusta, links the medical college with 44 sites throughout the state, including the Eisenhower Army Medical Center and Emory University Medical Center, according to Max Stachura, M.D., the network's executive director. Medical students in remote locations take classes at the university, doctors earn continuing medical education credits, and health information is communicated to the public.

FDA's Role

FDA's primary role with respect to telemedicine is to review the devices, or hardware, before clearing them for marketing and to conduct postmarketing surveillance—that is, to be aware of significant problems that occur after the devices are marketed.

In July 1996, the Center for Devices and Radiological Health issued the report "Telemedicine Related Activities." It reviews current and potential areas of telemedicine of interest to FDA and is available on the World Wide Web at http://www.fda.gov/cdrh/telemed.html.

Certain medical software products that may be used for diagnostic purposes also fall under FDA's jurisdiction. However, other government agencies—such as the Federal Communications Commission, which regulates some aspects of the communications technologies—are involved in telemedicine, as well. The Federal Joint Working Group on Telemedicine, of which FDA is a participant, includes representatives from various government agencies working together to clarify regulatory issues related to telemedicine.

Benefits

Telemedicine advocates believe the technology can make a critical difference in health-care delivery in rural communities, where access to specialized care is often sporadic and people may hesitate to travel long distances to see a doctor. With telemedicine, experts say, patients can benefit from the expertise of distant specialists and still receive treatment in the community.

Kansas doctor Cox notes, for instance, that his clinic has established a relationship with a hematologist/oncologist (a specialist in blood diseases and cancer) at the University of Kansas Medical Center. The specialist visits Hays twice a month, and also is available twice a week via telemedicine. "Thus, we have a specialist available in our town twice a week either in person or electronically," he says. "The result is that we're able to deliver more health-care services to the community. In addition, the level of quality at our local hospital is bolstered, so our staff feels better working here. Everyone benefits."

The community benefits financially, as well, Cox says, because medical tests and prescriptions generated by the specialist are handled locally.

The Georgia Telemedicine Network has brought similar benefits by "empowering local practitioners," network director Stachura says. An initial concern about telemedicine was that it would take patients away from local primary-care doctors by moving them to larger facilities. "But we've been able to demonstrate that 88 percent of patients seen by specialists via telemedicine never leave their hometown," he says.

Telemedicine also can be cost-effective. In Georgia, for example, telemedicine is used to provide services to prisoners who otherwise would have to be transferred to health-care facilities, a move that can be costly because of the need for guards to accompany prisoners and for transportation. Now, according to Stachura, a mobile telemedicine van comes to the prison on a regular basis, plugs in, and allows the health-care professionals to give medical check-ups to inmates on site.

A cable television health-care program that is being instituted in Georgia also can help cut health-care costs by serving as a type of "electronic house call," both in rural communities and underserved urban neighborhoods, Stachura notes. For example, in some instances, at-home monitoring can delay an older person's entry into a nursing home, resulting in improved quality of life, as well as significant cost savings.

As the technology becomes more accepted, telemedicine could be used for home-based follow-up care for the chronically ill, Stachura adds. Doctors could monitor patients with diabetes or asthma at home, thus avoiding hospitalization unless it is truly necessary. Similarly, high-risk patients with heart problems could have their electrocardiograms and blood pressure readings monitored at home, forestalling the onset of more serious problems and allowing for more cost-effective, early care.

A computerized service that could facilitate this type of care was developed to monitor various health signs, according to a December 1996 New York Times report. The service helps patients check their blood pressure and undergo an electrocardiogram at home, and then sends the results via modem to a health-care provider. According to the newspaper, the service is now in clinical trials to see whether its use can cut down on hospital stays and emergency visits by patients with congestive heart disease who are recovering at home.

Obstacles

Although telemedicine offers benefits, there still are obstacles to overcome before it becomes part of mainstream medicine, experts say.

One obstacle involves reimbursement. While Medicare and insurance companies pay for diagnostic services such as teleradiology, most do not yet pay for other consultative telemedicine services.

Cox joined the pediatric committee of a Kansas insurance company to help convince company officials to provide reimbursement for telemedicine. He argued that the technology allows doctors to take medical histories, review scans and x-rays, diagnose problems, schedule follow-ups, and prepare reports. "The company ultimately agreed that those components make the consultation a reimbursable event," Cox says, adding that he hopes other insurers will follow this precedent.

Medical licensing is another potential problem. Because telemedicine can cross state lines, some states could require an out-of-state doctor whose use of telemedicine crosses into their jurisdiction to get a license in their state, even if the doctor's practice is physically located elsewhere.

Stachura notes for instance that he sees patients from both Georgia and South Carolina because his Georgia clinic is near the South Carolina border. "If the patient comes to me, everything is fine,"

Stachura says. "But if I use telemedicine technology to see a patient in South Carolina—that is, if I were going to the patient, so to speak—then I would need a license to practice medicine in South Carolina."

The licensing issue is further complicated by laws some states have passed that prohibit out-of-state physicians from performing telemedicine in their states, he notes.

Medical liability is an issue, as well. For example, a remote specialist who does not perform a hands-on examination could be regarded as delivering less-than-adequate care. Or if compressed digital images are not reconstructed well, causing loss of valuable diagnostic information, a doctor could possibly face a malpractice suit.

And, as in other areas, telemedicine advocates admit, the use of technology often means that things may not run smoothly every time. Brick recalls a time when the West Virginia telemedicine program switched to another phone carrier. "We had people from the state licensing board there to view the equipment, and nothing worked. We discovered we had to reboot all the computers to make the new phone connection."

Another time, he recalls, lightning hit a small hospital nearby and shorted out all the computers. "It took several weeks to fix." Also, he says, "a couple of times in the four years that we've been running the program, the system went down while a patient was waiting on the other end."

These technical problems notwithstanding, experts advise patients to give telemedicine a try. "Go into it with an open mind," Brick says. "Expect to be able to see and hear the doctor on the other end. Expect the doctor to connect with you and personalize the experience for you. Talk to him, ask whatever questions you have, just as you would in an in-person consultation."

According to Stachura, it's only a matter of time before the obstacles are overcome, and doctors and the public become more accepting of telemedicine. "If 20 years ago, someone said you could walk up to a machine on the street, press a few buttons and get cash or have your financial portfolio displayed, you would have said, 'It's incredible.'" But, like automated teller machines, he says, telemedicine eventually will be accepted, too.

—Marilynn Larkin

Marilynn Larkin is a medical writer in New York City.

Chapter 77

Resources for Additional Help

Cancer Information Sources

The American Cancer Society
1599 Clifton Road, N.E.
Atlanta, GA 303329-4251
800-ACS-2345
http://www.cancer.org

National Cancer Institute
Building 82, Room 123
Bethesda, MD 20892
800-422-6237 (800-4-CANCER); 800-332-8615 TTY
http://www.nci.nih.gov/
http://cancernet.nci.gov
http://rex.nci.nih.gov

E-mail and fax services:

CancerMail: Includes NCI information about cancer treatment, screening, prevention, and supportive care. To obtain a contents list, send e-mail to cancermail@icicc.nci.nih.gov with the word "help" in the body of the message.

CancerFax: To obtain a contents list, dial 301-402-58-74 from a fax machine hand set and follow the recorded instructions.

National Prostate Cancer Coalition
1156 15th St., N.W.
Suite 905
Washington, DC 20005
202-463-9455
http://www.4npcc.org

National Coalition for Cancer Survivorship
1010 Wayne Ave.
7th Floor
Silver Spring, MD 20910-5600
301-650-8868

Patient Advocates for Advanced Cancer Treatment
1143 Parmalee, N.W.
Grand Rapids, MI 49504
616-453-1477

US Too International Inc.
930 N. York Road, Suite 50
Hinsdale, IL 60521-2993
800-808-7866
http://www.ustoo.com

American Foundation for Urologic Disease
300 W. Pratt St., Suite 401
Baltimore, MD 21201-2463
800-828-7866

Eye Tests and Diseases

Groups and agencies that offer information about counseling, training, and other special services are available. You may also want to contact a nearby school of medicine or optometry as well as a local agency devoted to helping the visually impaired.

American Academy of Ophthalmology
655 Beach Street, P.O. Box 7424
San Francisco, CA 94109-7424
(415) 561-8500
http://www.eyenet.org

American Optometric Association
243 Lindbergh Boulevard
St. Louis, MO 63141
(314) 991-4100
http://www.aoanet.org

American Diabetes Association
1660 Duke Street
Alexandria, VA 22314
(703) 549-1500
800-342-2383
http://www.diabetes.org

Juvenile Diabetes Foundation International
432 Park Avenue South
New York, NY 10016
(212) 889-7575
http://www.jdfcare.com

National Diabetes Information Clearinghouse of the
National Institute of Diabetes and Digestive and Kidney
Diseases
1 Information Way
Bethesda, MD 20892-3560

National Eye Institute
2020 Vision Place
Bethesda, MD 20892-3655
(301) 496-5248
http://www.nei.nih.gov

Prevent Blindness America
500 East Remington Road
Schamburg, IL 60173
800-331-2020
847-843-2020
http://www.prevent-blindness.org

American Foundation for the Blind
11 Penn Plaza, Suite 300
New York, NY 10001
800-232-5463
212-502-7600
E-mail: afbinfo@afb.org
http://www.afb.org

Council of Citizens with Low Vision International
5707 Brockton Drive, Suite 302
Indianapolis, IN 46220-5481
800-733-2258
317-254-1332

Lighthouse International
111 E. 59th Street
New York, NY 10022
800-334-5497
800-829-0500
212-281-9200
http://www.lighthouse.org

National Federation of the Blind
1800 Johnson Street
Baltimore, MD 21230
301-659-9314
http://www.nfb.org

Association for Macular Diseases
210 E. 64th Street
New York, NY 10021
212-605-3719

(The) Foundation Fighting Blindness
Executive Plaza 1, Suite 800
11350 McCormick Road
Hunt Valley, MD 21031-1014
800-683-5555
410-785-1414
http://www.blindness.org

Macular Degeneration International
6700 North Oracle Road, Suite 121
Tucson, AZ 85704
800-393-7634
520-797-2525

(The) Glaucoma Foundation
33 Maiden Lane
New York, NY 10038
800-452-8266
E-mail: glaucomafdn@mindspring.com
http://www.glaucoma-foundation.org/info

Glaucoma Research Foundation
200 Pine Street, Suite 200
San Francisco, CA 94104
800-826-6693
(415) 986-3162
http://www.glaucoma.org

Gene Testing Information

National Center for Human Genome Research
Office of Communications
301-402-0911

Geriatrics (Aging) Information

National Institute on Aging
Department of Health and Human Services
Federal Building, Room 6C12
9000 Rockville Pike
Bethesda, MD 20892
301-496-1752

Heart, Lung, and Blood Disease Information

National Heart, Lung, and Blood Institute
NHLBI Information Center
P.O. Box 30105
Bethesda, MD 20824-0105
301-251-1222
Fax: 301-251-1223
http://www.nhlbi.nih.gov/

Infectious Diseases (including Sexually Transmitted Diseases), Allergies, and Asthma Information

National Institute of Allergy and Infectious Diseases
National Institutes of Health
Bethesda, MD 20892
http://www.niaid.nih.gov

HIV/AIDS Program of the FDA
For questions about HIV Home test kits:
Office of Special Health Issues
301-827-4460

AIDS
http://www.niaid.nih.gov/factsheets/facts.htm

National Herpes Hotline
919/361-8488, 9 a.m. to 7 p.m. Eastern Time, Monday through Friday

Herpes Resource Center
American Social Health Association
P.O. Box 13827
Research Triangle Park, NC 27709-9940
800/230-6039

Health Advice Company
2515 East Highway 54
2200 Century Plaza
Durham, NC 27713
888/ADVICE-8 (888/238-4238), 9 a.m. to 5 p.m. Eastern Time, Monday through Friday
http://www.advicecenter.com

The American College of Obstetricians and Gynecologists
409 12th Street, S.W.
P.O. Box 96920
Washington, DC 20090-6920
202/863-2518
http://www.acog.org

Kidney Function

American Kidney Fund
6110 Executive Boulevard
Rockville, MD 20852
1-800-638-8299

National Kidney Foundation
30 East 33rd Street
New York, NY 10016
1-800-622-9010

National Kidney and Urologic Diseases Information Clearinghouse of the National Institute of Diabetes and Digestive and Kidney Diseases
3 Information Way
Bethesda, MD 20892-3580
E-mail: nkudic@info.niddk.nih.gov

Neurologic Diseases

National Institute of Neurological Disorders and Stroke
http://www.nih.gov/ninds/

Osteoporosis Information

National Osteoporosis Foundation
1150 17th St., N.W., Suite 500
Washington, DC 20036
(202) 223-2226
http://www.nof.org/
For locations of your nearest bone density testing sites, call
(800) 464-6700.

Osteoporosis and Related Bone Diseases
National Resource Center (ORBD-NRC)
(800) 624-BONE
TDD: (202) 223-0344

Older Women's League (OWL)
666 11th St., N.W., Suite 700
Washington, DC 20001
(202) 783-6686

North American Menopause Society
c/o University Hospitals of Cleveland
Department of Obstetrics and Gynecology
11100 Euclid Ave., Suite 7024
Cleveland, OH 44106
(216) 844-8748
http://www.menopause.org/

American Association of Retired Persons (AARP)
601 E St., N.W.
Washington, DC 20049
(202) 434-2277
http://www.aarp.org/

Scope Tests

National Digestive Diseases Information Clearinghouse
2 Information Way
Bethesda, MD 20892-3570
301-654-3810
Fax: 301-907-8906
E-mail: nddic@aerie.com

Endometriosis Association
8585 North 76th Place
Milwaukee, WI 53223
414-355-2200

The American College of Obstetricians and Gynecologists
409 12th Street, SW
Washington, DC 20024-2188
202-638-5577

American Fertility Society
2140-11th Avenue South
Suite 200
Birmingham, AL 35205-2800
205-933-8494

American Academy of Orthopaedic Surgeons
6300 N. River Road
Rosemont, IL 60018-4262
847-823-7186
800-346-2267
http://www.aaos.org

    The academy publishes several brochures on the knee. Single copies of "Arthroscopy" and "Total Joint Replacement," are available free to the public if a self-addressed, stamped envelope is provided.

Arthritis Foundation
1330 Peach Tree Street
Atlanta, GA 30309
404-872-7100
800-283-7800 or call your local chapter (listed in the local telephone directory)
http://www.arthritis.org

American College of Rheumatology/Association of Rheumatology Health Professionals
60 Executive Park South, Suite 150
Atlanta, GA 30329
404-633-3777
Fax: 404-633-1870
http://www.rheumatology.org

National Arthritis and Musculoskeletal and Skin Diseases Information Clearinghouse (NAMSIC)
National Institutes of Health
1 AMS Circle
Bethesda, MD 20892-3675
301-495-4484
TTY: 301-565-2966
Automated faxback system: 301-881-2731
http://www.nih.gov/niams

Ultrasound

American Institute of Ultrasound in Medicine
14750 Sweitzer Lane, Suite 100
Laurel, MD 20707-5906
301-498-4100
301-498-4450 Fax
http://www.aium.org

Urinary System Tests and Disease Information

American Foundation for Urologic Disease
300 W. Pratt St., Suite 401
Baltimore, MD 21201-2463
1-800-828-7866

American Foundation for Urologic Disease
1128 N. Charles St.
Baltimore MD 21201
1-800-242-2383 or 410-468-1800
E-mail: admin@afud.org
http://www.access.digex.net/~afud

American Kidney Fund
5110 Executive Boulevard
Suite 100
Rockville, MD 20852
800-638-8299 or 301-881-3052

American Society of Pediatric Nephrology
Department of Pediatrics
University of Wisconsin
Children's Hospital
600 Highland Avenue
Madison, WI 53792-4108
608-265-6020

American Uro-Gynecologic Society
401 North Michigan Avenue
Chicago, IL 60611-4267
312-644-661- ext. 4712

Interstitial Cystitis Association
P.O. Box 1553
Madison Square Station
New York, NY 10159
1-800-ICA-1626 or 212-979-6057
http://www.ichelp.com

National Association for Continence (NAFC)
P.O. Box 8310
Spartanburg, SC 29305-8310
864-5799-7900 or 1-800-BLADDER
http://www.nafc.org/

National Kidney Foundation
30 East 33rd Street
New York, NY 10016
800-622-9010
http://www.kidney.org/

The Prostatitis Foundation
Information Distribution Center
Parkway Business Center
2029 Ireland Grove Road
Bloomington, IL 61704
309-664-6222
E-mail: Mcapstone@aol.com
http://www.prostate.org/

The Simon Foundation for Continence
P.O. Box 835
Wilmette, IL 60091
800-23-SIMON or (847)-864-3913 (main office)
E-mail: simoninfo@simonfoundation.org
http://www.simonfoundation.org/

National Kidney and Urologic Diseases Information Clearinghouse
3 Information Way
Bethesda, MD 20892-3580
301-654-4415
Fax: 301-907-8906
E-mail: nkudic@info.niddk.nih.gov

Financial Assistance with Medical Bills

Check your phone directory for the offices listed under Medicaid, Social Services, Medical Assistance, Public Assistance, Human Services or Community Services or call 1-800-638-6833 to speak to a representative from HCFA that will help you in finding the phone number in your State.

For help in applying for or filing Medicaid claims contact your State Medical Assistance Office.

Table 77.1. State Medical Assistance Offices, continued on next page.

State Name	Phone Number(s)
Alabama	800-362-1504
Alaska	800-770-5650
American Samoa	011-684-633-4590
Arizona	602-417-4680
Arkansas	501-682-8487
California	800-952-5253
Colorado	303-866-2993
Connecticut	860-424-5008
Delaware	302-577-4901
District of Columbia	202-727-0735; 202-724-5506
Florida	850-488-3560
Georgia	800-282-4536
Guam	1-0-671-734-7264
Hawaii	808-586-5391
Idaho	208-334-5747
Illinois	800-252-8635
Indiana	317-232-4966
Iowa	515-281-8621
Kansas	785-296-3349
Kentucky	502-564-6885
Louisana	504-342-3855; 504-342-5716
Maine	207-624-5277
Maryland	410-767-1432
Massachusetts	800-841-2900
Michigan	800-642-3195
Minnesota	800-657-3739
Mississippi	601-359-6056
Missouri	573-751-3425

Hill-Burton Free Care Program

Free Hospital Care, Nursing Home Care and Care Provided in Other Types of Health Facilities Under the Hill-Burton Program.

Call the Hot Line Toll Free number:
1-800-638-0742
Maryland Residents 1-800-492-0359.
http://www.hrsa.dhhs.gov/bhrd/drcr/drcrmain.htm
Note: The Hill-Burton website continually updates the list of obligated facilities.

Table 77.1. State Medical Assistance Offices, continued from previous page.

State Name	Phone Number(s)
Montana	406-444-5900
Nebraska	402-471-9147
Nevada	702-687-4775
New Hampshire	603-271-4344
New Jersey	609-588-2600
New Mexico	505-827-3100
New York	518-486-4803
North Carolina	800-662-7030
North Dakota	800-755-2604
Northern Mariana Islands	011-670-234-8950 ext. 2905
Ohio	800-324-8680
Oklahoma	405-530-3439
Oregon	503-945-5811
Pennsylvania	717-787-1870
Puerto Rico	787-765-1230
Rhode Island	401-464-2121
South Carolina	803-253-6100
South Dakota	605-773-3495
Tennessee	615-741-0213
Texas	512-438-3219
Utah	801-538-6155
Vermont	802-241-2880
Virginia	804-786-7933
Virgin Islands	809-774-4624
Washington	800-562-3022
West Virginia	800-642-3607
Wisconsin	608-266-2522
Wyoming	307-777-5500

Index

Index

Page numbers followed by 'n' indicate a footnote. Page numbers in *italics* indicate a table or illustration

A

A. M. Best Company, insurance company rating publication 578
AAA *see* Audiology, American Academy of (AAA)
abdomen, computed tomography 243, 252–58
ABR *see* auditory brain stem response (ABR)
accuracy
  see also false negative test results
  see also false positive test results
  defined 132, 621
  HIV home test kits 144–45
  home cholesterol tests 153
  home glucose tests 138–39
  Pap tests 405–6
acoustic schwannoma, magnetic resonance imaging 309–10
ACS *see* Cancer Society, American (ACS)
acyclovir, genital herpes 553, 554
adolescents
  cholesterol levels 374

adolescents, continued
  drug abuse tests 149–50
  pelvic inflammatory disease 544
  testing recommendations 167–72
adrenal biopsy 264
adult polycystic kidney disease 473
advance directives 51–52
  see also living wills
AFDC *see* Aid to Families with Dependent Children (AFDC)
African Americans
  allergies 92
  diabetes risk 117
  glaucoma risk 102, 104
  hyptertension 27
  tuberculosis 72, 79
age charting, described 159–60
age factor
  see also adolescents
  see also children
  see also geriatrics
  see also infants
  see also young adults
  cancer tests 13–15
  causes of death 161, 167, 173, 179
  cholesterol levels 370, 372
  diabetes tests 116
  gestational diabetes 511
  glaucoma risk 102

age factor, continued
  hyptertension 27
  mammograms 13
  oral cancer 38
  prostate cancer 39
  sigmoidoscopy 7
  thyroid disease 43–44
  uterine cancer 40
age-related macular degeneration
  (AMD) 104–9
  diagnosis 106–7
  prevention 108–9
  symptoms 106
  types, described 105
Aging, National Institute on (NIA),
  contact information 639
AIDS (acquired immune deficiency
  syndrome)
  see also HIV (human immunodefi-
    ciency virus)
  blood tests 367–68
  home testing 143
  tuberculosis 73
Aid to Families with Dependent Children (AFDC) 603
  see also Temporary Assistance for
    Needy Families (TANF)
  income and resources requirements
    601
  Medicaid eligibility 600
airborne allergens 83
  see also allergies
airborne allergies 83–84
air-contrast barium enemas 7, 8
alanine aminotransferase (ALT) 381
Alaska Natives, test recommendations 165, 169, 175
alcohol abuse, pancreatitis 255
alleles, described 474
allergens, defined 621
  see also airborne allergens
allergic dermatitis, statistics 92
allergic drug reactions, statistics 93
allergic rhinitis 83
  statistics 92
allergic salute, described 83
allergic tension fatigue syndrome 90
allergies
  defined 621

allergies, continued
  described 81–82
  information sources 640–41
  statistics 91–93
  symptoms 83
  tests, described 83–93
Allergy and Infectious Diseases, National Institute of (NIAID)
  advances in tuberculosis diagnosis 77
  contact information 640
  sexually transmitted diseases 535
  yeast infection diagnosis 558
Alliance of Genetic Support Groups,
  web page address 484
alpha-1-antitrypsin deficiency 472
alpha-fetoprotein (AFP) 386, 517
  pregnancy tests 501
ALS *see* amyotrophic lateral sclerosis
  (ALS)
ALT *see* alanine aminotransferase
  (ALT)
alveoli, tuberculosis 75
Alzheimer disease, genetic testing
  480–81
AMA *see* Medical Association, American
AMD *see* age-related macular degeneration (AMD)
American Association of Retired Persons (AARP), contact information
  63, 642
American Indians *see* Native Americans
amniocentesis 501, 502, 517–22
Amplicor HIV-1 Monitor Test 540
Amsler grid, depicted 107–8
amyotrophic lateral sclerosis (ALS)
  472
anaphylaxis
  angiography 270
  food allergies 85
  statistics 93
ANA test, described 66
anemia 366–67
  genetic testing 472
anencephaly, pregnancy tests 501
aneuploidy 518
aneurysm, cerebral 282
Angelman syndrome 473

financial concerns
  medical bills assistance 646–47
  medical test payments 569–618
fine needle aspiration, defined 624
First Response test 151, 500
Flieger, Ken 8
fluorescein angiography test, described 108, 111
fluorescent treponemal antibody absorption test (FTA-ABS) 561
fluorescent treponemal antibody
  (FTA) test, described 66
fluoride, dental care 38
FMD *see* fibromuscular dysplasia
  (FMD)
folic acid 168, 174, 175
food additives, allergies 86–87
food allergies 84–91
  common, described 85–86
  diagnosis 87–91
    controversial methods 89–91
  symptoms 85
Food and Drug Administration (FDA)
  approvals
    Accumeter Cholesterol Self-Test
      153
    Amplicor HIV-1 Monitor Test 540
    bone density devices 59
    Coulter HIV-1 p24 Antigen Assay
      540
    HIV home test kits 146–47
    Home Access Express HIV-1 Test
      System 144, 539
    NTx test 60
    risks *versus* benefits 192–93
    Sahara Clinical Bone Sonometer
      60
    urine based HIV test 541
  certification of mammography fa-
    cilities 209–10
  chlamydial infection diagnosis 548
  contact information 147
  electronic fetal monitors 523
  genital herpes treatment 553
  HIV/AIDS Program, contact infor-
    mation 640
  Home Access Express HIV-1 Test
    System 143
  home pregnancy tests 151

Food and Drug Administration (FDA)
  approvals, continued
    Office of AIDS and Special Health
      Issues on the World Wide Web
      541
  over the counter tests 131–32
  pap test rescreening systems 405
  preventing and treating AIDS 539
  protein marker NMP22 420
  regulation of contrast agent drugs
    198
  revised labeling on foods and
    supplements 58
  routine annual physical 5
  sulfites ban 87
  telemedicine
    areas of interest 631
    regulation 630
  ultrasound safety 220
  unapproved HIV home test kits 145
food intolerances 84–85
food labels, bone strength 58
foot problems
  diabetes 141
  elderly persons 40–41
forced expiratory volume (FEV)
  asthma 464
  described 460
forced vital capacity (FVC)
  asthma 464
  described 460
forensic identity testing 477
fourier analysis 240
  see also computed tomography
fractures, osteoporosis 57
Fragile-X syndrome 472, 475
FTA-ABS test 561
FTA test, described 66
functional MRI test, described 68
functional reach test, described 42
fundoscopy 37
FVC *see* forced vital capacity (FVC)

G

gait testing, elderly persons 41–43
galactosemia 488, 494
gallbladder testing 290–91, 435–36

lumbar puncture (LP), continued
  described 69
  syphilis test 561
lung cancer
  CA 15-3 tumor marker 387
  CA 27-29 tumor marker 387
  computed tomography 245–46
  symptoms 18
  test recommendations 125
  tests 44–45
lung disorders
  see also pneumonia
  see also tuberculosis
  bronchoscopy 449–51
  collapsed lung 249
  information sources 640
  tests 459–66
lymphocytes 368
  see also white blood cells
lymphoma, computed tomography
  246–47

M

M. tuberculosis see *Mycobacterium tuberculosis*
macrocalcifications, defined 208, 624
macrophages, tuberculosis 75
macula, defined 105, 624
macular degeneration 36, 37
  see also age-related macular degeneration
Macular Degeneration International, contact information 113, 639
Macular Diseases, Association for, contact information 112, 638
macular edema, described 110
magnesium test, described 66
magnetic resonance imaging (MRI) 194–95, 300–328
  described 67, 300–304, 327–28
  functional, described 68
  patient preparations 188
  safety concerns 303–4
magnetic resonance spectroscopy (MRS), described 68
major medical health insurance, described 570

malnutrition, geriatrics 32–33
  see also diet and nutrition
  see also nutrition
mammograms 203–12
  defined 203–4, 625
  economic concerns 210
  legislation 209–10
  Medicare 587
  patient preparations 187, 189
  recommendations 8, 13, 46, 173, 210–11
  types, described 204
Mammography Quality Standards Act 209–10
managed care health insurance 570–71
Mantoux test 76
  see also tuberculin skin test
maple syrup urine disease, genetic testing 487
Marble, Michelle 136
Marfan syndrome, genetic testing 475
mast cells
  allergies 82, 83
  food allergies 88, 90
Matritech (Cambridge, MA) 420
Mayo Clinic Family Health Book (Larson) 440
McNeil, Caroline 421
MDR-TB *see under* tuberculosis (TB)
mediastinum 245, 247
Medicaid 599–607
  administered by Health Care Financing Administration 591
  amount and duration of services 605–6
  Hill-Burton Free Care Program 613
  Medically Needy (MN) program 602
  telemedicine services 595
  Title XIX 599
  "welfare reform" bill 603
Medical Assistance Offices, state listings 606–7, 646–47
Medical Association, American
  Pap test 46
  routine annual physical 4
  teleconsultation requirements 598
medical checkups *see* physical examinations

muscular dystrophy (MS) 472, 475
myasthenia gravis test, described 70
Mycobacterium bovis 79
Mycobacterium tuberculosis 71
    described 74
    drug resistance 72
Mycoplasma hominis 556
myelograms, described 68
myocardial infarction
    see also heart disease
    aspirin use 52–53
    cholesterol levels 370
Myotonic dystrophy, genetic testing
    473

N

National Health Interview Survey,
    cervical cancer 46
National Institutes of Health (NIH)
    see also *individual agencies and in-
        stitutes*
    Cholesterol Education Program,
        National (NCEP) 48, 154, 375
    neonatal screening 490
Native Americans
    diabetes risk 117
    test recommendations 165, 169, 175
    tuberculosis 79
NCV test, described 69
Neisseria gonorrhoeae 563
    see also gonorrhea
nerve conduction velocity (NCV) test,
    described 69
nerve regulators, described 430–31
neural tube defects
    genetic testing 475
    pregnancy tests 501
neurofibromatosis, genetic testing
    473
neurological diseases
    information sources 641
    tests, described 65–70
Neurological Disorders and Stroke,
    National Institute of, contact infor-
    mation 641
neuron-specific enolase (NSE) 388
neurosyphilis 560, 561

neutrophils 368
    see also white blood cells
newborn care 529–32
newborn screening 485–95
    see also infants
New Mexico, University of 495
nicotine patch 33
Nordenberg, Tamar 196
NSE *see* neuron-specific enolase
    (NSE)
NTx test, described 60
nuclear imaging 284–97
nuclear scanning, described 196
nuclear stress test, described 344–45
nucleic acid amplification, tuberculo-
    sis diagnosis 77
nursing home residents, tuberculosis
    73
nutrition, geriatrics 32–33

O

OAE test, described 99
OAG *see* open angle glaucoma (OAG)
obesity
    cholesterol levels 372
    gestational diabetes 511
obstetricians 501
Obstetricians and Gynecologists,
    American College of
    contact information 641, 642
    fetal monitoring 525–26
    HIV testing 502–3
Obstetrics and Gynecology, American
    College of, Papanicolaou (Pap)
    smear 46
OCG *see* oral cholecystogram (OCG)
ofloxacin
    chlamydial infection 548
    gonorrhea 565
OGTT *see* oral glucose tolerance test
    (OGTT)
Older Women's League (OWL), con-
    tact information 63, 642
O'Malley, Ann 160
Omnibus Budget and Reconciliation
    Act (1987) 52
open angle glaucoma (OAG) 36

Health Reference Series
COMPLETE CATALOG

AIDS Sourcebook, 1st Edition

Basic Information about AIDS and HIV Infection, Featuring Historical and Statistical Data, Current Research, Prevention, and Other Special Topics of Interest for Persons Living with AIDS, Along with Source Listings for Further Assistance

Edited by Karen Bellenir and Peter D. Dresser. 831 pages. 1995. 0-7808-0031-1. $78.

"One strength of this book is its practical emphasis. The intended audience is the lay reader ... useful as an educational tool for health care providers who work with AIDS patients. Recommended for public libraries as well as hospital or academic libraries that collect consumer materials." — *Bulletin of the MLA, Jan '96*

"This is the most comprehensive volume of its kind on an important medical topic. Highly recommended for all libraries." — *Reference Book Review, '96*

"Very useful reference for all libraries."
— *Choice, Oct '95*

"There is a wealth of information here that can provide much educational assistance. It is a must book for all libraries and should be on the desk of each and every congressional leader. Highly recommended."
— *AIDS Book Review Journal, Aug '95*

"Recommended for most collections."
— *Library Journal, Jul '95*

AIDS Sourcebook, 2nd Edition

Basic Consumer Health Information about Acquired Immune Deficiency Syndrome (AIDS) and Human Immunodeficiency Virus (HIV) Infection, Featuring Updated Statistical Data, Reports on Recent Research and Prevention Initiatives, and Other Special Topics of Interest for Persons Living with AIDS, Including New Antiretroviral Treatment Options, Strategies for Combating Opportunistic Infections, Information about Clinical Trials, and More; Along with a Glossary of Important Terms and Resource Listings for Further Help and Information

Edited by Karen Bellenir. 751 pages. 1999. 0-7808-0225-X. $78.

Allergies Sourcebook

Basic Information about Major Forms and Mechanisms of Common Allergic Reactions, Sensitivities, and Intolerances, Including Anaphylaxis, Asthma, Hives and Other Dermatologic Symptoms, Rhinitis, and Sinusitis, Along with Their Usual Triggers Like Animal Fur, Chemicals, Drugs, Dust, Foods, Insects, Latex, Pollen, and Poison Ivy, Oak, and Sumac; Plus Information on Prevention, Identification, and Treatment

Edited by Allan R. Cook. 611 pages. 1997. 0-7808-0036-2. $78.

Alternative Medicine Sourcebook

Basic Consumer Health Information about Alternatives to Conventional Medicine, Including Acupressure, Acupuncture, Aromatherapy, Ayurveda, Bioelectromagnetics, Environmental Medicine, Essence Therapy, Food and Nutrition Therapy, Herbal Therapy, Homeopathy, Imaging, Massage, Naturopathy, Reflexology, Relaxation and Meditation, Sound Therapy, Vitamin and Mineral Therapy, and Yoga, and More

Edited by Allan R. Cook. 720 pages. 1999. 0-7808-0200-4. $78.

Alzheimer's, Stroke & 29 Other Neurological Disorders Sourcebook, 1st Edition

Basic Information for the Layperson on 31 Diseases or Disorders Affecting the Brain and Nervous System, First Describing the Illness, Then Listing Symptoms, Diagnostic Methods, and Treatment Options, and Including Statistics on Incidences and Causes

Edited by Frank E. Bair. 579 pages. 1993. 1-55888-748-2. $78.

"Nontechnical reference book that provides reader-friendly information."
— *Family Caregiver Alliance Update, Winter '96*

"Should be included in any library's patient education section." — *American Reference Books Annual, '94*

"Written in an approachable and accessible style. Recommended for patient education and consumer health collections in health science center and public libraries." — *Academic Library Book Review, Dec '93*

"It is very handy to have information on more than thirty neurological disorders under one cover, and there is no recent source like it." — *RQ, Fall '93*

Alzheimer's Disease Sourcebook, 2nd Edition

Basic Consumer Health Information about Alzheimer's Disease, Related Disorders, and Other Dementias, Including Multi-Infarct Dementia, AIDS-Related Dementia, Alcoholic Dementia, Huntington's Disease, Delirium, and Confusional States; Along with Reports Detailing Current Research Efforts in Prevention and Treatment, Long-Term Care Issues, and Listings of Sources for Additional Help and Information

Edited by Karen Bellenir. 524 pages. 1999. 0-7808-0223-3. $78.

Arthritis Sourcebook

Basic Consumer Health Information about Specific Forms of Arthritis and Related Disorders, Including Rheumatoid Arthritis, Osteoarthritis, Gout, Polymyalgia Rheumatica, Psoriatic Arthritis, Spondyloarthropathies, Juvenile Rheumatoid Arthritis, and Juvenile Ankylosing Spondylitis; Along with Information about Medical, Surgical, and Alternative Treatment Options, and Including Strategies for Coping with Pain, Fatigue, and Stress

Edited by Allan R. Cook. 550 pages. 1998. 0-7808-0201-2. $78.

". . . accessible to the layperson."
— Reference and Research Book News, Feb '99

Back & Neck Disorders Sourcebook

Basic Information about Disorders and Injuries of the Spinal Cord and Vertebrae, Including Facts on Chiropractic Treatment, Surgical Interventions, Paralysis, and Rehabilitation, Along with Advice for Preventing Back Trouble

Edited by Karen Bellenir. 548 pages. 1997. 0-7808-0202-0. $78.

"The strength of this work is its basic, easy-to-read format. Recommended."
— Reference and User Services Quarterly, Winter '97

Blood & Circulatory Disorders Sourcebook

Basic Information about Blood and Its Components, Anemias, Leukemias, Bleeding Disorders, and Circulatory Disorders, Including Aplastic Anemia, Thalassemia, Sickle-Cell Disease, Hemochromatosis, Hemophilia, Von Willebrand Disease, and Vascular Diseases; Along with a Special Section on Blood Transfusions and Blood Supply Safety, a Glossary, and Source Listings for Further Help and Information

Edited by Karen Bellenir and Linda M. Shin. 554 pages. 1998. 0-7808-0203-9. $78.

"Recent and recommended reference source."
— Booklist, Feb '99

"An important reference sourcebook written in simple language for everyday, non-technical users. "
— Reviewer's Bookwatch, Jan '99

Brain Disorders Sourcebook

Basic Consumer Health Information about Strokes, Epilepsy, Amyotrophic Lateral Sclerosis (ALS/Lou Gehrig's Disease), Parkinson's Disease, Brain Tumors, Cerebral Palsy, Headache, Tourette Syndrome, and More; Along with Statistical Data, Treatment and

Rehabilitation Options, Coping Strategies, Reports on Current Research Initiatives, a Glossary, and Resource Listings for Additional Help and Information

Edited by Karen Bellenir. 481 pages. 1999. 0-7808-0229-2. $78.

Burns Sourcebook

Basic Consumer Health Information about Various Types of Burns and Scalds, Including Flame, Heat, Cold, Electrical, Chemical, and Sun Burns; Along with Information on Short-Term and Long-Term Treatments, Tissue Reconstruction, Plastic Surgery, Prevention Suggestions, and First Aid

Edited by Allan R. Cook. 604 pages. 1999. 0-7808-0204-7. $78.

Cancer Sourcebook, 1st Edition

Basic Information on Cancer Types, Symptoms, Diagnostic Methods, and Treatments, Including Statistics on Cancer Occurrences Worldwide and the Risks Associated with Known Carcinogens and Activities

Edited by Frank E. Bair. 932 pages. 1990. 1-55888-888-8. $78.

"Written in nontechnical language. Useful for patients, their families, medical professionals, and librarians."
— Guide to Reference Books, '96

"Designed with the non-medical professional in mind. Libraries and medical facilities interested in patient education should certainly consider adding the Cancer Sourcebook to their holdings. This compact collection of reliable information . . . is an invaluable tool for helping patients and patients' families and friends to take the first steps in coping with the many difficulties of cancer."
— Medical Reference Services Quarterly, Winter '91

"Specifically created for the nontechnical reader . . . an important resource for the general reader trying to understand the complexities of cancer."
— American Reference Books Annual, '91

"This publication's nontechnical nature and very comprehensive format make it useful for both the general public and undergraduate students."
— Choice, Oct '90

New Cancer Sourcebook, 2nd Edition

Basic Information about Major Forms and Stages of Cancer, Featuring Facts about Primary and Secondary Tumors of the Respiratory, Nervous, Lymphatic, Circulatory, Skeletal, and Gastrointestinal Systems, and Specific Organs; Statistical and Demographic Data; Treatment Options; and Strategies for Coping

Edited by Allan R. Cook. 1,313 pages. 1996. 0-7808-0041-9. $78.

"This book is an excellent resource for patients with newly diagnosed cancer and their families. The dialogue is simple, direct, and comprehensive. Highly recommended for patients and families to aid in their understanding of cancer and its treatment."
— *Booklist Health Sciences Supplement, Oct '97*

"The amount of factual and useful information is extensive. The writing is very clear, geared to general readers. Recommended for all levels."
— *Choice, Jan '97*

Cancer Sourcebook, 3rd Edition

Basic Consumer Health Information about Major Forms and Stages of Cancer, Featuring Facts about Primary and Secondary Tumors of the Respiratory, Nervous, Lymphatic, Circulatory, Skeletal, and Gastrointestinal Systems, and Specific Organs; Along with Statistical and Demographic Data, Treatment Options, Strategies for Coping, a Glossary, and a Directory of Sources for Additional Help and Information

Edited by Edward J. Prucha. 800 pages. 1999. 0-7808-0227-6. $78.

Cancer Sourcebook for Women

Basic Information about Specific Forms of Cancer That Affect Women, Featuring Facts about Breast Cancer, Cervical Cancer, Ovarian Cancer, Cancer of the Uterus and Uterine Sarcoma, Cancer of the Vagina, and Cancer of the Vulva; Statistical and Demographic Data; Treatments, Self-Help Management Suggestions, and Current Research Initiatives

Edited by Allan R. Cook and Peter D. Dresser. 524 pages. 1996. 0-7808-0076-1. $78.

". . . written in easily understandable, non-technical language. Recommended for public libraries or hospital and academic libraries that collect patient education or consumer health materials."
— *Medical Reference Services Quarterly, Spring '97*

"Would be of value in a consumer health library. . . . written with the health care consumer in mind. Medical jargon is at a minimum, and medical terms are explained in clear, understandable sentences."
— *Bulletin of the MLA, Oct '96*

"The availability under one cover of all these pertinent publications, grouped under cohesive headings, makes this certainly a most useful sourcebook."
— *Choice, Jun '96*

"Presents a comprehensive knowledge base for general readers. Men and women both benefit from the gold mine of information nestled between the two covers of this book. Recommended."
— *Academic Library Book Review, Summer '96*

"This timely book is highly recommended for consumer health and patient education collections in all libraries."
— *Library Journal, Apr '96*

Cancer Sourcebook for Women, 2nd Edition

Basic Consumer Health Information about Specific Forms of Cancer That Affect Women, Including Cervical Cancer, Ovarian Cancer, Endometrial Cancer, Uterine Sarcoma, Vaginal Cancer, Vulvar Cancer, and Gestational Trophoblastic Tumor; and Featuring Statistical Information, Facts about Tests and Treatments, a Glossary of Cancer Terms, and an Extensive List of Additional Resources

Edited by Edward J. Prucha. 600 pages. 1999. 0-7808-0226-8. $78.

Cardiovascular Diseases & Disorders Sourcebook

Basic Information about Cardiovascular Diseases and Disorders, Featuring Facts about the Cardiovascular System, Demographic and Statistical Data, Descriptions of Pharmacological and Surgical Interventions, Lifestyle Modifications, and a Special Section Focusing on Heart Disorders in Children

Edited by Karen Bellenir and Peter D. Dresser. 683 pages. 1995. 0-7808-0032-X. $78.

". . . comprehensive format provides an extensive overview on this subject."
— *Choice, Jun '96*

". . . an easily understood, complete, up-to-date resource. This well executed public health tool will make valuable information available to those that need it most, patients and their families. The typeface, sturdy non-reflective paper, and library binding add a feel of quality found wanting in other publications. Highly recommended for academic and general libraries."
— *Academic Library Book Review, Summer '96*

Communication Disorders Sourcebook

Basic Information about Deafness and Hearing Loss, Speech and Language Disorders, Voice Disorders, Balance and Vestibular Disorders, and Disorders of Smell, Taste, and Touch

Edited by Linda M. Ross. 533 pages. 1996. 0-7808-0077-X. $78.

"This is skillfully edited and is a welcome resource for the layperson. It should be found in every public and medical library."
— *Booklist Health Sciences Supplement, Oct '97*

Congenital Disorders Sourcebook

Basic Information about Disorders Acquired during Gestation, Including Spina Bifida, Hydrocephalus, Cerebral Palsy, Heart Defects, Craniofacial Abnormalities, Fetal Alcohol Syndrome, and More, Along with Current Treatment Options and Statistical Data

Edited by Karen Bellenir. 607 pages. 1997. 0-7808-0205-5. $78.

"Recent and recommended reference source."
— *Booklist, Oct '97*

Consumer Issues in Health Care Sourcebook

Basic Information about Health Care Fundamentals and Related Consumer Issues, Including Exams and Screening Tests, Physician Specialties, Choosing a Doctor, Using Prescription and Over-the-Counter Medications Safely, Avoiding Health Scams, Managing Common Health Risks in the Home, Care Options for Chronically or Terminally Ill Patients, and a List of Resources for Obtaining Help and Further Information

Edited by Karen Bellenir. 618 pages. 1998. 0-7808-0221-7. $78.

"Recent and recommended reference source."
— *Booklist, Dec '98*

Contagious & Non-Contagious Infectious Diseases Sourcebook

Basic Information about Contagious Diseases like Measles, Polio, Hepatitis B, and Infectious Mononucleosis, and Non-Contagious Infectious Diseases like Tetanus and Toxic Shock Syndrome, and Diseases Occurring as Secondary Infections Such as Shingles and Reye Syndrome, Along with Vaccination, Prevention, and Treatment Information, and a Section Describing Emerging Infectious Disease Threats

Edited by Karen Bellenir and Peter D. Dresser. 566 pages. 1996. 0-7808-0075-3. $78.

Death & Dying Sourcebook

Basic Consumer Health Information for the Layperson about End-of-Life Care and Related Ethical and Legal Issues, Including Chief Causes of Death, Autopsies, Pain Management for the Terminally Ill, Life Support Systems, Insurance, Euthanasia, Assisted Suicide, Hospice Programs, Living Wills, Funeral Planning, Counseling, Mourning, Organ Donation, and Physician Training; Along with Statistical Data, a Glossary, and Listings of Sources for Further Help and Information

Edited by Annemarie S. Muth. 630 pages. 1999. 0-7808-0230-6. $78.

Diabetes Sourcebook, 1st Edition

Basic Information about Insulin-Dependent and Noninsulin-Dependent Diabetes Mellitus, Gestational Diabetes, and Diabetic Complications, Symptoms, Treatment, and Research Results, Including Statistics on Prevalence, Morbidity, and Mortality, Along with Source Listings for Further Help and Information

Edited by Karen Bellenir and Peter D. Dresser. 827 pages. 1994. 1-55888-751-2. $78.

"... very informative and understandable for the layperson without being simplistic. It provides a comprehensive overview for laypersons who want a general understanding of the disease or who want to focus on various aspects of the disease." — *Bulletin of the MLA, Jan '96*

Diabetes Sourcebook, 2nd Edition

Basic Consumer Health Information about Type 1 Diabetes (Insulin-Dependent or Juvenile-Onset Diabetes), Type 2 (Noninsulin-Dependent or Adult-Onset Diabetes), Gestational Diabetes, and Related Disorders, Including Diabetes Prevalence Data, Management Issues, the Role of Diet and Exercise in Controlling Diabetes, Insulin and Other Diabetes Medicines, and Complications of Diabetes Such as Eye Diseases, Periodontal Disease, Amputation, and End-Stage Renal Disease; Along with Reports on Current Research Initiatives, a Glossary, and Resource Listings for Further Help and Information

Edited by Karen Bellenir. 688 pages. 1998. 0-7808-0224-1. $78.

"Recent and recommended reference source."
— *Booklist, Feb '99*

Diet & Nutrition Sourcebook, 1st Edition

Basic Information about Nutrition, Including the Dietary Guidelines for Americans, the Food Guide Pyramid, and Their Applications in Daily Diet, Nutritional Advice for Specific Age Groups, Current Nutritional Issues and Controversies, the New Food Label and How to Use It to Promote Healthy Eating, and Recent Developments in Nutritional Research

Edited by Dan R. Harris. 662 pages. 1996. 0-7808-0084-2. $78.

"Useful reference as a food and nutrition sourcebook for the general consumer."
— *Booklist Health Sciences Supplement, Oct '97*

"Recommended for public libraries and medical libraries that receive general information requests on nutrition. It is readable and will appeal to those interested in learning more about healthy dietary practices."
— *Medical Reference Services Quarterly, Fall '97*

"With dozens of questionable diet books on the market, it is so refreshing to find a reliable and factual reference book. Recommended to aspiring professionals, librarians, and others seeking and giving reliable dietary advice. An excellent compilation." — *Choice, Feb '97*

Diet & Nutrition Sourcebook, 2nd Edition

Basic Consumer Health Information about Dietary Guidelines, Recommended Daily Intake Values, Vitamins, Minerals, Fiber, Fat, Weight Control, Dietary Supplements, and Food Additives; Along with Special Sections on Nutrition Needs throughout Life and Nutrition for People with Such Specific Medical Concerns as Allergies, High Blood Cholesterol, Hypertension, Diabetes, Celiac Disease, Seizure Disorders, Phenylketonuria (PKU), Cancer, and Eating Disorders, and Including Reports on Current Nutrition Research and Source Listings for Additional Help and Information

Edited by Karen Bellenir. 650 pages. 1999. 0-7808-0228-4. $78.

Digestive Diseases & Disorders Sourcebook

Basic Consumer Health Information about Diseases and Disorders that Impact the Upper and Lower Digestive System, Including Celiac Disease, Constipation, Crohn's Disease, Cyclic Vomiting Syndrome, Diarrhea, Diverticulosis and Diverticulitis, Gallstones, Heartburn, Hemorrhoids, Hernias, Indigestion (Dyspepsia), Irritable Bowel Syndrome, Lactose Intolerance, Ulcers, and More; Along with Information about Medications and Other Treatments, Tips for Maintaining a Healthy Digestive Tract, a Glossary, and Directory of Digestive Diseases Organizations

Edited by Karen Bellenir. 300 pages. 1999. 0-7808-0327-2. $48.

Domestic Violence & Child Abuse Sourcebook

Basic Information about Spousal/Partner, Child, and Elder Physical, Emotional, and Sexual Abuse, Teen Dating Violence, and Stalking, Including Information about Hotlines, Safe Houses, Safety Plans, and Other Resources for Support and Assistance, Community Initiatives, and Reports on Current Directions in Research and Treatment; Along with a Glossary, Sources for Further Reading, and Governmental and Non-Governmental Organizations Contact Information

Edited by Helene Henderson. 600 pages. 1999. 0-7808-0235-7. $78.

Ear, Nose & Throat Disorders Sourcebook

Basic Information about Disorders of the Ears, Nose, Sinus Cavities, Pharynx, and Larynx, Including Ear Infections, Tinnitus, Vestibular Disorders, Allergic and Non-Allergic Rhinitis, Sore Throats, Tonsillitis, and Cancers That Affect the Ears, Nose, Sinuses, and Throat, Along with Reports on Current Research Initiatives, a Glossary of Related Medical Terms, and a Directory of Sources for Further Help and Information

Edited by Karen Bellenir and Linda M. Shin. 576 pages. 1998. 0-7808-0206-3. $78.

"Overall, this sourcebook is helpful for the consumer seeking information on ENT issues. It is recommended for public libraries."
— *American Reference Books Annual, '99*

"Recent and recommended reference source."
— *Booklist, Dec '98*

Endocrine & Metabolic Disorders Sourcebook

Basic Information for the Layperson about Pancreatic and Insulin-Related Disorders Such as Pancreatitis, Diabetes, and Hypoglycemia; Adrenal Gland Disorders Such as Cushing's Syndrome, Addison's Disease, and Congenital Adrenal Hyperplasia; Pituitary Gland Disorders Such as Growth Hormone Deficiency, Acromegaly, and Pituitary Tumors; Thyroid Disorders Such as Hypothyroidism, Graves' Disease, Hashimoto's Disease, and Goiter; Hyperparathyroidism; and Other Diseases and Syndromes of Hormone Imbalance or Metabolic Dysfunction, Along with Reports on Current Research Initiatives

Edited by Linda M. Shin. 574 pages. 1998. 0-7808-0207-1. $78.

"Recent and recommended reference source."
— *Booklist, Dec '98*

Environmentally Induced Disorders Sourcebook

Basic Information about Diseases and Syndromes Linked to Exposure to Pollutants and Other Substances in Outdoor and Indoor Environments Such as Lead, Asbestos, Formaldehyde, Mercury, Emissions, Noise, and More

Edited by Allan R. Cook. 620 pages. 1997. 0-7808-0083-4. $78.

"Recent and recommended reference source."
— *Booklist, Sept '98*

"This book will be a useful addition to anyone's library."
— *Choice Health Sciences Supplement, May '98*

". . . a good survey of numerous environmentally induced physical disorders . . . a useful addition to anyone's library."
— *Doody's Health Science Book Reviews, Jan '98*

". . . provide[s] introductory information from the best authorities around. Since this volume covers topics that potentially affect everyone, it will surely be one of the most frequently consulted volumes in the *Health Reference Series*."
— *Rettig on Reference, Nov '97*

Ethical Issues in Medicine Sourcebook

Basic Information about Controversial Treatment Issues, Genetic Research, Reproductive Technologies, and End-of-Life Decisions, Including Topics Such as Cloning, Abortion, Fertility Management, Organ Transplantation, Health Care Rationing, Advance Directives, Living Wills, Physician-Assisted Suicide, Euthanasia, and More; Along with a Glossary and Resources for Additional Information

Edited by Helene Henderson. 600 pages. 1999. 0-7808-0237-3. $78.

Fitness & Exercise Sourcebook

Basic Information on Fitness and Exercise, Including Fitness Activities for Specific Age Groups, Exercise for People with Specific Medical Conditions, How to Begin a Fitness Program in Running, Walking, Swimming, Cycling, and Other Athletic Activities, and Recent Research in Fitness and Exercise

Edited by Dan R. Harris. 663 pages. 1996. 0-7808-0186-5. $78.

"A good resource for general readers."
— *Choice, Nov '97*

"The perennial popularity of the topic . . . make this an appealing selection for public libraries."
— *Rettig on Reference, Jun/Jul '97*

Food & Animal Borne Diseases Sourcebook

Basic Information about Diseases That Can Be Spread to Humans through the Ingestion of Contaminated Food or Water or by Contact with Infected Animals and Insects, Such as Botulism, E. Coli, Hepatitis A, Trichinosis, Lyme Disease, and Rabies, Along with Information Regarding Prevention and Treatment Methods, and a Special Section for International Travelers Describing Diseases Such as Cholera, Malaria, Travelers' Diarrhea, and Yellow Fever, and Offering Recommendations for Avoiding Illness

Edited by Karen Bellenir and Peter D. Dresser. 535 pages. 1995. 0-7808-0033-8. $78.

"Targeting general readers and providing them with a single, comprehensive source of information on selected topics, this book continues, with the excellent caliber of its predecessors, to catalog topical information on health matters of general interest. Readable and thorough, this valuable resource is highly recommended for all libraries."
— *Academic Library Book Review, Summer '96*

"A comprehensive collection of authoritative information."
— *Emergency Medical Services, Oct '95*

Food Safety Sourcebook

Basic Consumer Health Information about the Safe Handling of Meat, Poultry, Seafood, Eggs, Fruit Juices, and Other Food Items, and Facts about Pesticides, Drinking Water, Food Safety Overseas, and the Onset, Duration, and Symptoms of Foodborne Illnesses, Including Types of Pathogenic Bacteria, Parasitic Protozoa, Worms, Viruses, and Natural Toxins; Along with the Role of the Consumer, the Food Handler, and the Government in Food Safety; a Glossary, and Resources for Additional Help and Information

Edited by Dawn D. Matthews. 320 pages. 1999. 0-7808-0326-4. $48.

Forensic Medicine Sourcebook

Basic Consumer Information for the Layperson about Forensic Medicine, Including Crime Scene Investigation, Evidence Collection and Analysis, Expert Testimony, Computer-Aided Criminal Identification, Digital Imaging in the Courtroom, DNA Profiling, Accident Reconstruction, Autopsies, Ballistics, Drugs and Explosives Detection, Latent Fingerprints, Product Tampering, and Questioned Document Examination; Along with Statistical Data, a Glossary of Forensics Terminology, and Listings of Sources for Further Help and Information

Edited by Annemarie S. Muth. 574 pages. 1999. 0-7808-0232-2. $78.

Gastrointestinal Diseases & Disorders Sourcebook

Basic Information about Gastroesophageal Reflux Disease (Heartburn), Ulcers, Diverticulosis, Irritable Bowel Syndrome, Crohn's Disease, Ulcerative Colitis, Diarrhea, Constipation, Lactose Intolerance, Hemorrhoids, Hepatitis, Cirrhosis, and Other Digestive Problems, Featuring Statistics, Descriptions of Symptoms, and Current Treatment Methods of Interest for Persons Living with Upper and Lower Gastrointestinal Maladies

Edited by Linda M. Ross. 413 pages. 1996. 0-7808-0078-8. $78.

". . . very readable form. The successful editorial work that brought this material together into a useful and understandable reference makes accessible to all readers information that can help them more effectively understand and obtain help for digestive tract problems."
— *Choice, Feb '97*

Genetic Disorders Sourcebook

Basic Information about Heritable Diseases and Disorders Such as Down Syndrome, PKU, Hemophilia, Von Willebrand Disease, Gaucher Disease, Tay-Sachs Disease, and Sickle-Cell Disease, Along with Information about Genetic Screening, Gene Therapy, Home Care, and Including Source Listings for Further Help and Information on More Than 300 Disorders

Edited by Karen Bellenir. 642 pages. 1996. 0-7808-0034-6. $78.

Head Trauma Sourcebook

Basic Information for the Layperson about Open-Head and Closed-Head Injuries, Treatment Advances, Recovery, and Rehabilitation, Along with Reports on Current Research Initiatives

Edited by Karen Bellenir. 414 pages. 1997. 0-7808-0208-X. $78.

Health Insurance Sourcebook

Basic Information about Managed Care Organizations, Traditional Fee-for-Service Insurance, Insurance Portability and Pre-Existing Conditions Clauses, Medicare, Medicaid, Social Security, and Military Health Care, Along with Information about Insurance Fraud

Edited by Wendy Wilcox. 530 pages. 1997. 0-7808-0222-5. $78.

Healthy Aging Sourcebook

Basic Consumer Health Information about Maintaining Health through the Aging Process, Including Advice on Nutrition, Exercise, and Sleep, Help in Making Decisions about Midlife Issues and Retirement, and Guidance Concerning Practical and Informed Choices in Health Consumerism; Along with Data Concerning the Theories of Aging, Different Experiences in Aging by Minority Groups, and Facts about Aging Now and Aging in the Future; and Featuring a Glossary, a Guide to Consumer Help, Additional Suggested Reading, and Practical Resource Directory

Edited by Jenifer Swanson. 536 pages. 1999. 0-7808-0390-6. $78.

Heart Diseases & Disorders Sourcebook, 2nd edition

Basic Consumer Health Information about Heart Attacks, Angina, Rhythm Disorders, Heart Failure, Valve Disease, Congenital Heart Disorders, and More, Including Descriptions of Surgical Procedures and Other Interventions, Medications, Cardiac Rehabilitation, Risk Identification, and Prevention Tips; Along with Statistical Data, Reports on Current Research Initiatives, a Glossary of Cardiovascular Terms, and Resource Directory

Edited by Karen Bellenir. 600 pages. 1999. 0-7808-0238-1. $78.

Immune System Disorders Sourcebook

Basic Information about Lupus, Multiple Sclerosis, Guillain-Barré Syndrome, Chronic Granulomatous Disease, and More, Along with Statistical and Demographic Data and Reports on Current Research Initiatives

Edited by Allan R. Cook. 608 pages. 1997. 0-7808-0209-8. $78.

Infant & Toddler Health Sourcebook

Basic Consumer Health Information about the Physical and Mental Development of Newborns, Infants, and Toddlers, Including Neonatal Concerns, Nutritional Recommendations, Immunization Schedules, Common Pediatric Disorders, Assessments and Milestones, Safety Tips, and Advice for Parents and Other Caregivers; Along with a Glossary of Terms and Resource Listings for Additional Help

Edited by Jenifer Swanson. 600 pages. 1999. 0-7808-0246-2. $78.

Kidney & Urinary Tract Diseases & Disorders Sourcebook

Basic Information about Kidney Stones, Urinary Incontinence, Bladder Disease, End Stage Renal Disease, Dialysis, and More, Along with Statistical and Demographic Data and Reports on Current Research Initiatives

Edited by Linda M. Ross. 602 pages. 1997. 0-7808-0079-6. $78.

Learning Disabilities Sourcebook

Basic Information about Disorders Such as Dyslexia, Visual and Auditory Processing Deficits, Attention Deficit/Hyperactivity Disorder, and Autism, Along with Statistical and Demographic Data, Reports on Current Research Initiatives, an Explanation of the Assessment Process, and a Special Section for Adults with Learning Disabilities

Edited by Linda M. Shin. 579 pages. 1998. 0-7808-0210-1. $78.

"Readable . . . provides a solid base of information regarding successful techniques used with individuals who have learning disabilities, as well as practical suggestions for educators and family members. Clear language, concise descriptions, and pertinent information for contacting multiple resources add to the strength of this book as a useful tool." — *Choice, Feb '99*

"Recent and recommended reference source."
— *Booklist, Sept '98*

Liver Disorders Sourcebook

Basic Consumer Health Information about the Liver and How It Works, Liver Diseases, Including Cancer, Cirrhosis, Hepatitis, and Toxic Drug Related Diseases; Tips for Maintaining a Healthy Liver; Laboratory Tests, Radiology Tests, and Facts about Liver Transplantation; Along with a Section on Support Groups, a Glossary, and Resource Listings

Edited by Joyce Brennfleck Shannon. 600 pages. 1999. 0-7808-0383-3. $78.

Medical Tests Sourcebook

Basic Consumer Health Information about Medical Tests, Including Periodic Health Exams, General Screening Tests, Tests You Can Do at Home, Findings of the U.S. Preventive Services Task Force, X-ray and Radiology Tests, Electrical Tests, Tests of Blood and Other Body Fluids and Tissues, Scope Tests, Lung Tests, Genetic Tests, Pregnancy Tests, Newborn Screening Tests, Sexually Transmitted Disease Tests, and Computer Aided Diagnoses; Along with a Section on Paying for Medical Tests, a Glossary, and Resource Listings

Edited by Joyce Brennfleck Shannon. 600 pages. 1999. 0-7808-0243-8. $78.

Men's Health Concerns Sourcebook

Basic Information about Health Issues That Affect Men, Featuring Facts about the Top Causes of Death in Men, Including Heart Disease, Stroke, Cancers, Prostate Disorders, Chronic Obstructive Pulmonary Disease, Pneumonia and Influenza, Human Immunodeficiency Virus and Acquired Immune Deficiency Syndrome, Diabetes Mellitus, Stress, Suicide, Accidents and Homicides; and Facts about Common Concerns for Men, Including Impotence, Contraception, Circumcision, Sleep Disorders, Snoring, Hair Loss, Diet, Nutrition, Exercise, Kidney and Urological Disorders, and Backaches

Edited by Allan R. Cook. 738 pages. 1998. 0-7808-0212-8. $78.

"Recent and recommended reference source."
— *Booklist, Dec '98*

Mental Health Disorders Sourcebook, 1st Edition

Basic Information about Schizophrenia, Depression, Bipolar Disorder, Panic Disorder, Obsessive-Compulsive Disorder, Phobias and Other Anxiety Disorders, Paranoia and Other Personality Disorders, Eating Disorders, and Sleep Disorders, Along with Information about Treatment and Therapies

Edited by Karen Bellenir. 548 pages. 1995. 0-7808-0040-0. $78.

"This is an excellent new book . . . written in easy-to-understand language."
— *Booklist Health Science Supplement, Oct '97*

". . . useful for public and academic libraries and consumer health collections."
— *Medical Reference Services Quarterly, Spring '97*

"The great strengths of the book are its readability and its inclusion of places to find more information. Especially recommended." — *RQ, Winter '96*

". . . a good resource for a consumer health library."
— *Bulletin of the MLA, Oct '96*

"The information is data-based and couched in brief, concise language that avoids jargon. . . . a useful reference source." — *Readings, Sept '96*

"The text is well organized and adequately written for its target audience." — *Choice, Jun '96*

". . . provides information on a wide range of mental disorders, presented in nontechnical language."
— *Exceptional Child Education Resources, Spring '96*

"Recommended for public and academic libraries."
— *Reference Book Review, '96*

Mental Health Disorders Sourcebook, 2nd Edition

Basic Consumer Health Information about Anxiety Disorders, Depression and Other Mood Disorders, Eating Disorders, Personality Disorders, Schizophrenia, and More, Including Disease Descriptions, Treatment Options, and Reports on Current Research Initiatives; Along with Statistical Data, Tips for Maintaining Mental Health, a Glossary, and Directory of Sources for Additional Help and Information

Edited by Karen Bellenir. 600 pages. 1999. 0-7808-0240-3. $78.

Ophthalmic Disorders Sourcebook

Basic Information about Glaucoma, Cataracts, Macular Degeneration, Strabismus, Refractive Disorders, and More, Along with Statistical and Demographic Data and Reports on Current Research Initiatives

Edited by Linda M. Ross. 631 pages. 1996. 0-7808-0081-8. $78.

Oral Health Sourcebook

Basic Information about Diseases and Conditions Affecting Oral Health, Including Cavities, Gum Disease, Dry Mouth, Oral Cancers, Fever Blisters, Canker Sores, Oral Thrush, Bad Breath, Temporomandibular Disorders, and other Craniofacial Syndromes, Along with Statistical Data on the Oral Health of Americans, Oral Hygiene, Emergency First Aid, Information on Treatment Procedures and Methods of Replacing Lost Teeth

Edited by Allan R. Cook. 558 pages. 1997. 0-7808-0082-6. $78.

"Unique source which will fill a gap in dental sources for patients and the lay public. A valuable reference tool even in a library with thousands of books on dentistry. Comprehensive, clear, inexpensive, and easy to read and use. It fills an enormous gap in the health care literature." — *Reference and User Services Quarterly, Summer '98*

"Recent and recommended reference source." — *Booklist, Dec '97*

Pain Sourcebook

Basic Information about Specific Forms of Acute and Chronic Pain, Including Headaches, Back Pain, Muscular Pain, Neuralgia, Surgical Pain, and Cancer Pain, Along with Pain Relief Options Such as Analgesics, Narcotics, Nerve Blocks, Transcutaneous Nerve Stimulation, and Alternative Forms of Pain Control, Including Biofeedback, Imaging, Behavior Modification, and Relaxation Techniques

Edited by Allan R. Cook. 667 pages. 1997. 0-7808-0213-6. $78.

"The text is readable, easily understood, and well indexed. This excellent volume belongs in all patient education libraries, consumer health sections of public libraries, and many personal collections." — *American Reference Books Annual, '99*

"A beneficial reference." — *Booklist Health Sciences Supplement, Oct '98*

"The information is basic in terms of scholarship and is appropriate for general readers. Written in journalistic style . . . intended for non-professionals. Quite thorough in its coverage of different pain conditions and summarizes the latest clinical information regarding pain treatment." — *Choice, Jun '98*

"Recent and recommended reference source." — *Booklist, Mar '98*

Pediatric Cancer Sourcebook

Basic Consumer Health Information about Leukemias, Brain Tumors, Sarcomas, Lymphomas, and Other Cancers in Infants, Children, and Adolescents, Including Descriptions of Cancers, Treatments, and Coping Strategies; Along with Suggestions for Parents, Caregivers, and Concerned Relatives, a Glossary of Cancer Terms, and Resource Listings

Edited by Edward J. Prucha. 580 pages. 1999. 0-7808-0245-4. $78.

Physical & Mental Issues in Aging Sourcebook

Basic Consumer Health Information on Physical and Mental Disorders Associated with the Aging Process, Including Concerns about Cardiovascular Disease, Pulmonary Disease, Oral Health, Digestive Disorders, Musculoskeletal and Skin Disorders, Metabolic Changes, Sexual and Reproductive Issues, and Changes in Vision, Hearing, and Other Senses; Along with Data about Longevity and Causes of Death, Information on Acute and Chronic Pain, Descriptions of Mental Concerns, a Glossary of Terms, and Resource Listings for Additional Help

Edited by Jenifer Swanson. 660 pages. 1999. 0-7808-0233-0. $78.

Pregnancy & Birth Sourcebook

Basic Information about Planning for Pregnancy, Maternal Health, Fetal Growth and Development, Labor and Delivery, Postpartum and Perinatal Care, Pregnancy in Mothers with Special Concerns, and Disorders of Pregnancy, Including Genetic Counseling, Nutrition and Exercise, Obstetrical Tests, Pregnancy Discomfort, Multiple Births, Cesarean Sections, Medical Testing of Newborns, Breastfeeding, Gestational Diabetes, and Ectopic Pregnancy

Edited by Heather E. Aldred. 737 pages. 1997. 0-7808-0216-0. $78.

"A well-organized handbook. Recommended." — *Choice, Apr '98*

"Recent and recommended reference source." — *Booklist, Mar '98*

"Recommended for public libraries." — *American Reference Books Annual, '98*

Public Health Sourcebook

Basic Information about Government Health Agencies, Including National Health Statistics and Trends, Healthy People 2000 Program Goals and Objectives, the Centers for Disease Control and Prevention, the Food and Drug Administration, and the National Institutes of Health, Along with Full Contact Information for Each Agency

Edited by Wendy Wilcox. 698 pages. 1998. 0-7808-0220-9. $78.

"Recent and recommended reference source."
— *Booklist, Sept '98*

"This consumer guide provides welcome assistance in navigating the maze of federal health agencies and their data on public health concerns."
— *SciTech Book News, Sept '98*

Rehabilitation Sourcebook

Basic Consumer Health Information about Rehabilitation for People Recovering from Heart Surgery, Spinal Cord Injury, Stroke, Orthopedic Impairments, Amputation, Pulmonary Impairments, Traumatic Injury, and More, Including Physical Therapy, Occupational Therapy, Speech/Language Therapy, Massage Therapy, Dance Therapy, Art Therapy, and Recreational Therapy, Along with Information on Assistive and Adaptive Devices, a Glossary, and Resources for Additional Help and Information

Edited by Dawn D. Matthews. 512 pages. 1999. 0-7808-0236-5. $78.

Respiratory Diseases & Disorders Sourcebook

Basic Information about Respiratory Diseases and Disorders, Including Asthma, Cystic Fibrosis, Pneumonia, the Common Cold, Influenza, and Others, Featuring Facts about the Respiratory System, Statistical and Demographic Data, Treatments, Self-Help Management Suggestions, and Current Research Initiatives

Edited by Allan R. Cook and Peter D. Dresser. 771 pages. 1995. 0-7808-0037-0. $78.

"Designed for the layperson and for patients and their families coping with respiratory illness. . . . an extensive array of information on diagnosis, treatment, management, and prevention of respiratory illnesses for the general reader."
— *Choice, Jun '96*

"A highly recommended text for all collections. It is a comforting reminder of the power of knowledge that good books carry between their covers."
— *Academic Library Book Review, Spring '96*

"This sourcebook offers a comprehensive collection of authoritative information presented in a nontechnical, humanitarian style for patients, families, and caregivers."
— *Association of Operating Room Nurses, Sept/Oct '95*

Sexually Transmitted Diseases Sourcebook

Basic Information about Herpes, Chlamydia, Gonorrhea, Hepatitis, Nongonoccocal Urethritis, Pelvic Inflammatory Disease, Syphilis, AIDS, and More, Along with Current Data on Treatments and Preventions

Edited by Linda M. Ross. 550 pages. 1997. 0-7808-0217-9. $78.

Skin Disorders Sourcebook

Basic Information about Common Skin and Scalp Conditions Caused by Aging, Allergies, Immune Reactions, Sun Exposure, Infectious Organisms, Parasites, Cosmetics, and Skin Traumas, Including Abrasions, Cuts, and Pressure Sores, Along with Information on Prevention and Treatment

Edited by Allan R. Cook. 647 pages. 1997. 0-7808-0080-X. $78.

". . . comprehensive easily read reference book."
— *Doody's Health Sciences Book Reviews, Oct '97*

Sleep Disorders Sourcebook

Basic Consumer Health Information about Sleep and Its Disorders, Including Insomnia, Sleepwalking, Sleep Apnea, Restless Leg Syndrome, and Narcolepsy; Along with Data about Shiftwork and Its Effects, Information on the Societal Costs of Sleep Deprivation, Descriptions of Treatment Options, a Glossary of Terms, and Resource Listings for Additional Help

Edited by Jenifer Swanson. 439 pages. 1998. 0-7808-0234-9. $78.

"Recent and recommended reference source."
— *Booklist, Feb '99*

Sports Injuries Sourcebook

Basic Consumer Health Information about Common Sports Injuries, Prevention of Injury in Specific Sports, Tips for Training, and Rehabilitation from Injury; Along with Information about Special Concerns for Children, Young Girls in Athletic Training Programs, Senior Athletes, and Women Athletes, and a Directory of Resources for Further Help and Information

Edited by Heather E. Aldred. 624 pages.1999. 0-7808-0218-7. $78.

Substance Abuse Sourcebook

Basic Health-Related Information about the Abuse of Legal and Illegal Substances Such as Alcohol, Tobacco, Prescription Drugs, Marijuana, Cocaine, and Heroin; and Including Facts about Substance Abuse Pre-

vention Strategies, Intervention Methods, Treatment and Recovery Programs, and a Section Addressing the Special Problems Related to Substance Abuse during Pregnancy

Edited by Karen Bellenir. 573 pages. 1996. 0-7808-0038-9. $78.

"A valuable addition to any health reference section. Highly recommended."
— The Book Report, Mar/Apr '97

". . . a comprehensive collection of substance abuse information that's both highly readable and compact. Families and caregivers of substance abusers will find the information enlightening and helpful, while teachers, social workers and journalists should benefit from the concise format. Recommended."
— Drug Abuse Update, Winter '96-'97

Women's Health Concerns Sourcebook

Basic Information about Health Issues That Affect Women, Featuring Facts about Menstruation and Other Gynecological Concerns, Including Endometriosis, Fibroids, Menopause, and Vaginitis; Reproductive Concerns, Including Birth Control, Infertility, and Abortion; and Facts about Additional Physical, Emotional, and Mental Health Concerns Prevalent among Women Such as Osteoporosis, Urinary Tract Disorders, Eating Disorders, and Depression, Along with Tips for Maintaining a Healthy Lifestyle

Edited by Heather Aldred. 567 pages. 1997. 0-7808-0219-5. $78.

"Handy compilation. There is an impressive range of diseases, devices, disorders, procedures, and other physical and emotional issues covered . . . well organized, illustrated, and indexed."
— Choice, Jan '98

Workplace Health & Safety Sourcebook

Basic Information about Musculoskeletal Injuries, Cumulative Trauma Disorders, Occupational Carcinogens and Other Toxic Materials, Child Labor, Workplace Violence, Histoplasmosis, Transmission of HIV and Hepatitis-B Viruses, and Occupational Hazards Associated with Various Industries, Including Mining, Confined Spaces, Agriculture, Construction, Electrical Work, and the Medical Professions, with Information on Mortality and Other Statistical Data, Preventative Measures, Reproductive Risks, Reducing Stress for Shiftworkers, Noise Hazards, Industrial Back Belts, Reducing Contamination at Home, Preventing Allergic Reactions to Rubber Latex, and More; Along with Public and Private Programs and Initiatives, a Glossary, and Sources for Additional Help and Information

Edited by Helene Henderson. 600 pages. 1999. 0-7808-0231-4. $78.

Health Reference Series Cumulative Index

A Comprehensive Index to 42 Volumes of the Health Reference Series, 1990-1998

1st ed. 1,500 pages. 0-7808-0382-5. $78.

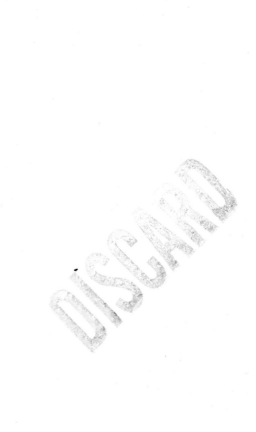